Workbook for Textbook of Diagnostic Sonography

Ninth Edition

Sandra L. Hagen-Ansert, MS, RDMS, RDCS, FASE, FSDMS
Cardiology Department
Manager, Echo Labs (retired)
Scripps Clinics and Scripps La Jolla Memorial Hospital
Torrey Pines, California

ELSEVIER

ELSEVIER

3251 Riverport Lane
St. Louis, Missouri 63043

WORKBOOK FOR TEXTBOOK OF DIAGNOSTIC
SONOGRAPHY, NINTH EDITION

ISBN: 978-0-323-82650-1

Notices

Practitioners and researchers must always rely on their own experience and knowledge in evaluating
and using any information, methods, compounds, or experiments described herein. Because of rapid
advances in the medical sciences, in particular, independent verification of diagnoses and drug dosages
should be made. To the fullest extent of the law, no responsibility is assumed by Elsevier, authors, editors,
or contributors for any injury and/or damage to persons or property as a matter of products liability,
negligence or otherwise, or from any use or operation of any methods, products, instructions, or ideas
contained in the material herein.

Content Strategist: Meg Benson
Content Development Specialist: Danielle Frazier
Project Manager: Andrew Riley

Printed in India

Last digit is the print number: 9 8 7 6 5 4 3

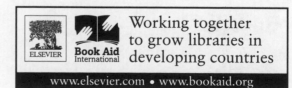

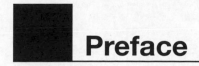

Preface

This workbook has been prepared to accompany Elsevier's *Textbook of Diagnostic Sonography*, Ninth Edition. The workbook chapters correlate with those in the primary textbook, and *Workbook for Textbook of Diagnostic Sonography* has been completely updated and expanded to keep pace with the ninth edition of the textbook.

The material serves both as a useful review of the textbook chapters and as a preparation tool for the national board examinations in diagnostic sonography. The workbook exercises provide the reader with a thorough review of terminology, anatomy, physiology, laboratory values, sonographic anatomy and technique, and pathology as it relates to diagnostic sonography. Each chapter begins with a review of the Key Terms that are bolded in the corresponding textbook chapter. A printable list of the key terms and their definitions may be found on the Evolve site. Each chapter also includes short answer questions, fill-in-the-blank exercises, and case reviews with images. Answers to all of the chapter exercises may be found at the back of the workbook.

Four Reviews—General Sonography, Pediatric, Cardiovascular Anatomy, and Obstetrics and Gynecology—are included at the end of the workbook. Students can test their knowledge here with the **hundreds of multiple choice questions**. Answers to these additional reviews and case studies may also be found on the Evolve site.

Sandra L. Hagen-Ansert, MS, RDMS, RDCS, FASE, FSDMS

Contents

1 **Foundations of Sonography**

EXERCISE 1: MATCHING KEY TERMS

Match the following sonography terms with their definitions.

_____ 1. angle of reflection

_____ 2. velocity

_____ 3. cycle

_____ 4. Fraunhofer zone

_____ 5. hertz (Hz)

_____ 6. kilohertz (kHz)

_____ 7. lateral resolution

_____ 8. pulse duration

_____ 9. Fresnel zone

_____ 10. slice thickness

A. Time interval required for generating the transmitted pulse
B. Sequence of events occurring at regular intervals
C. Speed of the ultrasound wave; determined by tissue density
D. Minimum distance between two objects at which they still can be displayed as separate objects
E. Unit for frequency; equal to 1 cycle per second
F. Field closest to the transducer during formation of the sound beam
G. Angle of incidence at which the sound beam strikes the interface
H. 1000 Hz
I. Field farthest from the transducer during formation of the sound beam
J. Thickness of the section in a patient that contributes to echo signals on any one image

EXERCISE 2: CROSSWORD PUZZLE

Read the clues and complete the puzzle.

Across

1. Region of increased particle denisty
2. Number of cycles per second that a periodic event or function undergoes
3. Any device that converts energy from one form to another
4. Passive force in opposition to another, active force; occurs when tissue exerts pressure against the flow.
5. Propagation of energy that moves back and forth or vibrates at a steady rate.

Down

6. Reduction in amplitude and intensity of a sound wave as it propagates through a medium
7. Special material in the transducer that has the ability to convert electric impulses into sound waves
8. Unit used to quantitatively express the ratio of two amplitudes or intensities.
9. Rate of energy flow over the entire beam of sound.
10. Ability of the transducer to distinguish between two structures adjacent to one another.

EXERCISE 3: MULTIPLE CHOICE: INSTRUMENTATION

Select the best answer that describes the term.

_____ 1. acoustic impedance
   a. Change in the direction of propagation of a sound wave transmitted across an interface where the speed of sound varies.
   b. Measure of a material's resistance to the propagation of sound; expressed as the product of acoustic velocity of the medium and density of the medium.
   c. Reduction in amplitude and intensity of a sound wave as it propagates through a medium.
   d. Ability of the transducer to distinguish between two structures adjacent to one another.

_____ 2. *angle of incidence*
   a. Special material in the transducer that has the ability to convert electric impulses into sound waves.
   b. Number of cycles per second that a periodic event or function undergoes.
   c. Generation of electric signals as the result of an incident sound beam on a material that has piezoelectric properties.
   d. Angle at which a sound beam strikes the interface between two types of tissue.

_____ 3. *axial resolution*
   a. Refers to the minimum distance between two structures positioned along the axis of the beam where both structures can be visualized as separate objects.
   b. Generation of electric signals as the result of an incident sound beam on a material that has piezoelectric properties.
   c. Region over which the effective width of the sound beam is within some measure of its width at the focal distance.
   d. Surface forming the boundary between media having different properties.

_____ 4. *piezoelectric effect*
   a. Rate of energy flow over the entire beam of sound.
   b. Ability of the transducer to distinguish between two structures adjacent to one another.
   c. Generation of electric signals as the result of an incident sound beam on a material that has piezoelectric properties.
   d. Distance over which a wave repeats itself during one period of oscillation.

_____ 5. *wavelength*
   a. Distance over which a wave repeats itself during one period of oscillation.
   b. Propagation of energy that moves back and forth or vibrates at a steady rate.
   c. Power per unit area.
   d. 1,000,000 Hz

EXERCISE 4: MATCHING

Match the following instrumentation terms with their definitions.

_____ 1. aliasing

_____ 2. amplitude

_____ 3. continuous wave (CW) Doppler

_____ 4. Doppler angle

_____ 5. Doppler shift

_____ 6. dynamic range

_____ 7. frame rate

_____ 8. gain

_____ 9. gray scale

_____ 10. laminar

_____ 11. Nyquist sampling limit

_____ 12. pulse repetition frequency (PRF)

_____ 13. pulsed wave (PW) Doppler

_____ 14. real time

_____ 15. spectral analysis

_____ 16. spectral broadening

_____ 17. temporal resolution

A. Sound transmitted and received intermittently with one transducer
B. Ability to compensate for attenuation of the transmitted beam as the sound wave travels through tissue in the body
C. Change in frequency of a reflected wave; caused by motion between the reflector and the transducer's beam
D. One transducer continuously transmits sound, and one continuously receives sound; used in high-velocity flow patterns
E. Normal pattern of vessel flow; flow in the center of the vessel is faster than it is at the edges
F. Rate at which images are updated on the display; dependent on transducer frequency and depth selection
G. Analysis of the entire frequency spectrum
H. Technical artifact that occurs when the frequency change is so great that it exceeds the sampling view and pulse repetition frequency
I. In pulse-echo instruments, it is the number of pulses launched per second by the transducer
J. Ability of the system to accurately depict motion
K. Ratio of the largest to the smallest signals that an instrument or a component of an instrument can respond to without distortion

Chapter **1** **Foundations of Sonography**

_____ 18. time gain compensation (TGC)

_____ 19. gate

_____ 20. frequency shift

L. In pulsed Doppler, the Doppler signal must be sampled at least twice for each cycle in the wave if Doppler frequencies are to be detected accurately

M. Strength of the ultrasound wave measured in decibels

N. Measure of strength of the ultrasound signal

O. Echo fill-in of the spectral window that is proportional to the severity of stenosis

P. Ultrasound instrumentation that allows the image to be displayed many times per second to achieve a "real-time" image of anatomic structures and their motion patterns

Q. B-mode scanning technique that permits the brightness of the B-mode dots to be displayed in various shades of gray to represent different echo amplitudes

R. Amount of change in the returning frequency compared with the transmitting frequency when the sound wave hits a moving target such as blood in an artery

S. Sample site from which the signal is obtained with pulsed Doppler

T. Angle that the reflector path makes with the ultrasound beam; the most accurate velocity is recorded when the beam is parallel to flow

EXERCISE 5: INSTRUMENTATION

Fill in the blank(s) with the word(s) that best completes the statements or provide a short answer about ultrasound instrumentation.

1. As the ceramic element vibrates, it periodically presses against and pulls away from the adjacent medium with resultant particle _____ and refaction in the medium.

2. A transducer converts _____ energy into _____ energy.

3. The time required to produce each cycle depends on the _____ of the transducer.

4. The distance between two peaks over a period of time is the _____.

5. Wavelength is inversely related to frequency, which means that the higher the frequency, the _____ the wavelength.

6. As frequencies become higher, the pulse duration _____, yielding a decrease in the depth of field.

7. If you double the power, the intensity _____.

8. The piezoelectric effect was first described by the _____ brothers in 1880.

9. Air-filled structures, such as lungs and stomach, or gas-filled structures, such as bowel, _____ sound transmission.

10. Bone conducts sound at a _____ speed than soft tissue.

11. Normal transmission of sound through soft tissue travels at _____ m/sec.

12. Acoustic impedance is the product of the velocity of _____ in a medium and the density of that medium.

13. The angle of reflection is equal to the angle of _____.

14. If specular reflectors are aligned _____ to the direction of the transmitted pulse, they reflect sound directly back to the active crystal elements in the transducer and produce a strong signal.

15. Lateral resolution is determined by beam _____.

16. _____ resolution refers to the ability to resolve objects that are the same distance from the transducer but are located perpendicular to the plane of imaging.

17. If the gain is set too _____, artifactual echo noise will be displayed throughout the image.

EXERCISE 5: IMAGE IDENTIFICATION

1. Answer the question using (horizontal/vertical) axis.

   a. Distance is found on the _____ axis.

   b. Time is found along the _____ axis.

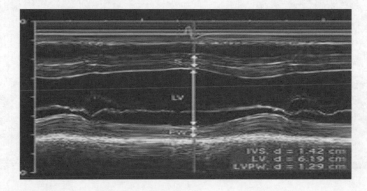

2. Which image demonstrates turbulent flow?

A   B

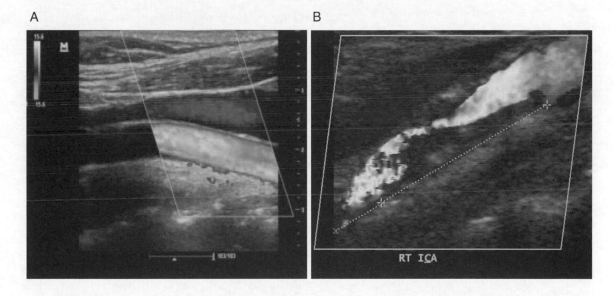

3. Does this image represent high resistance or low resistance:

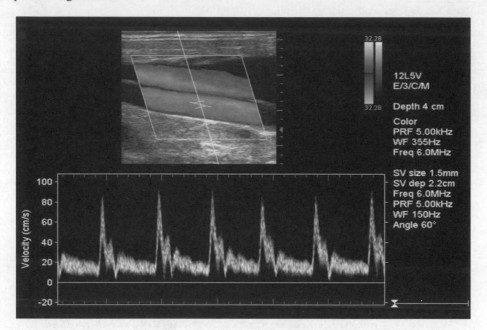

Chapter **1** **Foundations of Sonography**   Copyright © 2023 by Elsevier, Inc. All rights reserved.

2 Essentials of Patient Care for the Sonographer

KEY TERMS

Exercise 1

Match the following basic patient care term terms with their definitions.

_____ 1. patient-focused care (PFC)

_____ 2. vital signs

_____ 3. pulse

_____ 4. nasal cannula

_____ 5. bradycardia

_____ 6. oximetry

_____ 7. respiration

_____ 8. dyspnea

_____ 9. apnea

_____ 10. ostomy

_____ 11. isolated systolic hypertension

_____ 12. pulse pressure

_____ 13. intravenous (IV) therapy

_____ 14. body mechanics

_____ 15. standard precautions

_____ 16. nosocomial infection

A. An easy and effective way to measure heart rate; recorded as beats per minute (bpm)

B. Non-invasive method of monitoring oxygen levels in the blood

C. Refers to observable and measurable signs of life

D. Hospital-acquired infection

E. Shortness of breath or the feeling of not getting enough air, which may leave a person gasping

F. Difference between systolic and diastolic blood pressures

G. Spontaneous breathing that stops for any reason; it may be temporary, starting and stopping at intervals, or prolonged

H. Exists when systolic pressure is above 140 mmHg, while diastolic pressure remains below 90 mmHg

I. Represents a national movement to recapture the respect and goodwill of the American public

J. Heart rate of less than 60 bpm arising from disease in the heart's electrical conduction system

K. Process of inhaling and exhaling air

L. Surgical procedure to create an opening to allow passage of contents of the urinary bladder or bowel through the abdominal wall

M. The practice of giving liquid substances directly into a vein

N. Basic infection control guidelines used to reduce the risks of infection spread through these transmission modes: airborne infection, droplet infection, and contact infection

O. Refers to using the correct muscles to complete a task safely, efficiently, and without undue strain on any joints or muscles

P. Device for delivering oxygen by way of two small tubes inserted into the nostrils

BASIC PATIENT CARE

Exercise 2

Fill in the blank(s) with the word(s) that best completes the statements or provide a short answer.

1. Examples of vital signs include _____, _____, _____, and _____.

2. Strenuous exercise, coronary artery disease, and electrolyte imbalances in the blood can cause _____.

3. When a pulse is taken, which artery is usually palpated? _____

4. A normal pulse oximetry reading for a person breathing room air is _____.

5. Normal respiration occurs at a rate of 15 to _____ breaths per minute.

6. In measuring blood pressure, the higher number is the _____ pressure, which occurs when the ventricles contract to pump blood to the body; the lower number is the _____ pressure, which occurs near the end of the cardiac cycle when the ventricles are filling with blood.

7. True/False. The NG or nasogastric tube is placed through the mouth and esophagus into the stomach to drain the gastric contents.

8. When catheterized patients are transferred from wheelchairs or stretchers to the scanning table, where should the collecting bag be placed? (higher or lower than the patient).

PATIENT TRANSFER TECHNIQUES

Exercise 3

Fill in the blanks with the word(s) that best completes the statements or provide a short answer.

1. Identify the four basic principles of body mechanics.

    a. _____ Maintain a stable center of gravity

    b. _____ Keep center of gravity higher than the object

    c. _____ Keep your back straight

    d. _____ Bend your hips and knees

    e. _____ Keep feet together

2. Lifting should be done using the _____ muscles, by lifting straight upward in one smooth motion.

3. Idenitfy the method used to transfer a patient from a wheelchair to the bed when working alone:

    a. _____ First position and lock the wheelchair close to the bed and facing the foot of the bed.

    b. _____ Remove the armrest nearest the bed and swing away both leg rests.

    c. _____ Do not change the bed height position

    d. _____ Swing the patient's legs over the edge of the bed, helping him to sit up.

    e. _____ Ask the patient to scoot to the edge of the bed until his feet are on the floor.

INFECTION CONTROL

Exercise 4

Fill in the blanks with the word(s) that best completes the statements or provide a short answer.

1. The most important weapon against the spread of infection is proper _____.

2. You should wash your hands whenever you come in contact with these five substances:

    a. _____

    b. _____

    c. _____

    d. _____

    e. _____

3. Is it acceptable to not wash your hands if gloves were used? _____

4. What should be used to clean the transducer? _____

5. One of the most serious of the contact diseases is the methicillin-resistant *Staphylococcus aureus* (_____) infection.

8

Exercise 5

Reply to each question based on what you have learned in the chapter.

1. List three rights that patients have in the medical setting.

    a. _____

    b. _____

    c. _____

2. List three responsibilities that the patient has.

    a. _____

    b. _____

    c. _____

3. The Health Portability and Accountability Act of 1996 (_____) established new standards for the use of health care information.

4. The three standards created by this act are:

    a. _____

    b. _____

    c. _____

3 Ergonomics and Musculoskeletal Issues in Sonography

KEY TERMS

Exercise 1

Match the following terms with their definitions.

_____ 1. work-related musculoskeletal disorders (WRMSDs)

_____ 2. tendinitis and tenosynovitis

_____ 3. de Quervain's disease

_____ 4. ergonomics

_____ 5. carpal tunnel

_____ 6. cubital tunnel

_____ 7. epicondylitis (lateral and medial)

_____ 8. thoracic outlet syndrome

_____ 9. Occupational Safety and Health Act

_____ 10. trigger finger

_____ 11. bursitis (shoulder)

_____ 12. rotator cuff injury

_____ 13. spinal degeneration

_____ 14. Rotator cuff injury

A. Entrapment of the median nerve as it runs through the carpal bones of the wrist; results from repeated flexion and extension of the wrist and from mechanical pressure against the wrist

B. Nerve entrapment can occur at different levels, resulting in a variety of symptoms

C. The science of designing a job to fit the individual worker

D. Intervertebral disk degeneration resulting from bending and twisting and improper seating

E. Inflammation of the tendon and the sheath around the tendon; often occurs together.

F. Inflammation of the periosteum in the area of the insertion of the biceps tendon into the distal humerus; can result from repeated twisting of the forearm

G. Inflammation of the shoulder bursa from repeated motion

H. Specific type of tendinitis involving the thumb; can result from gripping the transducer

I. Entrapment of the ulnar nerve as it runs through the elbow; can result from repeated twisting of the forearm and mechanical pressure against the elbow when it is rested on the examination table during scanning

J. Repeated motion resulting in fraying of the rotator cuff muscle tendons; this injury increases with age and is even more prevalent when work-related stresses are added

K. Repeated arm abduction contributes to this injury by restricting blood flow to the soft tissues of the shoulder

L. Term currently used to describe occupational injury

M. Inflammation and swelling of the tendon sheath in a finger, entrapping the tendon and restricting motion of the finger

N. Federal law that ensures that every working man and woman in the United States has safe and healthful working conditions

RISK FACTORS FOR MUSCULOSKELETAL INJURY

Exercise 2

Complete the following comments regarding risk factors that may lead to musculoskeletal injury for sonographers.

1. Forceful _____

2. Awkward _____

3. Prolonged _____ postures

4. Repetitive _____

5. "Pinch" _____

6. Exposure to _____ factors

BEST PRACTICES

Exercise 3

Provide a short answer for the following questions.

1. Does the photo below demonstrate good or bad ergonomics? Explain your answer.

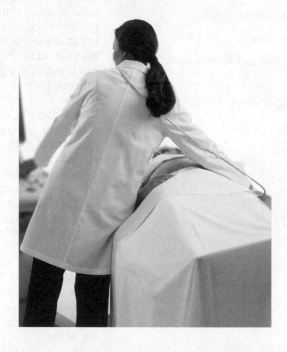

_____

_____

_____

2. Does the photo below demonstrate good or bad ergonomics? Explain your answer.

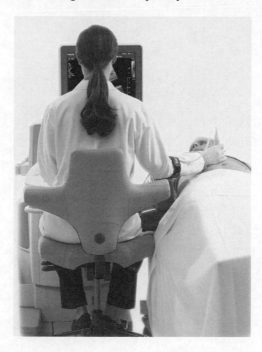

_____
_____
_____

3. Does the photo below demonstrate good or bad ergonomics? Explain your answer.

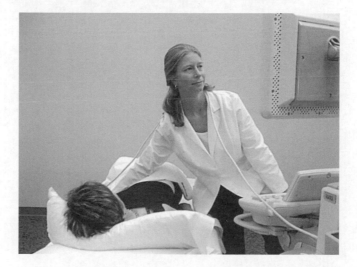

_____
_____
_____

Chapter **3 Ergonomics and Musculoskeletal Issues in Sonography**

4 Anatomic and Physiologic Relationships Within the Abdominal-Pelvic Cavity

EXERCISE 1: MATCHING KEY TERMS

Match the following general terms and terms related to abdominal planes with their definitions.

_____ 1. homeostasis

_____ 2. intertubercular plane

_____ 3. metabolism

_____ 4. subcostal plane

_____ 5. transpyloric plane

A. Physical and chemical changes that occur within the body
B. Maintenance of normal body physiology
C. Lowest horizontal imaginary line that joins the tubercles on the iliac crests
D. Horizontal plane that passes through the pylorus, the duodenal junction, the neck of the pancreas, and the hilum of the kidneys
E. Upper horizontal imaginary line that joins the lowest point of the costal margin on each side of the body

EXERCISE 2: CROSSWORD

Read the clues and complete the crossword puzzle.

Across

1. The internal organs.

2. Structures located toward the surface of the body are _____.

3. Nearest point of attachment, center of body, or point of reference.

4. The hepatic artery is _____ to the common bile duct.

5. Lower extremity from the knee to the foot.

Down

6. Broad muscle that separates the thoracic and abdominopelvic cavities and forms the floor of the thoracic cavity.

7. Refers to the back surface of the body.

8. Refers to the front surface of the body

9. The top of the head is the most _____ point of the body.

10. The structure is _____ if it is toward the side, away from the midline.

11. The bottom of the feet is the most _____ point of the body.

12. Toward the feet; sometimes used instead of inferior.

	6							9					12	
1						8		2				11		
			7				5							
									10					
				3										
					4									

EXERCISE 3: MATCHING

Match the following terms related to body cavities and abdominal structures with their definitions.

_____ 1. Peritoneal cavity

_____ 2. inguinal ligament

_____ 3. lateral arcuate ligament

_____ 4. left crus of the diaphragm

_____ 5. linea alba

_____ 6. linea semilunaris

_____ 7. medial arcuate ligament

_____ 8. pelvic cavity

_____ 9. rectouterine space

_____ 10. rectus abdominis muscle

_____ 11. right crus of the diaphragm

_____ 12. scrotal cavity

_____ 13. superficial inguinal ring

_____ 14. vesicouterine pouch

A. Arises from the sides of the bodies of the first two lumbar vertebrae

B. Thickened upper margin of the fascia covering the anterior surface of the psoas muscle

C. Slightly curved line on the ventral abdominal wall that marks the lateral border of the rectus abdominis

D. Ligament between the anterior superior iliac spine and the pubic tubercle

E. Area in the pelvic cavity between the rectum and the uterus where free fluid may accumulate

F. Arises from the sides of the bodies of the first three lumbar vertebrae

G. Fibrous band of tissue that stretches from the xiphoid to the symphysis pubis

H. Formed by the deflection of the peritoneum from the bladder to the uterus

I. Potential space between the parietal and visceral peritoneal layers.

J. Thickened upper margin of the fascia covering the anterior surface of the quadratus lumborum muscle

K. In the male, a small outpocket of the pelvic cavity containing the testes

L. Triangular opening in the external oblique aponeurosis

M. Lower portion of the abdominopelvic cavity that contains part of the large intestine, the rectum, urinary bladder, and reproductive organs

N. Muscle of the anterior abdominal wall

EXERCISE 4: MATCHING ABDOMINAL MEMBRANES AND LIGAMENTS

Match the following terms related to abdominal membranes and ligaments, potential spaces in the body, and the retro-peritoneum with their definitions.

_____ 1. anterior pararenal space

_____ 2. ascites

_____ 3. epiploic foramen

_____ 4. falciform ligament

_____ 5. gastrosplenic ligament

_____ 6. greater omentum

_____ 7. greater sac

_____ 8. lesser omentum

_____ 9. lesser sac

_____ 10. ligamentum teres

_____ 11. Morison's pouch

_____ 12. parietal peritoneum

_____ 13. perirenal space

_____ 14. posterior pararenal space

_____ 15. visceral peritoneum

A. Attaches the liver to the anterior abdominal wall and undersurface of the diaphragm

B. Located between the anterior surface of the renal fascia and the posterior area of the peritoneum

C. Primary compartment of the peritoneal cavity; extends across the anterior abdomen from the diaphragm to the pelvis

D. Ligament between the stomach and the spleen; helps support the stomach and spleen

E. Located directly around the kidney; completely enclosed by renal fascia

F. Accumulation of serous fluid in the peritoneal cavity

G. Membranous extension of the peritoneum that suspends the stomach and duodenum from the liver; helps support the lesser curvature of the stomach

H. Layer of the peritoneum that lines the abdominal wall

I. Found between the posterior renal fascia and the muscles of the posterior abdominal wall

J. Opening to the lesser sac

K. Double fold of the peritoneum attached to the duodenum, stomach, and large intestine; helps support the greater curve of the stomach

L. Right posterior subhepatic space located anterior to the kidney and inferior to the liver where fluid may accumulate

M. Layer of peritoneum that covers the abdominal

N. Peritoneal pouch located behind the lesser omentum and stomach organs

O. Termination of the falciform ligament; seen in the left lobe of the liver

ANATOMY AND PHYSIOLOGY

Exercise 5: Word Scramble Anatomy

Unscramble the following anatomy terms with their region.

_____ 1. rubaml

_____ 2. veilcp

_____ 3. olfeam

_____ 4. poalleitp

_____ 5. alicec

_____ 6. gnanliui

_____ 7. saltco

_____ 8. cariabhl

_____ 9. moiabldan

_____ 10. carichto

Loin; the region of the lower back and side, between the lowest rib and the pelvis

Pelvis; the bony ring that girdles the lower portion of the trunk

Thigh; the part of the lower extremity between the hip and the knee

Area behind the knee

Abdomen

Depressed region between the abdomen and the thigh

Ribs

Arm

Portion of trunk below the diaphragm

Chest; the part of the trunk below the neck and above the diaphragm

17

Exercise 6: Fill in the Blank About the Abdominal Cavity

Fill in the blank(s) with the word(s) that best completes the statements about the abdominal cavity.

1. The abdominal cavity is bounded superiorly by the _____; anteriorly by the _____ muscles; posteriorly by the vertebral column, ribs, and iliac fossa; and inferiorly by the _____.

2. The liver lies posterior to the lower ribs with the majority of the right lobe in the right _____ .

3. The right kidney lies slightly more (inferior/ superior) relative to the left kidney.

4. The aorta lies _____ to the spine, slightly to the _____ of the midline in the abdomen.

5. The inferior vena cava lies to the _____ of the spine.

6. The dome-shaped muscle that separates the thorax from the abdominal cavity is the _____.

7. The _____ crus of the diaphragm arises from the sides of the bodies of the first three lumbar vertebrae.

8. The fibrous band that stretches from the xiphoid to the symphysis pubis is the _____.

9. A sheath formed by the aponeuroses of the muscles of the lateral group is the _____ _____ muscle.

10. List the four organs contained within the pelvic cavity. _____, _____, _____, and _____.

11. The peritoneum passes from the bladder to the uterus to form the _____ pouch.

12. Between the uterus and the rectum the peritoneum forms the deep _____ pouch.

13. The _____ tubes extend laterally from the fundus of the uterus and are enveloped by a fold of peritoneum known as the broad ligament.

14. A muscular "sling" composed of the _____ and _____ muscles forms the inferior boundary of the true pelvis and separates it from the perineum.

15. The muscles that lie along the posterior and lateral margins of the pelvis major are the _____ and _____.

16. The _____ muscles form the posterior pelvic wall.

17. The _____ peritoneum is the portion that lines the abdominal wall, but does not cover a viscus; the _____ peritoneum is the portion that covers an organ.

18. The _____ omentum is attached to the greater curvature of the stomach and hangs down like an apron in the space between the small intestine and anterior abdominal wall.

19. An extensive peritoneal pouch located behind the lesser omentum and stomach is the _____ sac.

20. The opening to the lesser sac in the abdomen is the _____.

21. The liver is attached by the _____ ligament to the anterior abdominal wall and to the undersurface of the diaphragm.

Exercise 7: Fill in the Blank About Potential Spaces

Fill in the blank(s) with the word(s) that best completes the statements about the potential spaces in the body.

1. The right and left anterior _____ spaces lie between the diaphragm and the liver, one on each side of the falciform ligament.

2. The right posterior subphrenic space that lies between the right lobe of the liver, the right kidney, and the right colic flexure is also called _____.

3. The omental bursa normally has some empty places known as _____.

4. The _____ lateral paracolic gutter communicates with the right posterior subphrenic space.

5. The protrusion of part of the abdominal contents beyond the normal confines of the abdominal wall is called a _____.

Exercise 8: Differentiate

Differentiate between the peritoneal (P) and retroperitoneal (R) structures by placing the correct letter in front of the organ.

1. _____ Bladder
2. _____ Liver
3. _____ Kidneys
4. _____ Gallbladder
5. _____ Spleen
6. _____ Stomach
7. _____ Pancreas
8. _____ Inferior vena cava
9. _____ Ovaries
10. _____ Prostate gland
11. _____ Duodenum
12. _____ Aorta
13. _____ Ureters

Chapter **4** Anatomic and Physiologic Relationships Within the Abdominal-Pelvic Cavity

5 Comparative Sectional Anatomy of the Abdominal-Pelvic Cavity

KEY TERMS

Exercise 1

Match the following general terms and terms related to abdominal planes with their definitions.

_____ 1. Transverse

_____ 2. Sagittal

_____ 3. Longitudinal

_____ 4. Coronal

A. The plane is a lengthwise plane running from front to back. It divides the body or any of its parts into right and left sides, or two equal halves; this is known as the midsagittal plane.
B. The plane is a lengthwise plane running from side to side, dividing the body into anterior and posterior portions.
C. The plane is horizontal to the body
D. The plane is parallel to the long axis of the body or part.

ANATOMY AND PHYSIOLOGY

Exercise 2

Select the correct anatomical relationship for the following:

1. Superior mesenteric artery is (superior/inferior) to the celiac axis.

2. Splenic vein is (superior/inferior) to the splenic artery.

3. Right hepatic vein is seen as the (medial/lateral) drainage into the inferior vena cava.

4. Right renal vein is (anterior/posterior) to the right renal artery.

5. Pancreas is located (anterior/posterior) to the aorta.

6. Gallbladder is usually located in the (medial/lateral) aspect of the right lobe of the liver.

7. Endometrium is the (inner/outer) lining of the uterine cavity.

8. Falciform ligament is (superior/inferior) to the coronary sinus.

9. Right kidney is (superior/inferior) to the left kidney.

10. Inferior vena cava is (anterior/posterior) to the head of the pancreas.

Exercise 3

List the nine regions of the abdominal wall.

1	2	3
4	5	6
7	8	9

Exercise 4

Label the following illustrations.

a. Cross section of the abdomen at the level of the tenth intervertebral disk.

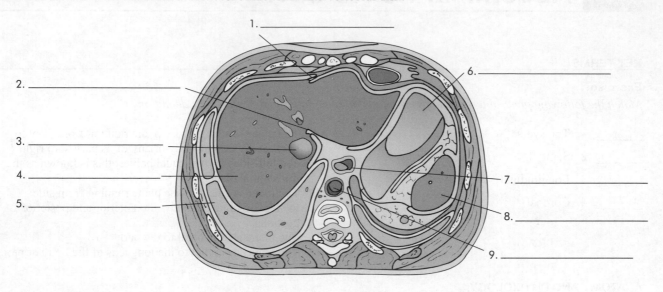

b. Cross section of the abdomen at the level of the eleventh thoracic disk.

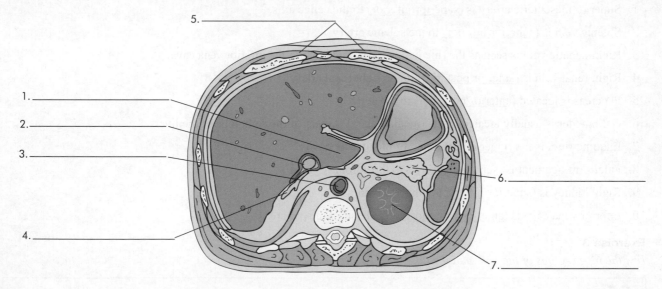

c. Cross section of the abdomen at the level of the twelfth thoracic vertebra.

3. _____

4. _____

1. _____

5. _____

6. _____

2. _____

7. _____

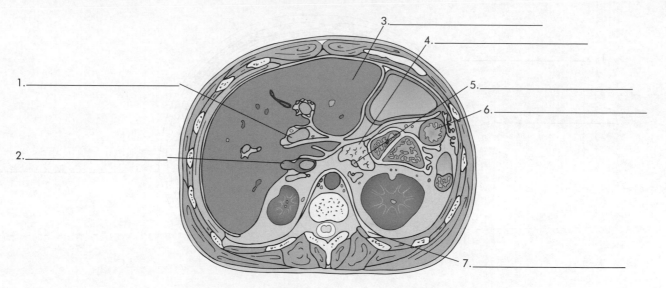

d. Cross section of the abdomen at the level of the second lumbar vertebra.

6. _____

1. _____

7. _____

2. _____

3. _____

8. _____

9. _____

4. _____

5. _____

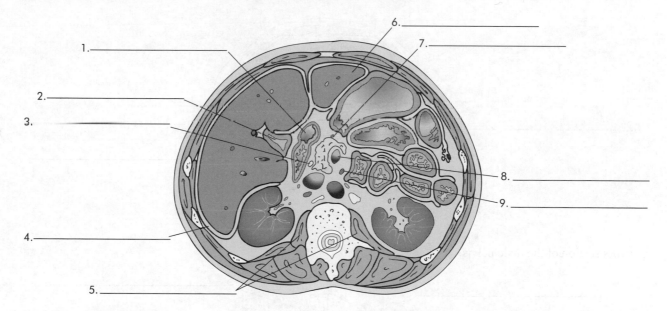

Chapter **5 Comparative Sectional Anatomy of the Abdominal-Pelvic Cavity**

e. Cross section of the abdomen at the level of the third lumbar vertebra.

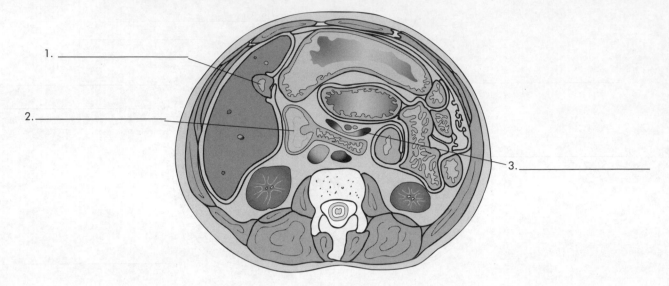

1. _____

2. _____

3. _____

f. Cross section of the pelvis.

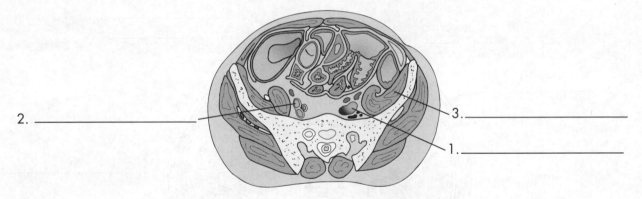

2. _____

3. _____

1. _____

g. Cross section of the male pelvis.

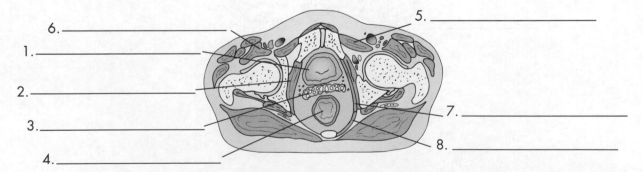

6. _____

1. _____

2. _____

3. _____

4. _____

5. _____

7. _____

8. _____

Chapter **5 Comparative Sectional Anatomy of the Abdominal-Pelvic Cavity**

h. Cross section of the female pelvis.

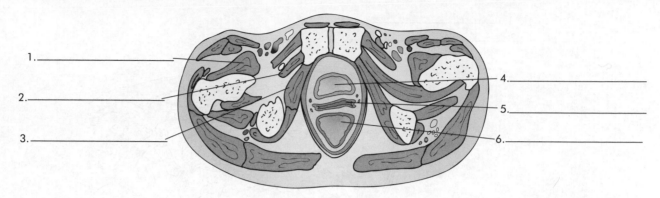

1. _____
2. _____
3. _____
4. _____
5. _____
6. _____

i. Sagittal section of the right abdomen 8 cm from the midline.

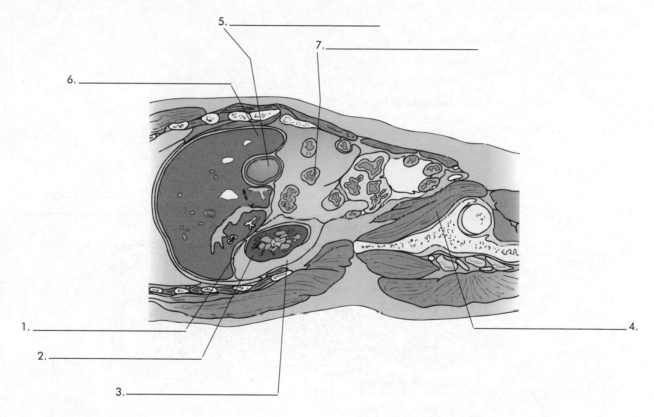

5. _____
7. _____
6. _____
1. _____
2. _____
3. _____
4. _____

j. Sagittal section of the right abdomen 6 cm from the midline.

1. _____

2. _____

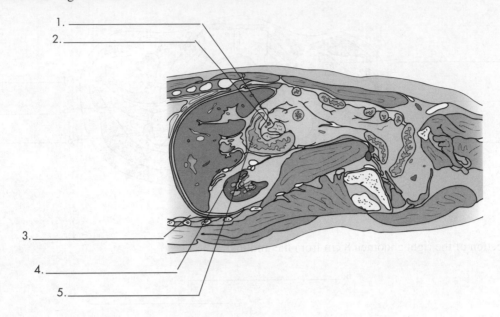

3. _____

4. _____

5. _____

k. Sagittal section of the abdomen just right of the midline.

1. _____

2. _____

3. _____

7. _____

8. _____

4. _____

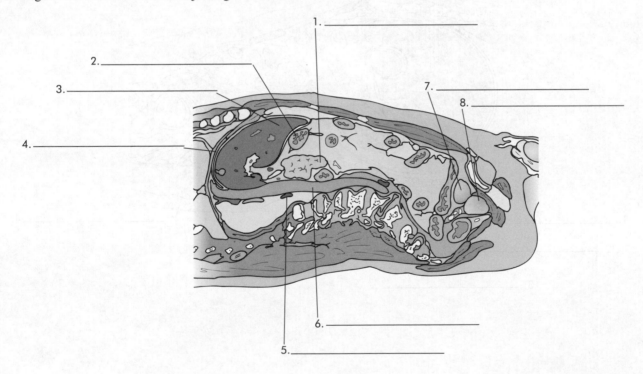

6. _____

5. _____

l. Sagittal section of the abdomen just left of the midline.

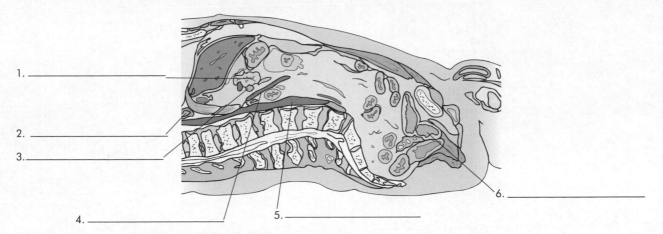

1. _____

2. _____

3. _____

4. _____

5. _____

6. _____

m. Sagittal section of the abdomen along the left abdominal border.

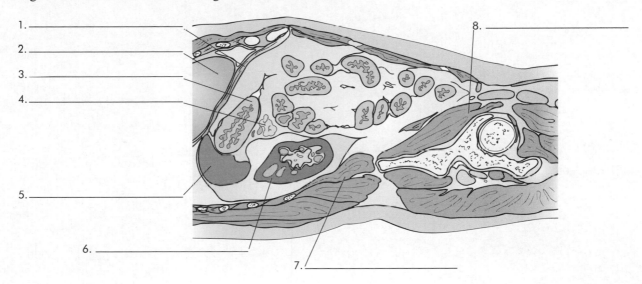

1. _____

2. _____

3. _____

4. _____

5. _____

6. _____

7. _____

8. _____

Chapter **5 Comparative Sectional Anatomy of the Abdominal-Pelvic Cavity**

6 Basic Ultrasound Imaging: Techniques, Terminology, and Tips

EXERCISE 1: TERMINOLOGY IDENTIFICATION

Match the following arterial terms with their definitions.

_____ 1. Curved array probe

_____ 2. Fan

_____ 3. Micro movement

_____ 4. Macro movement

_____ 5. Protocol

_____ 6. Rock

_____ 7. Rotate

_____ 8. Scan Window

_____ 9. Sector array probe

_____ 10. Slide

_____ 11. Sweep

A. standardization of specific anatomical structures that should be imaged in a complete or focused sonographic examination.

B. small face transducer that allows adequate intercostal visualization although the near field is reduced.

C. this movement of the probe is used with the sweep and slight motion in which the probe is moved less than one centimeter.

D. this motion is used when the probe is physically moved along the area of interest.

E. micro movement when the probe is minutely angled, pivoting on a point of interest.

F. motion used to navigate between the ribs or to change from transverse to longitudinal planes.

G. the probe remains in one area while using a large wrist motion with the probe perpendicular to the skin surface to sweep through the area of interest.

H. this movement of the probe is used with the sweep and slight motion in which the probe is moved greater than one centimeter.

I. large footprint that allows good near field and far field visualization with limited intercostal access.

J. probe is slowly angled back and forth in one place to image the area completely or to follow the anatomical structure.

K. areas in the body that allows the sound beam to penetrate without obstruction.

SONOGRAPHIC EVALUATION

Exercise 2: Fill in the blanks

Fill in the blank(s) with the word(s) that best completes the statements about abdominal scanning.

1. All transverse supine scans are oriented with the liver on the _____ of the screen.

2. Longitudinal scans present the patient's head to the _____ and feet to the _____ of the screen and use the xiphoid, umbilicus, or symphysis to denote the midline of the scan plane.

3. The position of the patient should be described in relation to the _____.

4. Variations in the patient's respiration may also help eliminate _____ interference and improve image quality.

5. Patients should be instructed not to eat or drink anything for _____ hours before the abdominal ultrasound procedure.

6. In Doppler imaging, flow toward the transducer is positive, or _____, whereas flow away from the transducer is negative, or _____.

7. Arterial flow pulsates with the cardiac cycle and shows its maximal peak during the _____ part of the cycle.

8. A phasic pattern may be seen in the _____ (near the heart) that is associated with overload of the right ventricle.

9. Identify the following patient positions for ultrasound examinations.

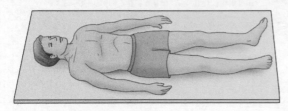

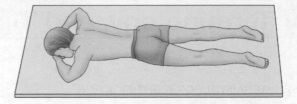

1. _____

2. _____

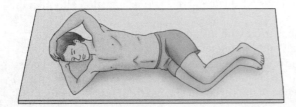

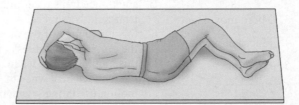

3. _____

4. _____

MEDICAL TERMS FOR THE SONOGRAPHER

Exercise 3: Matching

Match the following medical terms with their definitions.

_____ 1. anechoic or sonolucent

_____ 2. echogenic or hyperechoic

_____ 3. enhancement, increased through transmission

_____ 4. fluid-fluid level

_____ 5. heterogeneous

_____ 6. homogeneous

_____ 7. hypoechoic

_____ 8. infiltrating

_____ 9. irregular borders

_____ 10. isoechoic

_____ 11. loculated mass

_____ 12. shadowing

A. Not uniform in texture or composition
B. Usually refers to a diffuse disease process or metastatic disease
C. Echo-producing structure; reflects sound with a brighter intensity
D. Interface between two fluids with different acoustic characteristics. This level will change with patient position.
E. Very close to the normal parenchymal echogenicity pattern
F. Sound that travels through an anechoic (fluid-filled) substance and is not attenuated. There is increased brightness directly beyond the posterior border of the anechoic structure as compared with the surrounding area.
G. Completely uniform in texture or composition
H. Borders are not well defined, are ill-defined, or are not present.
I. Low-level echoes within a structure
J. Sound beam is attenuated by a solid or calcified object.
K. Well-defined borders with internal echoes; the septa may be thin (likely benign) or thick (likely malignant).
L. Without internal echoes; the structure is fluid filled and transmits sound easily.

Exercise 4: Multiple Choice

Identify the incorrect answer for each question about the criteria for identifying abnormalities.

_____1. The three terms are used to describe various textures of the border of a structure include all except:
   a. Smooth
   b. Echogenic
   c. Well-defined
   d. Irregular

_____2. Which term does not describe the transmission of sound.
   a. Increased
   b. Unchanged
   c. Slow
   d. Decreased

3. Match the five sonographic and medical terms that describe the characteristics of an organ or mass: anechoic, echogenic, hyperechoic, hypoechoic, isoechoic
   a. _____ Low-level echoes
   b. _____ Without internal echoes
   c. _____ Bright internal echoes, as in calcification
   d. _____ Same echo consistency as the organ
   e. _____ Increased level of echoes

_____4. The sonographic characteristics of a cystic mass include all except:
   a. Smooth well-defined border
   b. Anechoic
   c. Increased through-transmission
   d. Decreased through-transmission

_____5. The sonographic characteristics of a solid mass include all except:
   a. Increased through-transmission
   b. Decreased through-transmission
   c. Internal echoes
   d. Irregular borders

Exercise 5: Image Identification

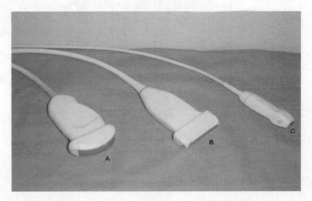

1. Identify the type of transducer:
   a. _____
   b. _____
   c. _____

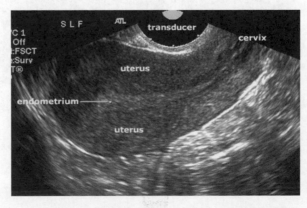

2. What sonographic term should be used to describe the texture of the myometrium? _____

Chapter **6 Basic Ultrasound Imaging: Techniques, Terminology, and Tips**

TRANSVERSE

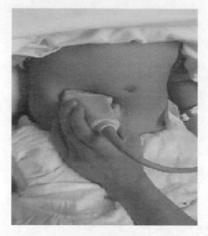

3. In the transverse plane, the liver would be seen on the (left/right) of the monitor?

LONGITUDINAL

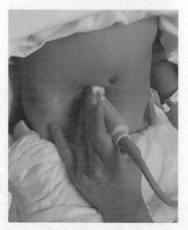

4. In the longitudinal plane, the head would be to the (left/right) of the monitor?

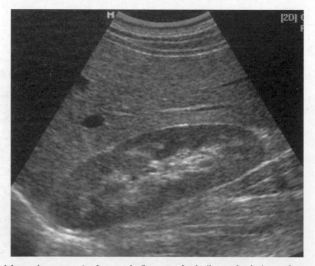

5. The parenchyma of the right kidney is more (<u>echogenic/hypoechoic/isoechoic/sonolucent</u>) than the liver?

KEY TERMS

Exercise 1

Match the following terms with their definitions.

_____ 1. aliasing

_____ 2. anechoic

_____ 3. baseline shift

_____ 4. comet tail

_____ 5. cross-talk

_____ 6. enhancement

_____ 7. hypoechoic

_____ 8. mirror image

_____ 9. multiple reflection

_____ 10. Nyquist limit

_____ 11. range ambiguity

_____ 12. resonance

_____ 13. reverberation

_____ 14. ring-down

_____ 15. section thickness

_____ 16. shadowing

_____ 17. speckle

_____ 18. speed error

A. Movement of the zero Doppler-shift frequency or zero flow speed line up or down on a spectral display

B. Increase in echo amplitude from reflectors that lie behind a weakly attenuating structure

C. Improper Doppler-shift information from a pulsed wave Doppler or color Doppler instrument when the true Doppler shift exceeds one half the pulse repetition frequency.

D. Series of closely spaced reverberation echoes

E. Artifact produced when echoes are placed too close to the transducer because a second pulse was emitted before they were received

F. Echo-free

G. Leakage of strong signals in one direction channel of a Doppler receiver into the other channel; can produce the Doppler mirror-image artifact

H. Artifact resulting from a continuous stream of sound emanating from an anatomic site

I. Having relatively weak echoes

J. Condition where a driven mechanical vibration is of a frequency similar to a natural vibration frequency of the structure

K. Several reflections produced by a pulse encountering a pair of reflectors; reverberation

L. Artifactual gray-scale, color flow, or Doppler signal appearing on the opposite side (from the real structure or flow) of a strong reflector

M. Doppler-shift frequency above which aliasing occurs; one half the pulse repetition frequency

N. Multiple reflections can occur between the transducer and a strong reflector (such as ribs).

O. Granular appearance of images and spectral displays that is caused by the interference of echoes from the distribution of scatterers in tissue

P. Thickness of the scanned tissue volume perpendicular to the scan plane; also called slice thickness

Q. Propagation speed that is different from the assumed value (1.54 mm/ms)

R. Reduction in echo amplitude from reflectors that lie behind a strongly reflecting or attenuating structure

Exercise 2

Use each of the following terms once to describe the artifacts shown in the sonographic images.

aliasing
banding
comet-tail
edge shadows
enhancement
grating lobe duplication
high gain produces a mirror image
mirror image

range-ambiguity
refraction
reverberation
ring-down
shadowing
slice thickness
speckle

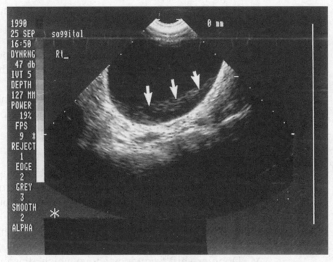

1. _____

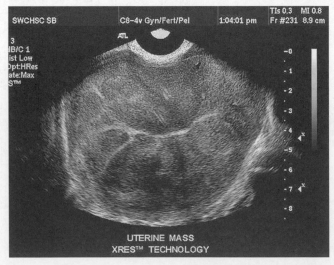

2. _____

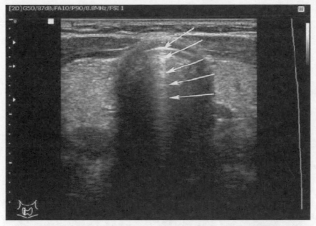

3. _____

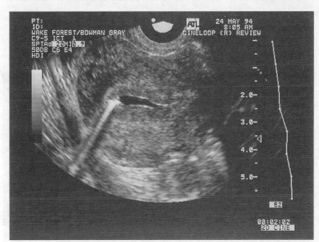

4. _____

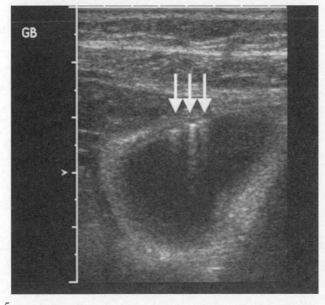

5. _____

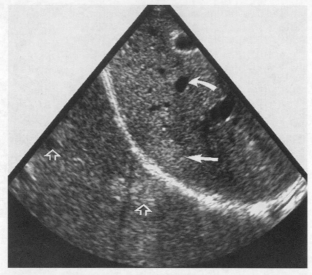

6. _____

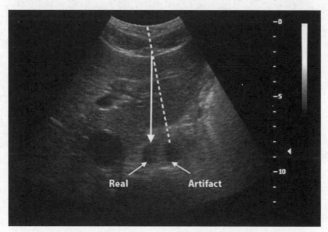

Real   Artifact

7. _____

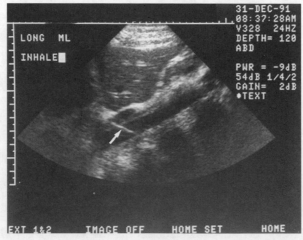

8. _____

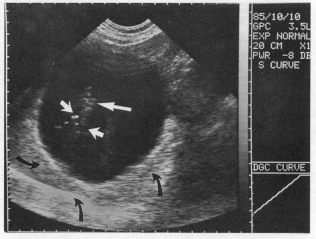

9. _____

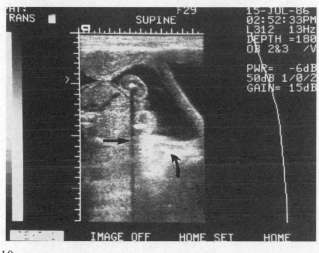

10. _____

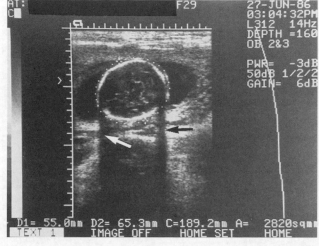

11. _____

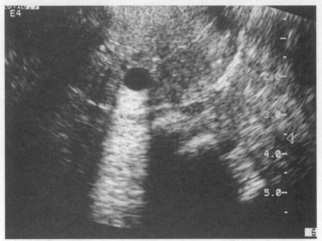

12. _____

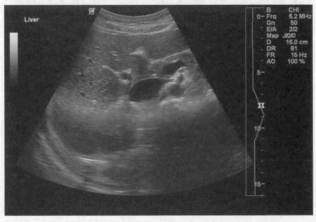

13. _____

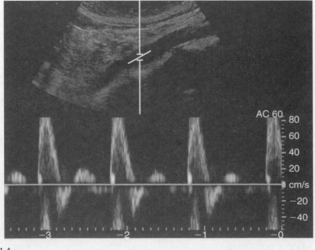

14. _____

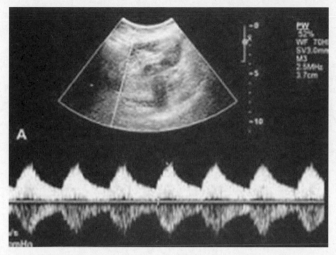

15. _____

8 The Vascular System

The Vascular System

KEY TERMS

Exercise 1 Matching

Match the following structural terms with their definitions.

_____ 1. vasa vasorum	A. Tiny arteries and veins that supply the walls of blood vessels
_____ 2. tunica media	B. Inner layer of the vascular system
_____ 3. tunica adventitia	C. Minute vessels that connect the arterial and venous systems
_____ 4. tunica intima	D. Communication between two blood vessels without any intervening capillary network
_____ 5. anastomosis	E. Outer layer of the vascular system, contains the vasa vasorum
_____ 6. capillaries	F. Middle layer of the vascular system; veins have thinner tunica media than arteries
_____ 7. arteries	G. Largest arterial structure in the body; arises from the left ventricle to supply blood to the body
_____ 8. aorta	H. Vascular structures that carry blood away from the heart.

Exercise 2 Identify

Match the origin of the following arteries.

_____ 1. superior mesenteric artery	A. Aorta
_____ 2. splenic artery	B. Celiac axis
_____ 3. left hepatic artery	C. Common hepatic artery
_____ 4. common iliac arteries	D. Splenic artery
_____ 5. right renal artery	
_____ 6. gastroduodenal artery	
_____ 7. left gastric artery	
_____ 8. inferior mesenteric artery	
_____ 9. left renal artery	
_____ 10. great pancreatic artery	
_____ 11. common hepatic artery	
_____ 12. right hepatic artery	

Exercise 3 Matching

Match the following venous terms with their definitions.

_____ 1. splenic vein	A. Formed by the union of the superior mesenteric vein and splenic vein near the porta hepatis of the liver
_____ 2. hepatic veins	B. Collapsible vascular structures that carry blood back to the heart
_____ 3. portal vein	C. Drains the spleen; travels horizontally across abdomen (posterior to the pancreas) to join the superior mesenteric vein to form the portal vein
_____ 4. right renal vein	D. Drains the left third of the colon and upper colon and joins the splenic vein
_____ 5. veins	E. Drains the proximal half of the colon and small intestine, travels vertically (anterior to the inferior vena cava) to join the splenic vein to form the portal veins
_____ 6. inferior mesenteric vein	F. Three large veins that drain the liver and empty into the inferior vena cava at the level of the diaphragm

_____ 7. left renal vein

_____ 8. superior mesenteric vein

_____ 9. inferior vena cava

G. Leaves the renal hilum, travels anterior to the aorta and posterior to the superior mesenteric artery to enter the lateral wall of the inferior vena cava

H. Largest venous abdominal vessel that conveys blood from the body below the diaphragm to the right atrium of the heart

I. Leaves the renal hilum to enter the lateral wall of the inferior vena cava

Exercise 4 Crossword

Use the definitions below to complete the puzzle

ACROSS

1. _Permanent localized dilatation of an artery, with an increase of 1.5 times its normal diameter._
2. _Condition in which the aortic wall becomes irregular from plaque formation, athero _____._
3. _Pulsatile hematoma that results from leakage of blood into soft tissue abutting the punctured artery with fibrous encapsulation and failure of the vessel wall to heal is called a _____ aneurysm._
4. _Peak systole minus peak diastole divided by peak systole is called the resistive _____._
5. _Increased turbulence is seen within the spectral tracing that indicates flow disturbance._

DOWN

6. _Transjugular intrahepatic portosystemic shunt_
7. _Vessels that have little or reversed flow in diastole and supply organs that do not need a constant blood supply (i.e., external carotid artery and brachial arteries)_
8. _Flow toward the liver._
9. _Vessels that have high diastolic component and supply organs that need constant perfusion (i.e., internal carotid artery, hepatic artery, and renal artery)._
10. _Flow away from the liver._

Exercise 5

Match the following pathology terms with their definitions.

_____ 1. cystic medial necrosis

_____ 2. Budd-Chiari syndrome

_____ 3. fusiform aneurysm

_____ 4. saccular aneurysm

_____ 5. cavernous transformation of the portal vein

A. Tear in the intima or media of the abdominal aorta

B. Periportal collateral channels in patients with chronic portal vein obstruction

C. Circumferential enlargement of a vessel with tapering at both ends

D. Weakening of the arterial wall

E. Most commonly results from intrinsic liver disease; however, also results from obstruction of the portal vein, hepatic veins, inferior vena cava, or prolonged congestive heart failure

_____ 6. dissecting aneurysm
_____ 7. arteriovenous fistula
_____ 8. portal venous hypertension
_____ 9. Marfan syndrome
_____ 10. true aneurysm

F. Communication between an artery and a vein
G. Localized dilatation of the vessel
H. Permanent dilation of an artery that forms when tensile strength of the arterial wall decreases
I. Hereditary disorder of connective tissue, bones, muscles, ligaments, and skeletal structures
J. Thrombosis of the hepatic veins

Exercise 6: Anatomy Identification

Label the following illustrations.

A. The abdominal arterial vascular system and its tributaries.

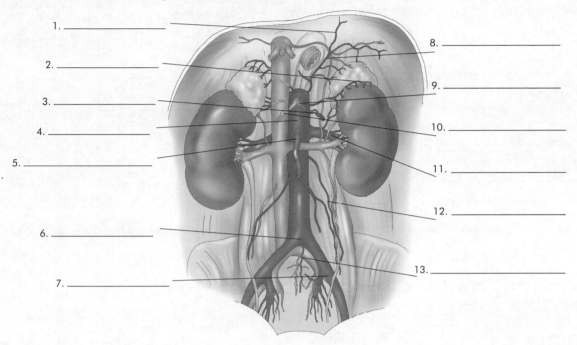

1. _____
2. _____
3. _____
4. _____
5. _____
6. _____
7. _____
8. _____
9. _____
10. _____
11. _____
12. _____
13. _____

B. The celiac artery and its branches.

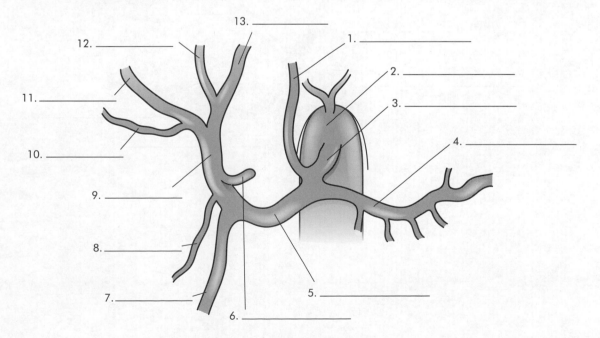

13. _____
12. _____
11. _____
10. _____
9. _____
8. _____
7. _____
6. _____
5. _____
1. _____
2. _____
3. _____
4. _____

C. The abdominal venous system and its tributaries.

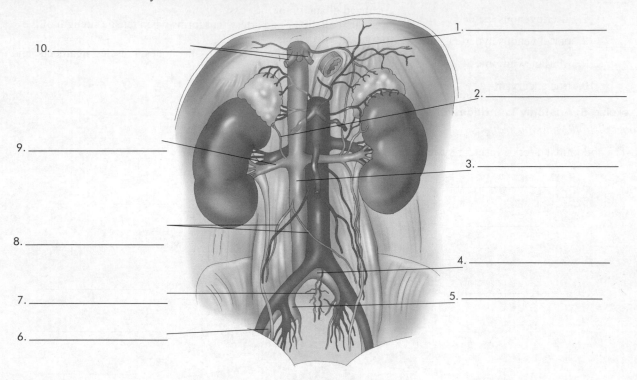

10. _____

9. _____

8. _____

7. _____

6. _____

1. _____

2. _____

3. _____

4. _____

5. _____

D. The portal vein.

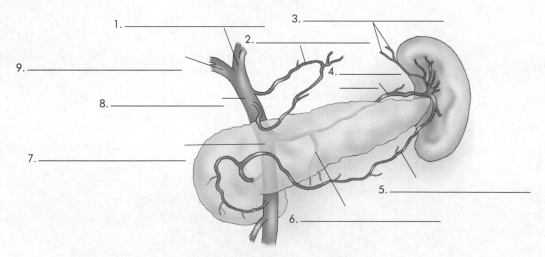

1. _____

9. _____

8. _____

7. _____

3. _____

2. _____

4. _____

5. _____

6. _____

Exercise 7 Short Answers

Fill in the blank(s) with the word(s) that best completes the statements about the arterial and venous structures.

1. The _____ hepatic artery supplies the gallbladder via the cystic artery and the liver.

2. The _____ trunk is the first anterior branch of the aorta, arising 1 to 2 cm inferior to the diaphragm.

3. The _____ flows from the kidney posterior to the superior mesenteric artery and anterior to the aorta to enter the lateral wall of the inferior vena cava.

4. The _____ is the second anterior branch, arising approximately 2 cm from the celiac trunk.

5. Portal veins become _____ as they progress into the liver from the porta hepatis.

6. The _____ renal artery courses from the aorta posterior to the inferior vena cava and anterior to the vertebral column in a posterior and slightly caudal direction to enter the hilum of the kidney.

7. The _____ artery courses along the upper border of the head of the pancreas, behind the posterior layer of the peritoneal bursa, to the upper margin of the superior part of the duodenum, which forms the lower boundary of the epiploic foramen.

8. The _____ vein is formed posterior to the pancreas by the union of the superior mesenteric vein and splenic veins at the level of L2.

9. The _____ artery takes a somewhat tortuous course horizontally to the left as it forms the superior border of the pancreas.

10. The _____ veins originate in the liver and drain into the inferior vena cava at the level of the diaphragm.

SONOGRAPHIC EVALUATION

Exercise 8: Short Answers

Fill in the blank(s) with the word(s) that best completes the statements or provide a short answer about the vascular and abdominal sonographic evaluations.

1. Describe how Doppler is used to distinguish the presence or absence of flow in a vessel from nonvascular structures.

_____

_____

_____

_____

2. Describe the technique that should be used to image the inferior vena cava.

_____

_____

_____

_____

3. Nonresistive vessels have a high _____ component and supply organs that need constant perfusion, such as the internal carotid artery, the hepatic artery, and the renal artery.

4. Explain how to differentiate the inferior vena cava from the aorta.

_____

_____

_____

_____

5. Doppler only records accurate velocity patterns when the beam is _____ to the flow.

6. The main renal artery has a(n) _____ impedance (nonresistive) pattern with significant diastolic flow—usually 30% to 50% of peak systole.

7. The portal vein shows a relatively _____ flow at low velocities, which may vary slightly with respirations.

8. Cavernous transformation of the portal vein demonstrates _____ collateral channels in patients with chronic portal vein obstruction.

9. With a recanalized _____ vein, the main portal vein and the left portal vein show normal flow, but the flow in the right portal vein is reversed.

PATHOLOGY

Exercise 9

Fill in the blank(s) with the word(s) that best completes the statements or provide a short answer about vascular pathology.

1. The most common causes of aneurysms are _____ and _____.

2. The large aneurysm may rupture into the peritoneal cavity or retroperitoneum, causing _____ and a drop in _____.

3. The normal measurement for an adult abdominal aorta is less than 3 cm, measuring from _____ to _____ walls.

4. Thrombus usually occurs along the _____ or _____ wall.

5. A(n) _____ is a pulsatile hematoma that results from the leakage of blood into the soft tissue abutting the punctured artery, with subsequent fibrous encapsulation and failure of the vessel wall defect to heal.

6. What are the clinical findings in a patient with a dissecting aneurysm?

_____

_____

_____

_____

7. Describe the three locations where a dissection of the aorta may occur.

_____

_____

_____

_____

8. Describe other pseudopulsatile abdominal masses that may simulate an aortic aneurysm.

_____

_____

_____

_____

Exercise 10

Provide a short answer for each question after evaluating the images.

1. *Complete the questions:*

   a. *What sonographic view is this?*

   b. *Structure A is* _____.

   c. *Structure B is* _____.

   d. *Structure C is* _____.

e. Structure D is _____.

f. Structure E is _____.

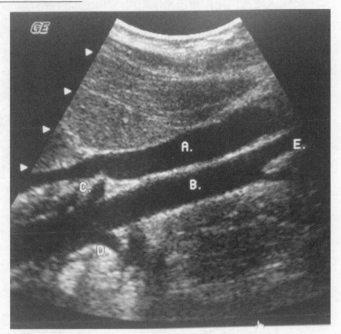

2. *Identify the vascular structures:*

   a. long arrow: _____.

   b. short arrow: _____.

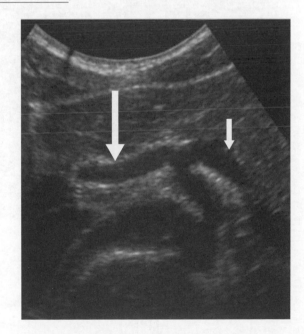

47

3. *The arrow is pointing to the* _____.

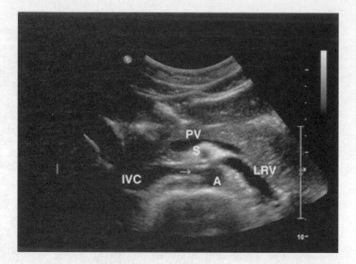

4. *The arrow is pointing to the* _____.

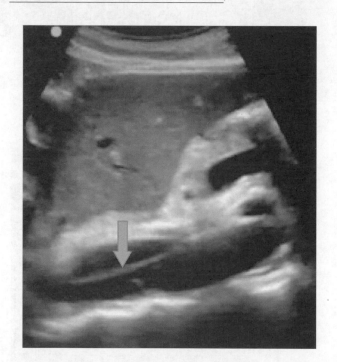

5. a) *The arrow is pointing to what structure?* _____.

    b) *The arrowhead is pointing to what structure?* _____.

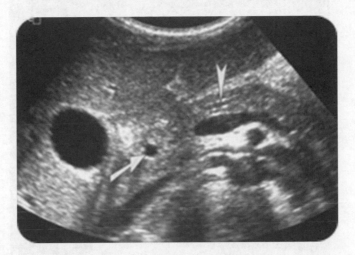

6. *The arrow is pointing to what structure?* _____.

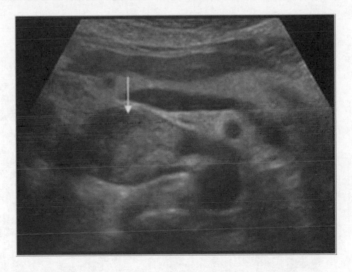

7. What structure is the arrow pointing to? _____.

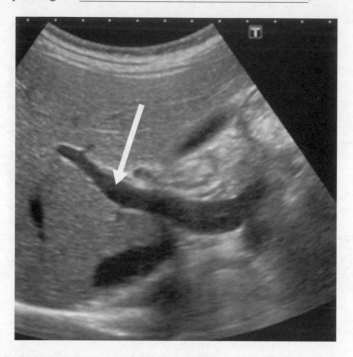

8. What structure is anterior to the common bile duct? _____

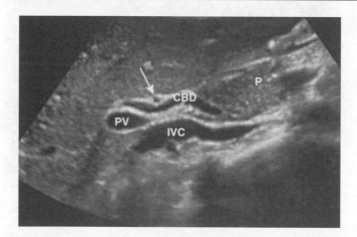

9 The Liver

KEY TERMS

Exercise 1: Matching

Match the following anatomy terms with their definitions.

_____ 1. bare area

_____ 2. caudate lobe

_____ 3. epigastrium

_____ 4. falciform ligament

_____ 5. left hypochondrium

_____ 6. left lobe of the liver

_____ 7. left portal vein

_____ 8. ligamentum teres

_____ 9. ligamentum venosum

_____ 10. main lobar fissure

_____ 11. main portal vein

_____ 12. right hypochondrium

_____ 13. right lobe of the liver

_____ 14. right portal vein

A. Smallest lobe of the liver situated on the posterosuperior surface of the left lobe; the ligamentum venosum is the anterior border

B. Separates left lobe from caudate lobe; shown as echogenic line on the transverse and sagittal images

C. Area superior to the liver that is not covered by peritoneum so that inferior vena cava may enter the chest

D. Lies in the epigastrium and left hypochondrium

E. Largest lobe of the liver

F. Boundary between the right and left lobes of the liver; seen as hyperechoic line on the sagittal image extending from the portal vein to the neck of the gallbladder

G. Extends from the umbilicus to the diaphragm in a sagittal plane and contains the ligamentum teres

H. Supplies the left lobe of the liver

I. Appears as bright echogenic foci on transverse image; along with falciform ligament, it divides medial and lateral segments of left lobe of the liver

J. Enters the liver at the porta hepatis

K. Right upper quadrant of the abdomen that contains the liver and gallbladder

L. Supplies the right lobe of the liver; branches into anterior and posterior segments

M. Left upper quadrant of the abdomen that contains the left lobe of the liver, spleen, and stomach

N. Area between the right and left hypochondrium

Exercise 2: Matching

Match the following physiology and laboratory terms with their definitions.

_____ 1. alkaline phosphatase

_____ 2. ALT

_____ 3. AST

_____ 4. bilirubin

_____ 5. BUN

_____ 6. hepatocellular disease

_____ 7. hepatocyte

_____ 8. liver function tests

_____ 9. obstructive diseas

_____ 10. hyperglycemia

_____ 11. hypoglycemia

A. Yellow pigment in bile formed by the breakdown of red blood cells; excreted by liver and stored in the gallbladder

B. Deficiency in blood glucose levels

C. Specific laboratory tests that look at liver function (aspartate or alanine aminotransferase, lactic acid dehydrogenase, alkaline phosphatase, and bilirubin)

D. Aspartate aminotransferase—enzyme of the liver

E. Alanine aminotransferase—enzyme of the liver

F. Parenchymal liver cell that performs all functions ascribed to the liver

G. Uncontrolled increase in blood glucose levels

H. Enzyme of the liver

I. Classification of liver disease where hepatocytes are the primary problem

J. Blood urea nitrogen; laboratory measurement of the amount of nitrogenous waste and creatinine in the blood

K. Classification of liver disease where the main problem is blocked bile excretion within the liver or biliary system

Exercise 3: Crossword

Read the clues and complete the crossword puzzle.

Across

1. *Disease affects hepatocytes and interferes with liver function.*
2. *Hypoechoic mass with an echogenic central core (abscess, metastases).*
3. *Within the liver*
4. *Most common form of neoplasm of the liver; primary sites are from colon, breast, and lung.*
5. *Pus-forming collection of fluid*

Down

6. *Outside the liver*
7. *Abbreviation for one of the liver enzymes.*
8. *Any new growth (benign or malignant)*
9. *Alanine aminotransferase*
10. *Smallest lobe of the liver*

Exercise 4: Identify the Anatomy

Label the following illustrations.

A. Anterior view of the liver.

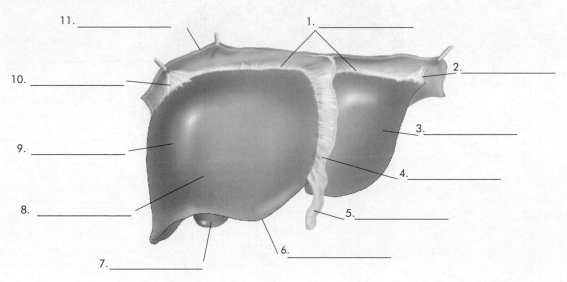

B. Superior view of the liver.

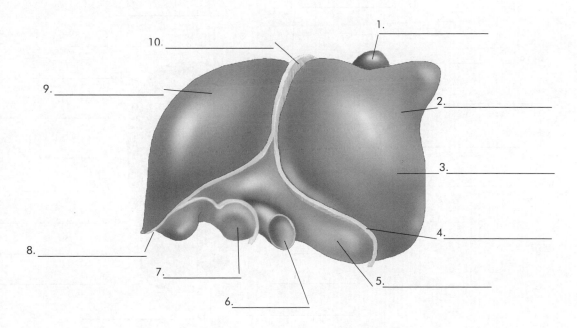

C. Interior view of the visceral surface of the liver.

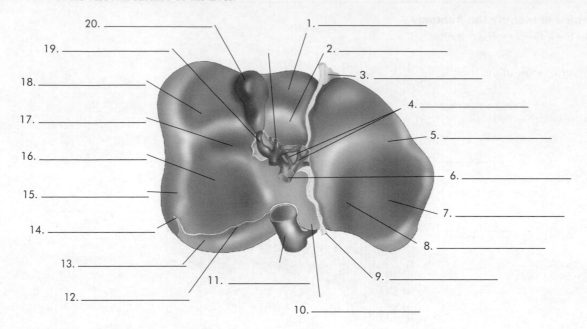

20. _____   1. _____
19. _____   2. _____
18. _____   3. _____
17. _____   4. _____
16. _____   5. _____
15. _____   6. _____
14. _____   7. _____
13. _____   8. _____
11. _____   9. _____
12. _____
                                    10. _____

D. Posterior view of the diaphragmatic surface of the liver.

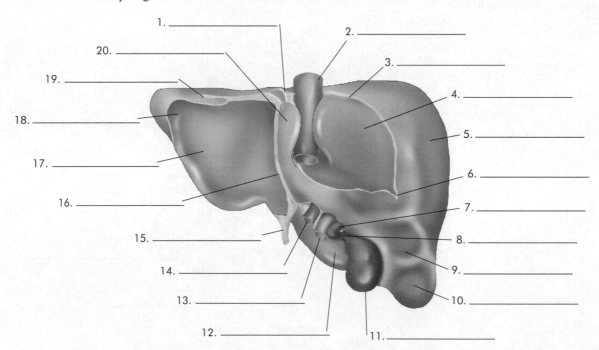

1. _____   2. _____
20. _____   3. _____
19. _____   4. _____
18. _____   5. _____
17. _____   6. _____
16. _____   7. _____
15. _____   8. _____
14. _____   9. _____
13. _____   10. _____
12. _____   11. _____

Exercise 5: Short Answer

Fill in the blank(s) with the word(s) that best completes the statements about the anatomy and physiology of the liver.

1. A congenital variant, _____ lobe, can sometimes be seen as an anterior projection of the liver and may extend inferiorly as far as the iliac crest.

2. The liver is covered by a thin connective tissue layer called _____ capsule.

3. The _____ fissure is the boundary between the right and left lobes of the liver.

4. The _____ ligament extends from the umbilicus to the diaphragm in a parasagittal plane and contains the ligamentum teres.

5. The ligamentum_____ appears as a bright echogenic focus on the sonogram and is seen as the rounded termination of the falciform ligament.

6. The fissure for the ligamentum_____ separates the left lobe from the caudate lobe.

7. The hepatic veins are divided into three components: _____, _____, and _____.

8. The liver is a major center of _____, which may be defined as the physical and chemical process whereby foodstuffs are synthesized into complex elements.

9. A pigment released when the red blood cells are broken down is _____.

10. The liver is also a center for _____ of the waste products of metabolism accumulated from other sources in the body and foreign chemicals that enter the body.

11. Sugars may be absorbed from the blood in several forms, but only _____ can be used by cells throughout the body as a source of energy.

12. The accompanying loss of oncotic pressure in the vascular system allows fluid to migrate into the interstitial space, resulting in _____ in dependent areas.

13. Hemoglobin released from the red cells is converted to _____ within the reticuloendothelial system and is then released into the bloodstream.

14. Elevation of serum bilirubin results in _____, which is a yellow coloration of the skin, sclerae, and body secretions.

Exercise 6: Multiple Choice

Select the false statement for each anatomy and physiology question.

1. The landmarks of the liver include all except:
   a. Right hypochondrium
   b. Greater part of the epigastrium
   c. Left hypochondrium
   d. Right hypogastrium

2. Which characteristic of the right lobe of the liver is untrue:
   a. The right lobe exceeds the left lobe by a ratio of 2:1.
   b. The falciform ligament borders its upper surface
   c. The inferior and posterior surfaces are marked by three fossae: the porta hepatis, the gallbladder fossa, and the inferior vena cava fossa.
   d. The left sagittal fossa borders the posterior surface

3. Which characteristic of the left lobe of the liver is incorrect:
   a. The upper surface is convex and molded onto the diaphragm.
   b. The undersurface includes the gastric impression and omental tuberosity.
   c. The porta hepatis is the anterior border.
   d. The fossa for the gallbladder is on the right of the medial segment.

4. Which ligament and fissure is not found within the hepatic parenchyma.
   a. Main lobar fissure
   b. Transverse fissure
   c. Falciform ligament
   d. Ligamentum teres

5. Which statement is incorrect to distinguish hepatic veins from portal veins.
   a. Hepatic veins flow into the inferior vena cava
   b. Splenic veins flow into the inferior vena cava
   c. Hepatic veins course between hepatic lobes and segments
   d. Portal veins are larger at their origin as they emanate from the porta hepatis

SONOGRAPHIC EVALUATION

Exercise 7

Fill in the blank(s) with the word(s) that best completes the statements or provide a short answer about the sonographic techniques used for liver examination.

1. The portal flow is shown to be _____ (toward the liver), whereas the hepatic venous flow is _____ (away from the liver).

2. Generally a wider pie sector or curved linear array transducer is the most appropriate to optimally image the _____ of the abdomen.

3. To image the far field better, a(n) _____ array transducer with a longer focal zone is used.

4. Fatty infiltration implies increased _____ accumulation in the hepatocytes and results from significant injury to the liver or a systemic disorder leading to impaired or excessive metabolism of fat.

5. On ultrasound examination, the liver parenchyma in chronic hepatitis is _____ with _____ brightness of the portal triads, but the degree of attenuation is not as great as seen in fatty infiltration.

6. Glycogen storage disease is associated with _____, focal nodular _____, and hepatomegaly.

7. A(n) _____ is any new growth of new tissue, either benign or malignant.

8. The liver is the third most common organ injured in the abdomen after the _____ and the _____.

9. An increase in portal venous pressure or hepatic venous gradient is defined as _____.

10. The umbilical vein may become _____ secondary to portal hypertension.

11. The pulse repetition frequency allows one to record lower velocities as the PRF is _____.

12. The Doppler sample volume should be _____ than the diameter of the lumen.

13. Acute abdominal pain, massive ascites, and hepatomegaly secondary to thrombosis of the hepatic veins or inferior vena cava characterize _____ syndrome, which has a poor prognosis.

Exercise 8: Image Identification

Identify the abnormality for each question after evaluating the images.

1. _____

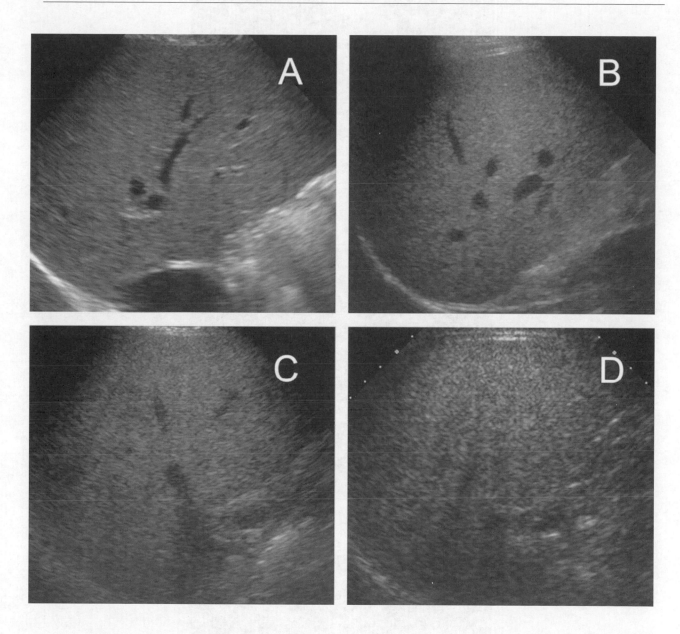

2. _____

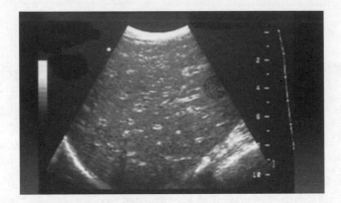

3. _____

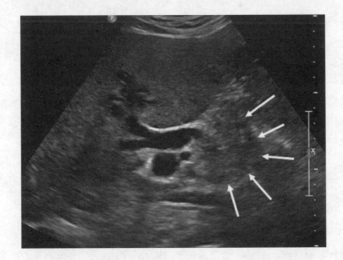

4. _____

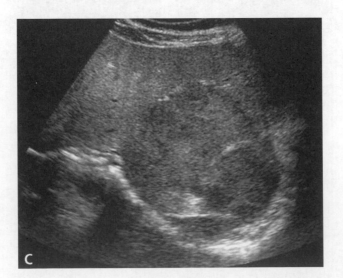

5. _____

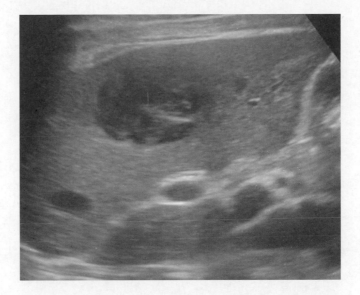

6. _____

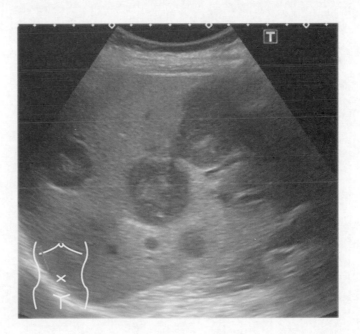

10 The Gallbladder and the Biliary System

Exercise 1

Match the following anatomy and physiology terms with their definitions.

_____ 1. ampulla of Vater
_____ 2. bilirubin
_____ 3. cholecystectomy
_____ 4. common bile duct
_____ 5. common duct
_____ 6. common hepatic duct
_____ 7. cystic duct
_____ 8. gallbladder
_____ 9. Hartmann's pouch
_____ 10. Heister's valve
_____ 11. hydrops
_____ 12. pancreatic duct
_____ 13. phrygian cap
_____ 14. porta hepatis
_____ 15. sphincter of Oddi

A. Extends from the point where the common hepatic duct meets the cystic duct; drains into the duodenum after it joins with the main pancreatic duct

B. Storage pouch for bile

C. Small opening in the duodenum in which the pancreatic and common bile duct enter to release secretions

D. Massive enlargement of the gallbladder

E. Tiny valves found within the cystic duct

F. Refers to common bile and hepatic ducts when cystic duct is not seen

G. Connects the gallbladder to the common hepatic duct

H. Central area of the liver where the portal vein, common duct, and hepatic artery enter

I. Small part of the gallbladder that lies near the cystic duct where stones may collect

J. Travels horizontally through the pancreas to join the common bile duct at the ampulla of Vater

K. Small muscle that guards the ampulla of Vater

L. Yellow pigment in bile formed by the breakdown of red blood cells

M. Removal of the gallbladder

N. Gallbladder variant in which part of the fundus is bent back on itself

O. Bile duct system that drains the liver into the common bile duct

Exercise 2

Match the following sonographic evaluation and pathology terms with their definitions.

_____ 1. adenomyomatosis
_____ 2. cholangitis
_____ 3. cholecystitis
_____ 4. cholecystokinin
_____ 5. choledochal cyst
_____ 6. choledocholithiasis
_____ 7. cholelithiasis
_____ 8. cholesterolosis
_____ 9. jaundice
_____ 10. junctional fold
_____ 11. Klatskin's tumor
_____ 12. Murphy's sign
_____ 13. polyp

A. Gallstones in the gallbladder

B. Calcification of the gallbladder wall

C. Inflammation of the bile duct

D. Excessive bilirubin accumulation causes yellow pigmentation of the skin; first seen in the whites of the eyes

E. Small polypoid projections from the gallbladder wall

F. Sonographic pattern found when the gallbladder is packed with stones

G. Cancer at the bifurcation of the hepatic ducts; may cause asymmetrical obstruction of the biliary tree

H. Low-level echoes found along the posterior margin of the gallbladder; move with change in position

I. Hormone secreted into the blood by the mucosa of the upper small intestine; stimulates contraction of the gallbladder and pancreatic secretion of enzymes

J. Variant of adenomyomatosis; cholesterol polyps

K. Inflammation of the gallbladder; may be acute or chronic

L. Cystic growth on the common duct that may cause obstruction

M. Small septum within the gallbladder, usually arising from the posterior wall

_____14. porcelain
                   gallbladder

_____15. sludge

_____16. wall echo shadow
                   (WES) sign

N. Small, well-defined soft tissue projection from the gallbladder wall

O. Stones in the bile duct

P. Positive sign implies exquisite tenderness over the area of the gallbladder upon palpation

ANATOMY AND PHYSIOLOGY

Exercise 3

Label the following illustrations.

A. Gallbladder and biliary system.

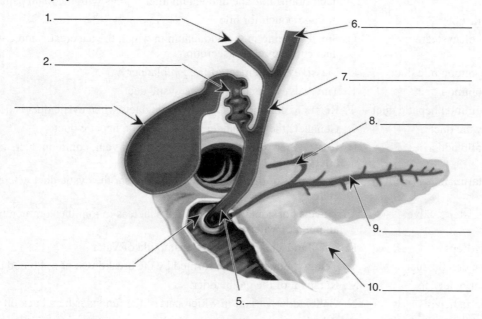

B. Relationships within the porta hepatis.

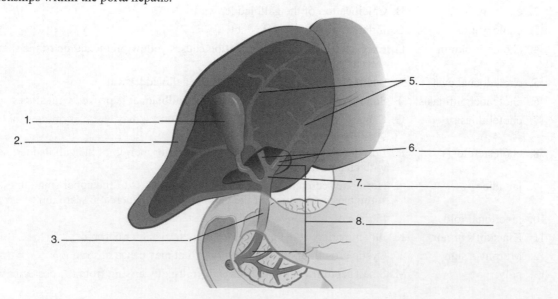

Exercise 4

Fill in the blank(s) with the word(s) that best completes the statements or provide a short answer about the anatomy and physiology of the gallbladder.

1. The gallbladder serves as a reservoir for _____ that is drained from the hepatic ducts in the liver.

2. The common hepatic duct is joined by the cystic duct to form the _____ duct.

3. The main pancreatic duct joins the common bile duct, and together they open through a small ampulla (the ampulla of _____) into the duodenal wall.

4. The end parts of the common bile duct and main pancreatic duct and the ampulla are surrounded by circular muscle fibers known as the sphincter of _____.

5. The arterial supply of the gallbladder is from the _____ artery, which is a branch of the right hepatic artery.

6. Bile is the principal medium for excretion of bilirubin _____.

7. The sign that indicates an extrahepatic mass compressing the common bile duct, which can produce an enlarged gallbladder, is called _____.

8. Sonographically, the common duct lies _____ and to the _____ of the portal vein in the region of the porta hepatis and gastrohepatic ligament.

9. The hepatic artery lies _____ and to the _____ of the portal vein.

SONOGRAPHIC EVALUATION

Exercise 5: Crossword

Use the description to complete the puzzle.

ACROSS

1. *The patient is initially examined with ultrasound in full _____.*

2. *The gallbladder may be identified as a(n) _____ oblong structure located anterior to the right kidney, lateral to the head of the pancreas and duodenum.*

3. *A small _____ fold has been reported to occur along the posterior wall of the gallbladder at the junction of the body and infundibulum.*

4. *To obtain a cross section of the portal triad, the transducer must be directed in a slightly _____ path from the left shoulder to the right hip.*

5. *The common duct is seen just _____ to the portal vein before it dips posteriorly to enter the head of the pancreas.*

DOWN

6. *The patient should also be rolled into a steep _____ or upright position in an attempt to separate small stones from the gallbladder wall or cystic duct.*

7. *The gallbladder commonly resides in _____ on the medial aspect of the liver.*

8. *Because of _____ tissue within the main lobar fissure of the liver, this bright linear reflector is a reliable indicator of the location of the gallbladder.*

9. *On sagittal scans, the right branch of the hepatic artery usually passes _____ to the common duct.*

10. *The right branch of the* _____ *artery can be seen between the duct and the portal vein as a small circular structure on the right subcostal transverse image.*

PATHOLOGY

Exercise 6

Fill in the blank(s) with the word(s) that best completes the statements or provide a short answer about the pathology of the gallbladder and biliary system.

1. The most classic symptom of gallbladder disease is _____ pain, usually occurring after ingestion of greasy foods.

2. A gallbladder attack may cause pain in the _____ shoulder.

3. The normal wall thickness of the gallbladder is less than _____ mm.

4. The _____ sign is described as a contracted bright gallbladder with posterior shadowing caused by a packed bag of stones.

5. A fairly rare complication of acute cholecystitis associated with the presence of gas-forming bacteria in the gallbladder wall and lumen with extension into the biliary ducts is called _____cholecystitis.

6. _____ cysts may be the result of pancreatic juices refluxing into the bile duct because of an anomalous junction of the pancreatic duct into the distal common bile duct, causing duct wall abnormality, weakness, and outpouching of the ductal walls.

7. A hyperplastic change in the gallbladder wall is _____.

8. An uncommon cause for extrahepatic biliary obstruction as a result of an impacted stone in the cystic duct creating extrinsic mechanical compression of the common hepatic duct is _____ syndrome.

9. _____ causes increasing pressure in the biliary tree with pus accumulation.

10. On ultrasound, multiple cystic structures that converge toward the porta hepatis are seen in _____ disease.

Exercise 7: Image Identification

Provide a short answer to identify the pathology after evaluating the images.

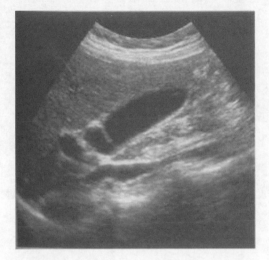

1. _____

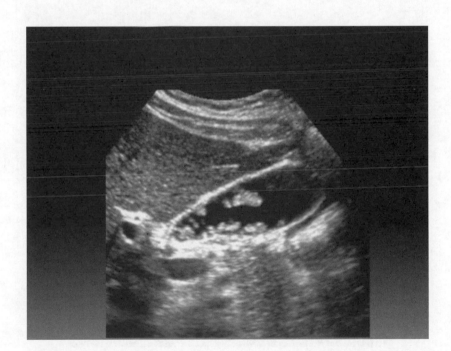

2. _____

Chapter **10** **The Gallbladder and the Biliary System**

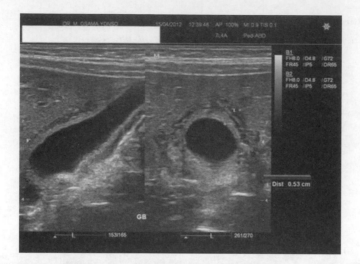

3. _____

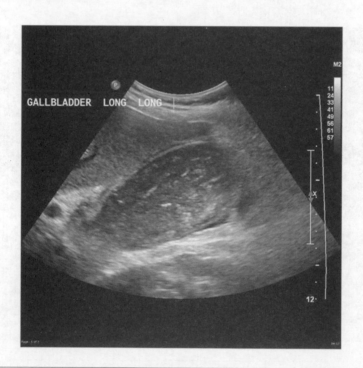

4. _____

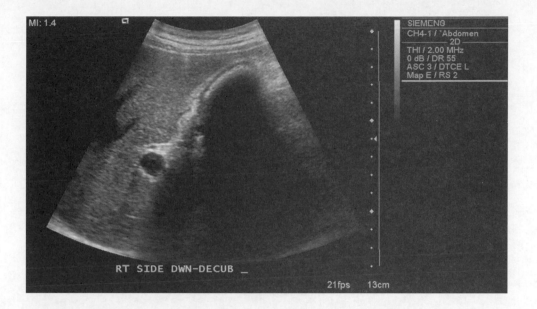

RT SIDE DWN-DECUB

5. _____

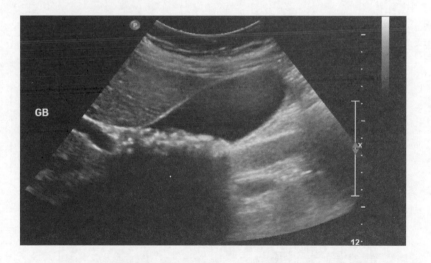

6. _____

Chapter **10** **The Gallbladder and the Biliary System**

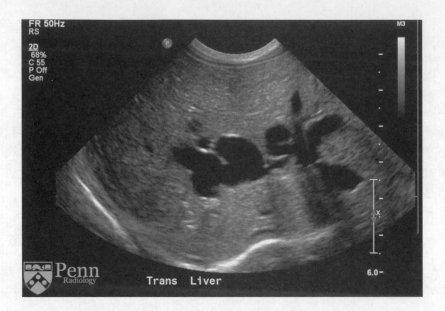

7. _____

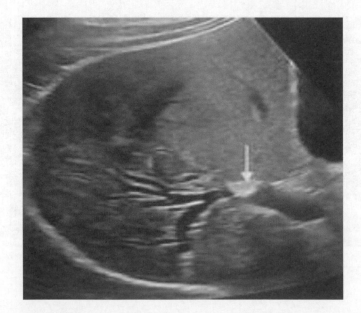

8. _____

Chapter **10 The Gallbladder and the Biliary System**

11 The Spleen

KEY TERMS

Exercise 1

Match the following anatomy terms with their definitions.

_____ 1. accessory spleen

_____ 2. gastrosplenic ligament

_____ 3. intraperitoneal

_____ 4. left hypochondrium

_____ 5. lienorenal ligament

_____ 6. leukopenia

_____ 7. phrenocolic ligament

_____ 8. pitting

_____ 9. reticuloendothelial

_____ 10. splenic agenesis

_____ 11. splenic artery

_____ 12. splenic hilum

_____ 13. splenic vein

_____ 14. wandering spleen

A. Process by which the spleen removes nuclei from blood cells without destroying the erythrocytes
B. Within the peritoneal cavity
C. Complete absence of the spleen
D. Ligament between the spleen and colon
E. Results from the failure of fusion of separate splenic masses forming on the dorsal mesogastrium; most commonly found in the splenic hilum or along the splenic vessels or associated ligaments
F. Leaves the splenic hilum, travels transversely through the upper abdomen to join with the superior mesenteric vein to form the main portal vein; serves as the posterior medial border of the pancreas
G. Located in the middle of the spleen; site where vessels and lymph nodes enter and exit the spleen
H. Spleen that has migrated from its normal location in the left upper quadrant
I. One of the ligaments between the stomach and spleen that helps to hold the spleen in place
J. Abnormal decrease of white blood corpuscles; may be drug induced
K. Ligament between the spleen and kidney that helps support the greater curvature of the stomach
L. Certain phagocytic cells (found in the liver and spleen) make up the reticuloendothelial system (RES); plays a role in the synthesis of blood proteins and hematopoiesis
M. Left upper quadrant of the abdomen that contains the left lobe of the liver, spleen, and stomach
N. Branch of the celiac axis; tortuous course toward the spleen; serves as the superior border of the pancreas

Exercise 2: CROSSWORD

Use the definitions to complete the puzzle.

ACROSS

1. Blood cell production
2. Process by which the spleen removes abnormal red blood cells as they pass through.
3. Oxygen-binding protein found in red blood cells
4. Follicles in the white pulp of the spleen, containing many lymphocytes
5. Alkaline fluid found in the lymphatic vessels
6. Condition in which there is more than one spleen is called _____ splenia.

DOWN

7. Consists of reticular cells and fibers (cords of Billroth); surrounds the splenic sinuses.
8. Red blood cell
9. Process by which the red pulp destroys the degenerating red blood cells
10. Long irregular channels lined by endothelial cells or flattened reticular cells. The crossword puzzle below had all the answers. I changed this to indicate the corresponding numbers. The letters should be removed and shaded out.

[Crossword puzzle grid with numbered clues: 1, 2, 3, 4, 5, 6, 7, 8, 9, 10]

Exercise 3

Match the following pathology terms with their definitions.

_____ 1. amyloidosis

_____ 2. autoimmune hemolytic anemia

_____ 3. Gaucher's disease

_____ 4. hemolytic anemia

_____ 5. Hodgkin disease

_____ 6. infarction

_____ 7. mononucleosis

_____ 8. non-Hodgkin lymphoma

_____ 9. polycythemia

_____ 10. polycythemia vera

_____ 11. sickle cell anemia

_____ 12. sickle cell crisis

_____ 13. spherocytosis

_____ 14. splenomegaly

_____ 15. thalassemia

A. Interruption in the blood supply to an area that may lead to necrosis of the area

B. Chronic, life-shortening condition of unknown cause involving bone marrow elements; characterized by an increase in red blood cell mass and hemoglobin concentration

C. Acute infection caused by the Epstein-Barr virus that most commonly affects teenagers and young adults; symptoms include fever, sore throat, enlarged lymph nodes, abnormal lymphocysts, and hepatosplenomegaly

D. Malignant disease of lymphoid tissue seen in increased frequency in individuals more than 50 years of age

E. Group of hereditary anemias occurring in Asian and Mediterranean populations

F. Hereditary condition in which erythrocytes assume a spheroid shape

G. One of the storage diseases in which fat and proteins are deposited abnormally in the body

H. Excess of red blood cells

I. Malignant disease that involves lymphoid tissue

J. Condition in sickle cell anemia in which the sickled cells interfere with oxygen transport, obstruct capillary blood flow, and cause fever and severe pain in the joints and abdomen

K. Metabolic disorder marked by amyloid deposits in organs and tissue

L. Enlargement of the spleen

M. Inherited disorder transmitted as an autosomal recessive trait that causes an abnormality of the globin genes in hemoglobin

N. Anemia resulting from hemolysis of red blood cells

O. Anemia caused by antibodies produced by the patient's own immune system

Exercise 4

Label the following illustrations.

A. Sagittal plane of the spleen and left kidney.

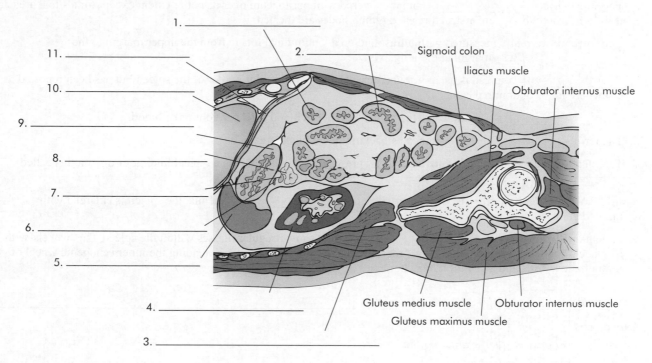

B. Anterior view of the spleen as it lies in the left hypochondrium.

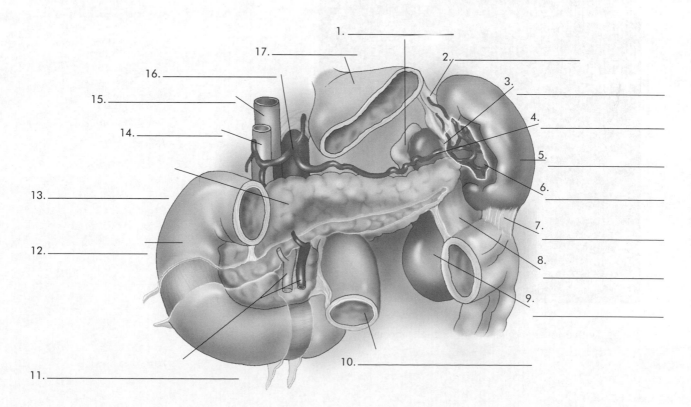

Fill in the blank(s) with the word(s) that best completes the statements about the anatomy and physiology of the spleen.

1. The spleen is part of the reticuloendothelial system and is the largest single mass of _____ tissue in the body.

2. The spleen is a(n) _____ organ, covered with peritoneum over its entire extent except for a small area at its hilum, where the vascular structures and lymph nodes are located.

3. The spleen is normally measured with ultrasound on a longitudinal image from the upper margin to the _____ margin at the long axis.

4. A(n) _____ spleen is usually found near the hilum or inferior border of the spleen but has been reported elsewhere in the abdominal cavity.

5. The _____ indicates the percentage of red blood cells per volume of blood.

6. The term _____ indicates bacteria in the bloodstream.

7. The increase in the number of white blood cells present in the blood that is a typical finding of infection is called _____.

8. In infants and children in crisis, the earlier stage of _____ anemia, the spleen is enlarged with marked congestion of the red pulp.

9. Patients with hepatosplenic _____ may show irregular masses within the spleen, the "wheels-with-in-wheels" pattern, with the outer wheel representing the ring of fibrosis surrounding the inner echogenic wheel of inflammatory cells and a central hypoechoic area.

PATHOLOGY

Exercise 6

Provide a short answer after evaluating the images.

1.

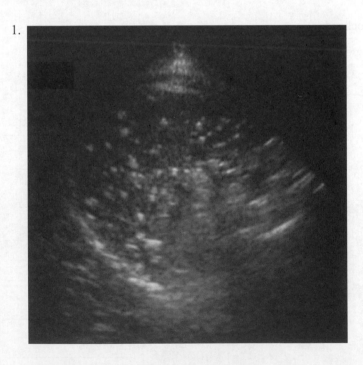

Patient with a fever and history of histoplasmosis. _____

2.

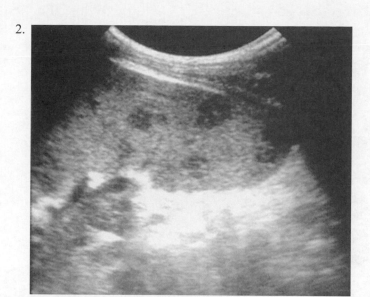

Clinical history included recent dental work followed by fever and LUQ pain. _____

3.

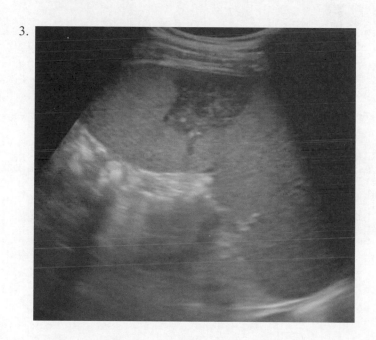

Patient recovering from septic emboli had this appearance. _____

4.

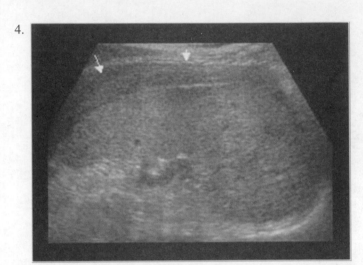

High school football player suffered traumatic injury to the back. _____

5.

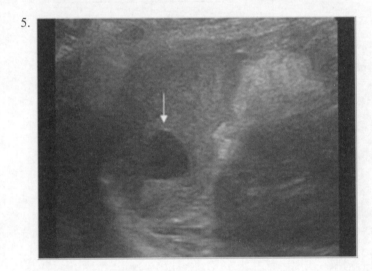

This finding was noted on an abdominal ultrasound. _____.

12 The Pancreas

Exercise 1

Match the following anatomy terms with their definitions.

_____ 1. body of the pancreas

_____ 2. caudal pancreatic artery

_____ 3. C-loop of the duodenum

_____ 4. common hepatic artery

_____ 5. dorsal pancreatic artery

_____ 6. duct of Santorini

_____ 7. duct of Wirsung

_____ 8. head of the pancreas

_____ 9. neck of the pancreas

_____ 10. pancreaticoduodenal arteries

_____ 11. portal-splenic confluence

_____ 12. superior mesenteric artery

_____ 13. superior mesenteric vein

_____ 14. tail of the pancreas

_____ 15. uncinate process

A. Branch of splenic artery that supplies the tail of the pancreas

B. Tapered end of the pancreas that lies in the left hypochondrium near the hilus of the spleen and upper pole of the left kidney

C. Junction of the splenic and main portal vein; posterior border of the body of the pancreas

D. Help supply blood to the pancreas along with the splenic artery

E. Lies in the midepigastrium anterior to the superior mesenteric artery and vein, aorta, and inferior vena cava

F. Small, curved tip of the pancreatic head that lies posterior to the superior mesenteric vein

G. Forms the lateral border of the head of the pancreas

H. Small area of the pancreas between the head and the body; anterior to the superior mesenteric vein

I. Lies posterior to the neck or body of the pancreas and anterior to the uncinate process of the gland

J. Forms the right superior border of the body and head of the pancreas and gives rise to the gastroduodenal artery

K. Largest duct of the pancreas that drains the tail, body, and head of the gland; it joins the common bile duct to enter the duodenum through the ampulla of Vater

L. Lies in the C-loop of the duodenum; the gastroduodenal artery is the anterolateral border, and the common bile duct is the posterolateral border

M. Serves as the posterior border to the body of the pancreas

N. Small accessory duct of the pancreas found in the head of the gland

O. Branch of the splenic artery that supplies the body of the pancreas

Exercise 2 CROSSWORD

Use the following definitions to complete the puzzle.

ACROSS

1. *Enzyme secreted by the pancreas to aid in the digestion of carbohydrates.*
2. *Portion of the pancreas that has an endocrine function and produces insulin, glucagon, and somatostatin.*
3. *Hormone that causes glycogen formation from glucose in the liver and that allows circulating glucose to enter tissue cells.*
4. *Dilated loops of bowel without peristalsis; associated with various abdominal problems, including pancreatitis, sickle cell crisis, and bowel obstruction.*

5. *Pancreatic enzyme that breaks down fats; enzyme is elevated in pancreatitis and remains increased longer than amylase.*
6. *Cells that perform exocrine function.*
7. *Pancreatic enzyme that is elevated during pancreatitis.*
8. *The kind of pancreatic function that involves the production of the hormone insulin.*
9. *The kind of pancreatic function that involves the production and digestion of pancreatic juice.*
10. *Stimulates the liver to convert the glycogen to glucose; produced by alpha cells*

Exercise 3

Match the following pathology terms with their definitions.

_____ 1. Courvoisier's gallbladder

_____ 2. cystic fibrosis

_____ 3. hypercalcemia

_____ 4. hyperlipidemia

_____ 5. ileus

_____ 6. leukocytosis

_____ 7. lymphoma

_____ 8. obstructive jaundice

A. Congenital condition in which elevated fat levels cause pancreatitis
B. Excessive bilirubin in the bloodstream caused by an obstruction of bile from the liver; characterized by a yellow discoloration of the sclera of the eye, skin, and mucous membranes
C. Malignant neoplasm that arises from the lymphoid tissues
D. Dilated loops of bowel without peristalsis; associated with various abdominal problems, including pancreatitis, sickle cell crisis, and bowel obstruction
E. Space or cavity that contains fluid but has no true endothelial lining membrane
F. Inflammation of the pancreas; may be acute or chronic
G. "Sterile abscess" collection of pancreatic enzymes that accumulate in the available space in the abdomen, usually in or near the pancreas
H. Abnormal increase in white blood cells caused by infections

_____ 9. pancreatic ascites

_____ 10. pancreatic pseudocyst

_____ 11. pancreatitis

_____ 12. pseudocyst

I. Enlargement of the gallbladder caused by a slow, progressive obstruction of the distal common bile duct from an external mass, such as adenocarcinoma of the pancreatic head

J. Elevated levels of calcium in the blood

K. Fluid accumulation caused by a rupture of a pancreatic pseudocyst into the abdomen; free-floating pancreatic enzymes are very dangerous to surrounding structures

L. Hereditary disease that causes excessive production of thick mucus by the endocrine glands

ANATOMY AND PHYSIOLOGY

Exercise 4

Label the following illustrations.

A. Sagittal plane of the pancreas.

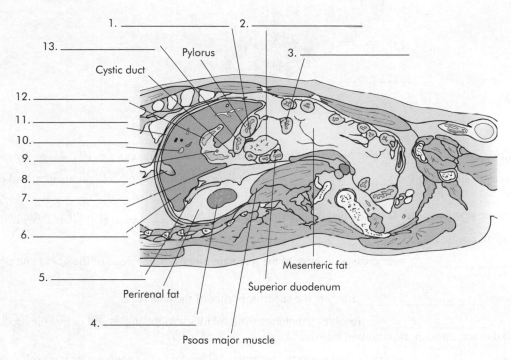

1. _____

2. _____

13. _____

Pylorus

3. _____

Cystic duct

12. _____

11. _____

10. _____

9. _____

8. _____

7. _____

6. _____

Mesenteric fat

5. _____

Superior duodenum

Perirenal fat

4. _____

Psoas major muscle

B. The portal venous system is the posterior border of the pancreas.

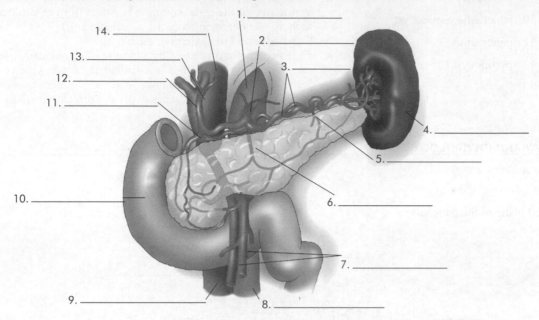

Exercise 5

Fill in the blank(s) with the word(s) that best completes the statements about the anatomy of the pancreas.

1. The pancreas is located in the _____ cavity posterior to the stomach, duodenum, and proximal jejunum of the small bowel.

2. The pancreatic gland appears sonographically isoechoic to slightly more _____ than the hepatic parenchyma.

3. The head of the pancreas lies _____ to the inferior vena cava.

4. The _____ vein crosses anterior to the uncinate process of the head of the gland and posterior to the neck and body.

5. The tortuous _____ artery is the superior border of the pancreas.

6. The duct of _____ receives tributaries from lobules at right angles and enters the medial second part of the duodenum with the common bile duct at the ampulla of Vater.

7. The _____ artery is seen along the anterolateral border of the pancreas as it travels a short distance along the anterior aspect of the pancreatic head.

8. The _____ duct crosses the anterior aspect of the portal vein to the right of the proper hepatic artery.

9. The portal vein is _____ to the inferior vena cava.

Exercise 6

Fill in the blank(s) with the word(s) that best completes the statements about the physiology of the pancreas.

1. The pancreas is both a digestive (_____) and a hormonal (_____) gland.

2. Failure of the pancreas to furnish sufficient insulin leads to _____.

3. Exocrine function is performed by _____ cells of the pancreas.

4. The sphincter of _____ is a muscle surrounding the ampulla of Vater that relaxes to allow pancreatic juice and bile to empty into the duodenum.

5. The endocrine function is located in the islets of _____ in the pancreas.

6. There are specific enzymes of the pancreas that may become altered in pancreatic disease, namely

_____ and _____.

7. Both amylase and lipase rise at the same rate, but the elevation in _____ concentration persists for a longer period in pancreatitis.

8. _____ controls the blood sugar level in the body.

PATHOLOGY

Exercise 7

Fill in the blank(s) with the word(s) that best completes the statements or provide a short answer about the pathology of the pancreas.

1. When the pancreas becomes damaged and malfunctions as a result of increased secretion and blockage of ducts,

_____ occurs.

2. Fluid collections around the pancreatic bed, along the pararenal spaces, within the _____ pouch, and around the duodenum may be present in a patient with acute pancreatitis.

3. Necrosis of the blood vessels results in the development of hemorrhagic areas referred to as _____ sign.

4. An inflammatory process that spreads along fascial pathways, causing localized areas of diffuse inflammatory edema

of soft tissue, is known as _____.

5. The _____ ducts become obstructed with a buildup of protein plugs with resultant calcifications along the duct in chronic pancreatitis.

6. The most common location of a pseudocyst is in the _____, anterior to the pancreas and posterior to the stomach.

7. A pseudocyst develops when pancreatic _____ escape from the gland and break down tissue to form a sterile abscess somewhere in the abdomen.

8. The most common primary neoplasm of the pancreas is _____.

Exercise 8: IMAGE IDENTIFICATION

Provide a short answer for each question.

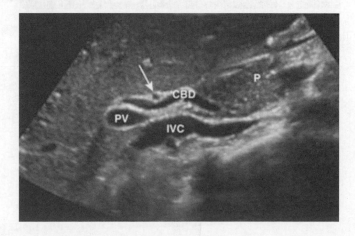

1. To which vascular structure is the arrow pointing in this image?

_____.

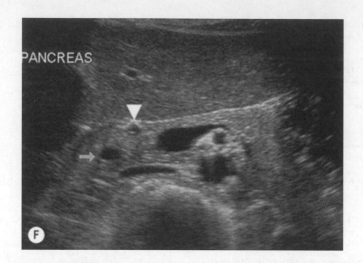

2. Identify the anatomy the arrows are pointing to.

Short arrow _____ Arrowhead _____

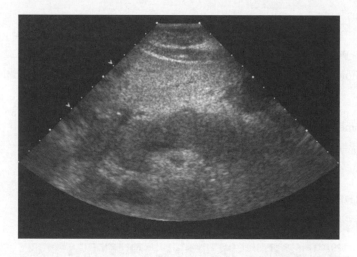

3. Patient presents to ED with severe mid-abdominal pain and elevated amylase levels.

_____,

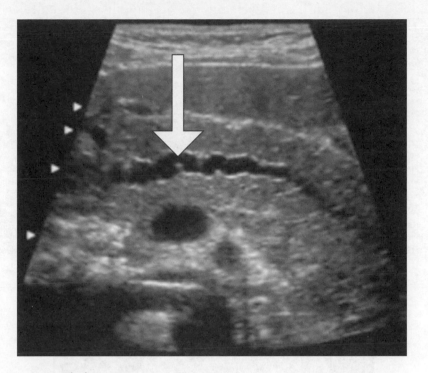

4. What structure is the arrow pointing to? _____.

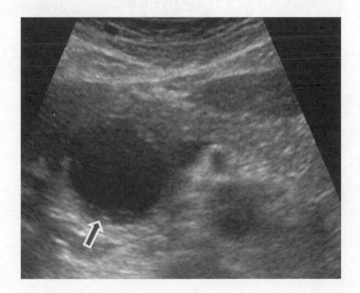

5. Patient presents with previous admissions of acute pancreatitis.

_____.

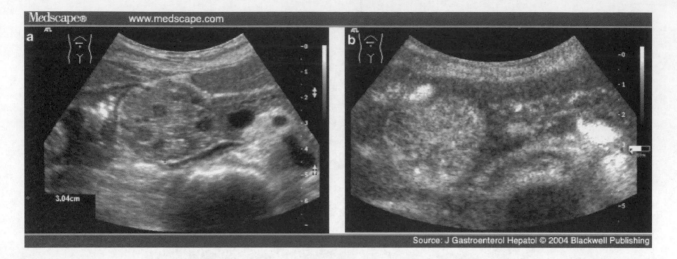

Source: J Gastroenterol Hepatol © 2004 Blackwell Publishing

6. Elderly female presents with abdominal discomfort and pain. _____

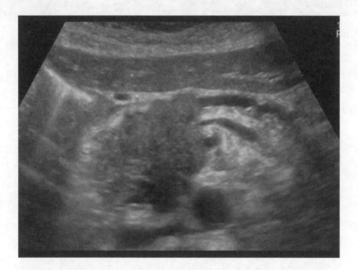

7. Patient presents with six-month history of weight loss, decreased appetite, and jaundice.

_____

13 The Gastrointestinal Tract

KEY TERMS

Exercise 1

Match the following anatomy terms with their definitions.

_____ 1. alimentary canal

_____ 2. cardiac orifice

_____ 3. duodenal bulb

_____ 4. gastrohepatic ligament

_____ 5. gastrophrenic, gastrosplenic, and lienorenal ligaments

_____ 6. greater omentum

_____ 7. haustra

_____ 8. hepatic flexure

_____ 9. lesser omentum

_____ 10. mesentery

_____ 11. mesothelium

_____ 12. mucosa

_____ 13. muscularis

_____ 14. pyloric canal

_____ 15. rugae

_____ 16. serosa

_____ 17. splenic flexure

_____ 18. submucosa

_____ 19. valvulae conniventes

_____ 20. villi

A. Ascending colon arises from the right lower quadrant to bend at this point to form the transverse colon

B. First part of the duodenum

C. Double fold of the peritoneum attached to the duodenum, stomach, and large intestine; helps support the greater curvature of the stomach; known as the "fatty apron"

D. Help support the greater curvature of the stomach

E. Fold from the parietal peritoneum that attaches to the small intestine, anchoring it to the posterior abdominal wall

F. Also known as the digestive tract; includes the mouth, pharynx, esophagus, stomach, duodenum, and small and large intestine

G. Inner folds of the small intestine

H. Entrance of the esophagus into the stomach

I. First layer of bowel

J. Helps support the lesser curvature of the stomach

K. The transverse colon travels horizontally across the abdomen and bends at this point to form the descending colon

L. One of the layers of the bowel, under the mucosal layer; contains blood vessels and lymph channels

M. Normal segmentation of the wall of the colon

N. Suspends the stomach and duodenum from the liver; helps to support the lesser curvature of the stomach

O. Muscle that connects the stomach to the proximal duodenum

P. Fourth layer of bowel; thin, loose layer of connective tissue, surrounded by mesothelium covering the intraperitoneal bowel loops

Q. Third layer of bowel

R. Normal segmentation of the small bowel

S. Inner folds of the stomach wall

T. Fifth layer of bowel

Exercise 2: CROSSWORD

Use the following definitions to complete the puzzle.

ACROSS

1. *Hormone secreted into the blood by the mucosa of the upper small intestine; stimulates contraction of the gallbladder and pancreatic secretion of enzymes.*
2. *Endocrine hormone released from the stomach; stimulates secretion of gastric acid.*
3. *Released from small bowel as antacid; stimulates secretion of bicarbonate.*
4. *Localized collection of pus surrounded by inflamed tissue.*

DOWN
5. *This point is located by drawing a line from the right anterosuperior iliac spine to the umbilicus.*
6. *Rhythmic dilation and contraction of the gastrointestinal tract as food is propelled through it.*
7. *Process of nutrient molecules passing through the wall of the intestine into the blood or lymph system.*

Exercise 3

Match the following pathology terms with their definitions.

_____ 1. appendicolith

_____ 2. ascites

_____ 3. Crohn's disease

_____ 4. diverticulum

_____ 5. fecalith

_____ 6. hemorrhage

_____ 7. lymphoma

_____ 8. McBurney's sign

_____ 9. Meckel's diverticulum

_____ 10. paralytic ileus

_____ 11. polyp

_____ 12. target sign

A. Calcified deposit within the appendix; appendicitis can develop when the appendix becomes blocked by hard fecal matter

B. Pouchlike herniation through the muscular wall of a tubular organ that occurs in the stomach, the small intestine or, most commonly, the colon

C. Malignancy of the lymph nodes, spleen, or liver

D. Dilated fluid-filled bowel loops without peristalsis

E. Characteristic of gastrointestinal wall thickening consisting of an echogenic center and a hypoechoic rim

F. Collection of blood

G. Site of maximal tenderness in the right lower quadrant; usually with appendicitis

H. Accumulation of serous fluid in the abdomen

I. Congenital sac or blind pouch found in the lower portion of the ileum

J. Fecalith or calcification located in the appendix

K. Small tumor-like growth that projects from a mucous membrane surface

L. Inflammation of the bowel, accompanied by abscess and bowel wall thickening

Exercise 4

Label the following illustrations.

A. The digestive system.

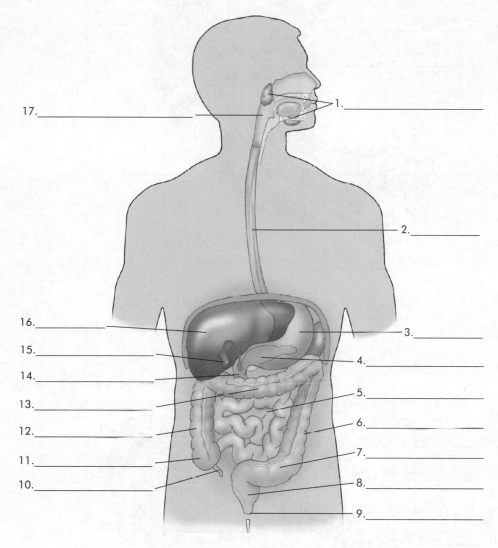

17. _____ 1. _____

2. _____

16. _____ 3. _____

15. _____ 4. _____

14. _____ 5. _____

13. _____ 6. _____

12. _____ 7. _____

11. _____ 8. _____

10. _____ 9. _____

B. The stomach.

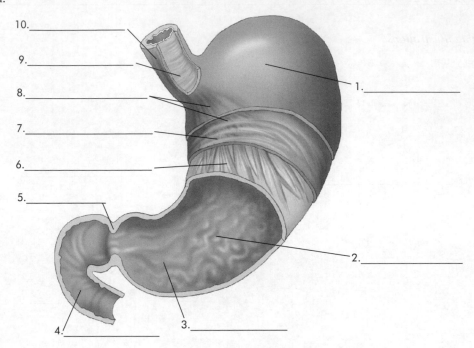

10._____

9._____

8._____

7._____

6._____

5._____

4._____

3._____

2._____

1._____

C. Vascular supply to the stomach.

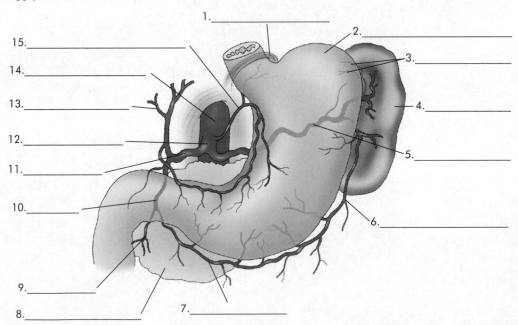

1._____

15._____

14._____

13._____

12._____

11._____

10._____

9._____

8._____

7._____

2._____

3._____

4._____

5._____

6._____

Exercise 5

Fill in the blank(s) with the word(s) that best completes the statements or provide a short answer about the anatomy and physiology of the gastrointestinal tract.

1. The pylorus is further subdivided into the _____, the _____ canal, and the pyloric sphincter.

2. The duodenal bulb is peritoneal, supported by the hepatoduodenal ligament, and passes _____ to the common bile duct, gastroduodenal artery, common hepatic artery, hepatic portal vein, and head of the pancreas.

3. The common bile duct joins the pancreatic duct to enter the ampulla of _____.

4. The _____ outlines the small intestine and contains the superior mesenteric vessels, nerves, lymphatic glands, and fat between its two layers.

5. The three layers of smooth muscle in the wall enable the stomach to mash and churn food and move it along with

   _____.

6. The hormone _____, which is released by the stomach mucosa, stimulates gastric acid secretion.

7. _____ within the large intestine devour the chyme and in turn produce vitamins that can be absorbed and used by the body.

8. The most common laboratory data the sonographer may come across in a patient with gastrointestinal disease relate

   to the presence of _____ in the stool.

9. As a result of chronic blood loss, _____ may be present.

SONOGRAPHIC EVALUATION

Exercise 6

Fill in the blank(s) with the word(s) that best completes the statements or provide a short answer about the sonographic evaluation of the gastrointestinal tract.

1. The _____ junction is seen on the sagittal scan to the left of the midline as a bull's-eye or target-shaped structure anterior to the aorta, posterior to the left lobe of the liver, and inferior to the hemidiaphragm.

2. The gastric _____ can be seen as a target shape in the midline.

3. Describe the measures that should be taken if a patient presents with a "cystic" mass in the left upper quadrant.

   _____

   _____

   _____

4. The small bowel valvulae conniventes may be seen as linear echo densities spaced 3 to 5 mm apart that are called

   the "_____" sign and can be seen in the duodenum and jejunum.

PATHOLOGY

Exercise 7

Fill in the blank(s) with the word(s) that best completes the statements about pathology of the gastrointestinal tract.

1. Movable intraluminal masses of congealed ingested materials that are seen on upper gastrointestinal radiographs are

   known as gastric _____.

2. A gastric _____ is an outgrowth of tissue from the wall.

3. The most common tumor of the stomach is the _____.

4. Acute _____ is the result of luminal obstruction and inflammation, leading to ischemia of the vermiform appendix.

5. The normal appendix can occasionally be visualized with gradual _____ on sonography.

6. The ultrasound pattern of acute appendicitis is characterized by a _____ shaped appearance of the appendix in transverse view.

7. A _____ designates gross enlargement of the appendix from accumulation of mucoid substance within the lumen.

8. _____ disease is regional enteritis, a recurrent granulomatous inflammatory disease that affects the terminal ileum, colon, or both at any level.

Exercise 8: Image Identification

Provide a short answer for each question after evaluating the images.

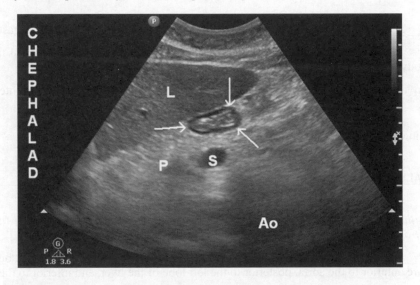

1. Identify the internal structures that are demonstrated in these images of the stomach.

_____

_____

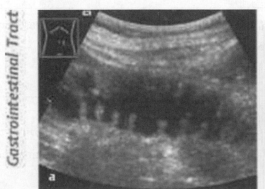
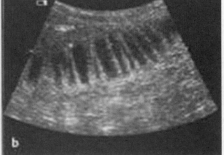

Gastrointestinal Tract

2. Identify the anatomic structure.

_____

_____

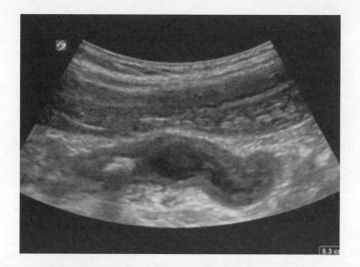

3. Identify the anatomy that is demonstrated in these images of the appendix.

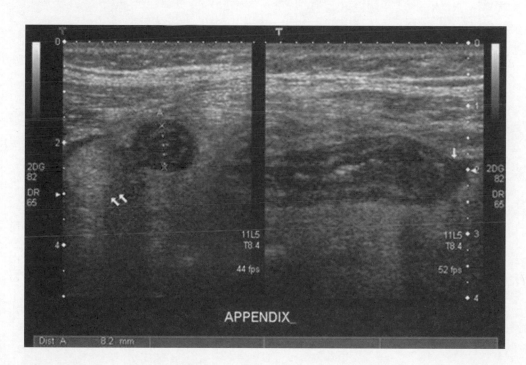

APPENDIX

4. Young patient presents with exquisite tenderness over the right lower quadrant.

14 The Peritoneal Cavity and Abdominal Wall

KEY TERMS

Exercise 1

Match the following anatomy terms with their definitions.

_____ 1. mesentery

_____ 2. Morison's pouch

_____ 3. omentum

_____ 4. subhepatic

_____ 5. subphrenic

A. Loops of the digestive tract are anchored to the posterior wall of the abdominal cavity by this large double fold of peritoneal tissue

B. Inferior to the liver

C. Pouchlike extension of the visceral peritoneum from the lower edge of the stomach, part of the duodenum, and the transverse colon

D. Below the diaphragm

E. Space anterior to the right kidney and posterior to the inferior border of the liver where ascites or fluid may accumulate or an abscess may develop

Exercise 2

Use the definitions to solve the puzzle.

ACROSS

1. *Infection in the blood*
2. *Collection of blood*
3. *Accumulation of serous fluid in the peritoneal cavity*
4. *Pus producing*
5. *Cyst containing urine*
6. *Inflammation of the peritoneum*
7. *Spread of an infection from its initial site to the bloodstream*

DOWN

3. *Describes the congenital absence or closure of a normal body opening or tubular structure.*
8. *Most dependent areas in the flanks of the abdomen and pelvis where fluid collections may accumulate.*
9. *Sonographic sign that you see when a vessel or an organ is surrounded by a tumor on either side.*
10. *Increase in the number of leukocytes (white blood cells).*
11. *Localized collection of pus*

Exercise 3

Label the following illustrations.

A. Transverse view of the subphrenic spaces.

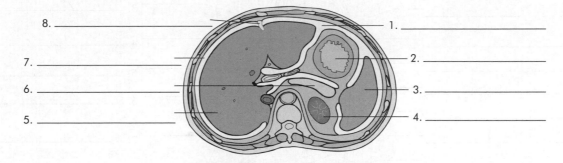

8. _____
7. _____
6. _____
5. _____

1. _____
2. _____
3. _____
4. _____

B. Transverse view of the retroperitoneal space.

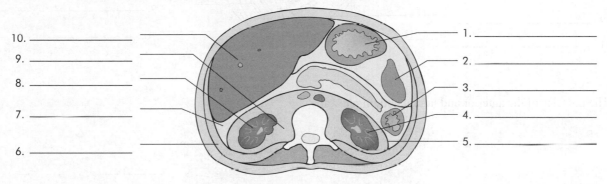

10. _____
9. _____
8. _____
7. _____
6. _____

1. _____
2. _____
3. _____
4. _____
5. _____

C. Transverse view of the subhepatic spaces and Morison's pouch.

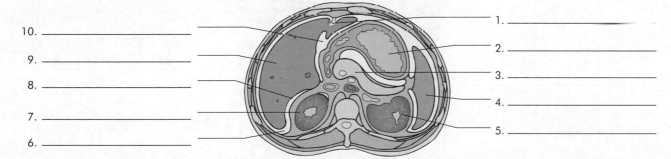

10. _____
9. _____
8. _____
7. _____
6. _____

1. _____
2. _____
3. _____
4. _____
5. _____

D. Sagittal view of the abdomen delineating the peritoneal cavity.

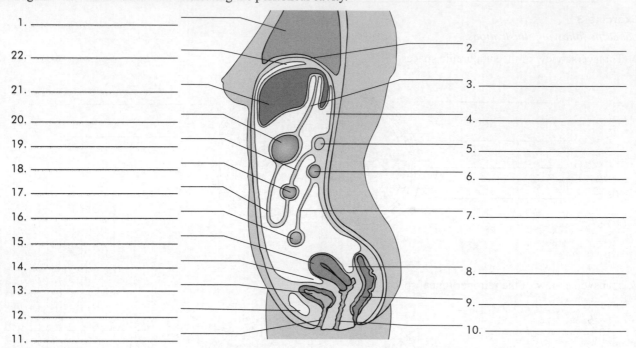

1. _____
22. _____
21. _____
20. _____
19. _____
18. _____
17. _____
16. _____
15. _____
14. _____
13. _____
12. _____
11. _____

2. _____
3. _____
4. _____
5. _____
6. _____
7. _____
8. _____
9. _____
10. _____

E. The muscles of the anterior and lateral abdominal walls.

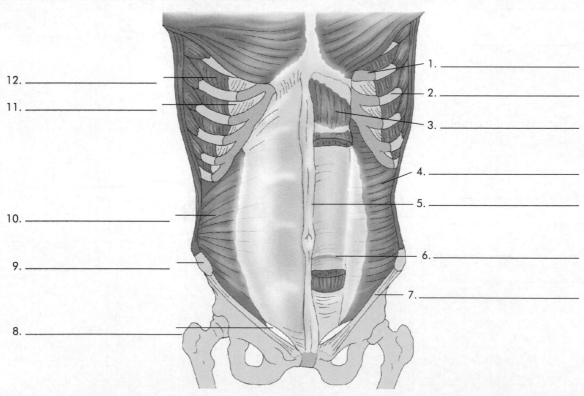

12. _____
11. _____
10. _____
9. _____
8. _____

1. _____
2. _____
3. _____
4. _____
5. _____
6. _____
7. _____

Exercise 4

Fill in the blank(s) with the word(s) that best completes the statements about the determination of intraperitoneal location.

1. Because of the _____ ligament attachments, collections in the right posterior subphrenic space cannot extend between the bare area of the liver and the diaphragm.

2. The pleural fluid tends to distribute _____ in the chest.

3. Subcapsular liver and splenic collections are seen when they are _____ to the diaphragm unilaterally and conform to the shape of an organ capsule.

4. Retroperitoneal lesions displace echoes _____ and cranially.

5. Hepatic and subhepatic lesions produce _____ and posterior displacement.

6. A large, right-sided retroperitoneal mass rotates the intrahepatic portal veins to the _____.

Exercise 5

Fill in the blank(s) with the word(s) that best completes the statements about the anatomy and sonographic evaluation of the peritoneal cavity and abdominal wall.

1. Within the cavity are found the lesser and greater _____, the mesenteries, and multiple fluid spaces (lesser sac, perihepatic and subphrenic spaces).

2. The _____ is a smooth membrane that lines the entire abdominal cavity and is reflected over the contained organs.

3. The structure that lines the walls of the cavity is the _____ peritoneum, whereas the structure covering the abdominal organs to a greater or lesser extent is the _____ peritoneum.

4. With the development of the stomach and the spleen, a smaller sac, called the _____ sac (omental bursa), is the peritoneal recess posterior to the stomach.

5. This sac communicates with the greater sac through a small vertical opening known as the _____ foramen.

6. When the patient is lying supine, the lowest part of the body is the _____.

7. A double layer of peritoneum extending from the liver to the lesser curvature of the stomach is known as the _____ omentum.

8. The _____ omentum is an apron-like fold of peritoneum that hangs from the greater curvature of the stomach.

9. The subphrenic space is divided into right and left components by the _____ ligaments.

10. The paired _____ abdominis muscles are delineated medially in the midline of the body by the linea alba.

PATHOLOGY

Exercise 6

Fill in the blank(s) with the word(s) that best completes the statements or provide a short answer about the pathology of the peritoneal cavity.

1. The ascitic fluid first fills the pouch of _____, then the lateral paravesical recesses before it ascends to both paracolic gutters.

2. Name the five major pathways through which bacteria can enter the liver and cause abscess formation.

   a.

   b.

   c.

   d.

   e.

3. Extrahepatic loculated collections of bile that may develop because of iatrogenic, traumatic, or spontaneous rupture of the biliary tree are _____.

4. An abscess that forms within the renal parenchyma is a renal _____. Clinical symptoms vary from none to fever, leukocytosis, and flank pain.

5. The most common abdominal pathologic process is (acute or chronic) pancreatitis which requires immediate surgery.

Exercise 7

Fill in the blank(s) with the word(s) that best completes the statements or provide a short answer about the pathology of the mesentery, omentum, and peritoneum.

1. An incomplete regression of the urachus during development is a(n) _____ cyst.

2. An encapsulated collection of urine, or _____, may result from a closed renal injury, from surgical intervention, or it may arise spontaneously secondary to an obstructing lesion.

3. The most common primary sites of peritoneal metastases are the stomach, colon, and _____.

4. The _____ sign of lymphoma represents a mass infiltrating the mesenteric leaves and encasing the superior mesenteric artery.

5. A collection of fluid that occurs after surgery in the pelvis, retroperitoneum, or recess cavities is known as a(n)

_____.

6. Extraperitoneal rectus sheath _____ are acute or chronic collections of blood lying either within the rectus muscle or between the muscle and its sheath.

7. An abdominal _____ is the protrusion of a peritoneal-lined sac through a defect in the weakened abdominal wall.

Exercise 8

Provide a short answer for each question after evaluating the images.

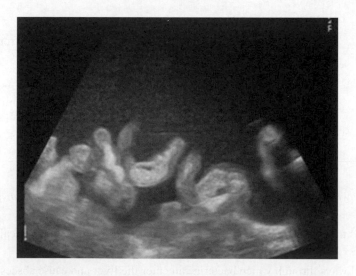

1. What is this fluid collection?

_____

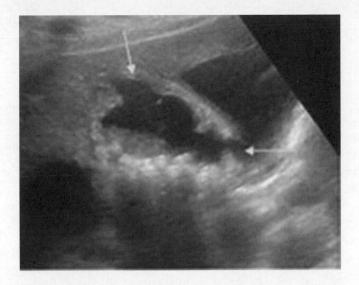

2. Which abnormality does this longitudinal image demonstrate in this patient post op from gallbladder surgery?

_____

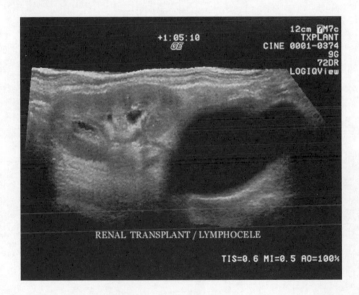

3. A patient 2 days after surgery for a renal transplant was imaged post op. Describe what this image shows.

_____

_____

_____

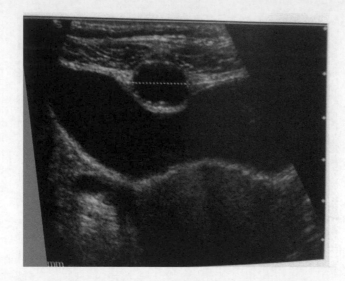

4. This mass was noted between the umbilicus and the bladder and most likely represents a

_____.

15 | The Urinary System

KEY TERMS

Exercise 1

Match the following anatomy terms with their definitions.

_____ 1. afferent arteriole

_____ 2. Bowman's capsule

_____ 3. cortex

_____ 4. Gerota's fascia

_____ 5. hilus

_____ 6. major calyces

_____ 7. minor calyces

_____ 8. nephron

_____ 9. renal corpuscle

_____ 10. renal pelvis

_____ 11. retroperitoneum

_____ 12. urethra

A. Area of kidney where vessels, ureter, and lymphatics enter and exit

B. Another term for the renal fascia; the kidney is covered by the renal capsule, perirenal fat, Gerota's fascia, and pararenal fat

C. Functional unit of the kidney; includes a renal corpuscle and a renal tubule

D. Carries blood into the glomerulus of the nephron

E. Receive urine from the renal pyramids; form the border of the renal sinus

F. Part of the nephron that consists of Bowman's capsule and the glomerulus

G. Area in the midportion of the kidney that collects urine before entering the ureter

H. Site of filtration in the kidney; contains water, salts, glucose, urea, and amino acids

I. Receives urine from the minor calyces to convey to the renal pelvis

J. Outer parenchyma of the kidney that contains the renal corpuscle and proximal and distal convoluted tubules of the nephron

K. Small, membranous canal that excretes urine from the urinary bladder

L. Space behind the peritoneal lining of the abdominal cavity

Exercise 2

Match the following anatomy and physiology terms with their definitions.

_____ 1. arcuate arteries

_____ 2. blood urea nitrogen (BUN)

_____ 3. calyx

_____ 4. creatinine

_____ 5. efferent arteriole

_____ 6. glomerulus

_____ 7. homeostasis

_____ 8. loop of Henle

_____ 9. medulla

_____ 10. Morison's pouch

_____ 11. renal pyramid

A. Portion of a renal tubule lying between the proximal and distal convoluted portions; reabsorption of fluid, sodium, and chloride occurs here and in the proximal convoluted tubule

B. One of several conical masses of tissue that form the kidney medulla; each consists of the loops of Henle and the collecting tubules of the nephrons

C. Retroperitoneal structures that exit the kidney to carry urine to the urinary bladder

D. Inner portion of the renal parenchyma that contains the loop of Henle

E. Small vessels found at the base of the renal pyramids; appear as echogenic structures

F. Muscular retroperitoneal organ that serves as a reservoir for urine

G. Part of the collecting system adjacent to the pyramid that collects urine and is connected to the major calyx

H. Network of capillaries that are part of the filtration process in the kidney

I. Central area of the kidney that includes the calyces, renal pelvis, renal vessels, fat, nerves, and lymphatics

J. Right posterior subhepatic space located anterior to the kidney and inferior to the liver where fluid may accumulate

K. Small vessel that carries blood from the glomerulus of the nephron and conducts blood to the peritubular capillaries that surround the renal tubule

_____12. renal hilum

_____13. renal sinus

_____14. specific gravity

_____15. ureters

_____16. urinary bladder

L. Area in the midportion of the kidney where the renal vessels and ureter enter and exit

M. Laboratory measurement of the amount of nitrogenous waste and creatinine in the blood

N. A product of metabolism; laboratory test that measures the ability of the kidney to get rid of waste

O. Maintenance of normal body physiology

P. Laboratory tests that measure how much dissolved material is present in the urine

Exercise 3

Match the following terms related to pathology and sonographic evaluation with their definitions.

_____ 1. columns of Bertin

_____ 2. dromedary hump

_____ 3. ectopic kidney

_____ 4. horseshoe kidney

_____ 5. hydronephrosis

_____ 6. renal agenesis

_____ 7. renal capsule

_____ 8. urolithiasis

A. Normal variant that occurs on the left kidney as a bulge on the lateral border

B. Located outside of the normal position, most often in the pelvic cavity

C. Stone within the urinary system

D. First layer adjacent to the kidney that forms a tough, fibrous covering

E. Bands of cortical tissue that separate the renal pyramids; may mimic a renal mass on ultrasound

F. Dilation of the renal collecting system

G. Congenital malformation in which both kidneys are joined together by an isthmus, most commonly at the lower poles

H. Interruption in the normal development of the kidney resulting in absence of the kidney; may be unilateral or bilateral

ANATOMY AND PHYSIOLOGY

Exercise 4

Label the following illustrations.

A. The kidney cut longitudinally.

1. _____

2. _____

3. _____

4. _____

5. _____

6. _____

7. _____

8. _____

9. _____

10. _____

11. _____

12. _____

13. _____

14. _____

15. _____

16. _____

17. _____

18. _____

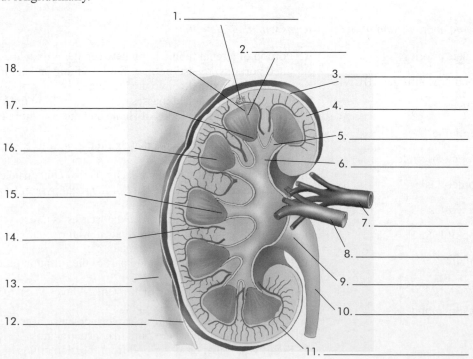

B. Anatomic structures related to the anterior surfaces of the kidneys.

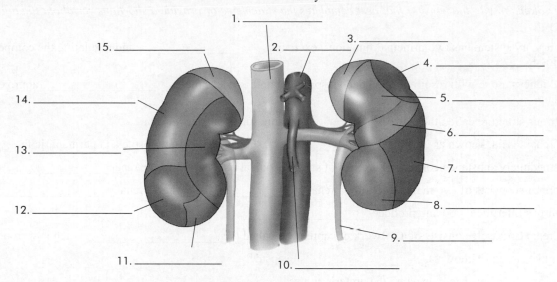

1. _____
2. _____
3. _____
4. _____
5. _____
6. _____
7. _____
8. _____
9. _____
10. _____
11. _____
12. _____
13. _____
14. _____
15. _____

C. Vascular relationship of the great vessels and their tributaries to the kidneys.

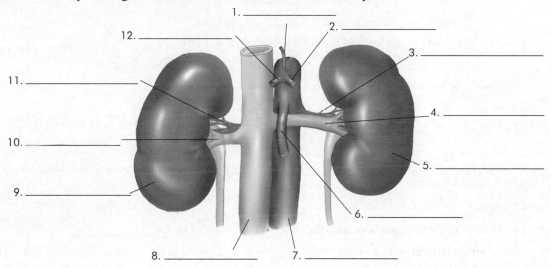

1. _____
2. _____
3. _____
4. _____
5. _____
6. _____
7. _____
8. _____
9. _____
10. _____
11. _____
12. _____

101

Exercise 5

Fill in the blank(s) with the word(s) that best completes the statements or provide a short answer about the anatomy of the kidney.

1. The urinary system has two principal functions: excreting _____ and regulating the composition of blood.

2. The kidneys move with respiration; on deep inspiration, both kidneys move _____ approximately 1 inch.

3. A fibrous structure called the _____ capsule surrounds the kidney.

4. The renal fascia, known as _____ fascia, surrounds the true capsule and perinephric fat.

5. The medullary substance consists of a series of striated conical masses, called the renal _____.

6. A nephron consists of two main structures, a renal _____ and a renal _____.

7. Nephrons filter the blood and produce _____.

8. The renal corpuscle consists of a network of capillaries, called the _____, which is surrounded by a cuplike structure known as _____ capsule.

9. There are three constrictions along the ureter's course:

   (a)_____,

   (b)_____, and

   (c)_____.

10. The main renal artery is a lateral branch of the aorta and arises just inferior to the _____ artery.

Exercise 6

Fill in the blank(s) with the word(s) that best completes the statements or provide a short answer about the physiology of the kidney.

1. The urinary system is located posterior to the peritoneum lining the abdominal cavity in an area called the

   _____.

2. The kidneys adjust the amounts of water and _____ leaving the body so that these equal the amounts of substances entering the body.

3. The principal metabolic waste products are water, _____ _____, and nitrogenous wastes.

4. Both urea and uric acid are carried away from the liver into the kidneys by the _____ system.

5. The presence of an acute infection causes _____, which is red blood cells in the urine; pyuria means there is _____ in the urine.

6. The pH refers to the strength of the urine as a partly _____ or _____ solution.

7. The _____ _____ is the measurement of the kidney's ability to concentrate urine.

8. The specific gravity is especially _____ in cases of renal failure, glomerular nephritis, and pyelonephritis.

9. A decreased _____ occurs with acute hemorrhagic processes secondary to disease or blunt trauma.

10. Impairment of renal function and increased protein catabolism result in BUN _____ that is relative to the degree of renal impairment and rate of urea nitrogen excreted by the kidneys.

Exercise 7

Fill in the blank(s) with the word(s) that best completes the statements or provide a short answer about the sonographic evaluation of the kidney.

1. The _____ is the area from the renal sinus to the outer renal surface.

2. The _____ arteries and interlobar arteries and are best demonstrated as intense specular echoes in cross section or oblique section at the corticomedullary junction.

3. The _____ generally is echo producing, whereas the medullary pyramids are

   _____.

4. The cortex and medullary pyramids are separated from each other by bands of cortical tissue, called

   _____, that extend inward to the renal sinus.

5. The _____ lie posterior to the renal arteries and should be identified by their lack of pulsations and absence of Doppler flow.

6. The _____ of the pyramid points toward the sinus, and the _____ lies adjacent to the renal cortex.

7. The _____ is a cortical bulge that occurs on the lateral border of the kidney, typically more on the left side.

8. A(n) _____ is a triangular, echogenic area in the upper pole of the renal parenchyma that can be seen during normal scanning.

9. In a patient with a(n) _____ kidney, there is fusion of the kidneys during fetal development that almost invariably involves the _____ poles.

10. A cystlike enlargement of the lower end of the ureter is called a(n) _____.

PATHOLOGY

Exercise 8

Fill in the blank(s) with the word(s) that best completes the statements or provide a short answer about the pathology of the kidney.

1. The parapelvic cyst is found in the _____ but does not communicate with the renal collecting system.

2. Usually a(n) _____ renal contour is the first finding that a mass may be present and requires further investigation.

3. One of the most common benign renal tumors is called _____.

4. An uncommon benign renal tumor composed mainly of fat cells and commonly found in the renal cortex is

   _____.

5. A(n) _____ appears as a well-defined echogenic mass, found more often in females.

6. Sonographic findings include one or more fluid spaces at the _____ junction that corresponds to the distribution of the renal pyramids.

7. The most common medical renal disease that produces acute renal failure is _____

   _____.

8. _____ is when the dilated pyelocalyceal system appears as separation of the renal sinus echoes by fluid-filled areas that conform anatomically to the infundibula, calyces, and renal pelvis.

9. Hydronephrosis with a dilated ureter and bladder indicates obstruction of the _____ junction or of the urethra.

10. If hydronephrosis is suspected, the sonographer should evaluate the _____.

11. Ureteral jets are best visualized by _____ imaging.

12. When pus is found within the obstructed renal system, the condition is called _____.

13. A renal _____ occurs when part of the tissue undergoes necrosis after the cessation of the blood supply, usually as a result of artery occlusion.

14. The initial clinical sign of a kidney stone is extreme _____, typically followed by cramping on the side where the stone is located; nausea and vomiting may also occur.

15. If the stone causes obstruction, there will be _____ and, depending on the location of the stone, the ureter may be dilated _____ to the level of obstruction.

Exercise 9

Fill in the blank(s) with the word(s) that best completes the statements or provide a short answer about renal transplantation.

1. The major problem encountered with renal transplantation is _____.

2. _____ rejection occurs within hours of transplantation and is caused by vasculitis leading to thrombosis and usually the loss of the graft.

3. _____ rejection occurs within days to months after transplant.

4. The incidence of acute tubular necrosis is usually higher in _____ transplants than in _____ transplants.

5. Early signs of obstruction are _____ or severe oliguria in a patient with satisfactory renal volumes.

6. Renal artery stenosis exhibits a(n) _____ jet with distal turbulence.

Exercise 10

Provide a short answer for each question after evaluating the images.

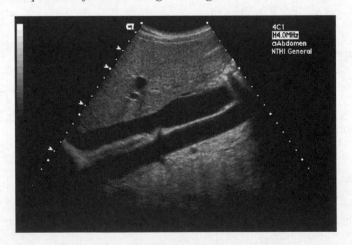

1. List the anatomic structures shown to arise from the inferior vena cava in this coronal image.

_____

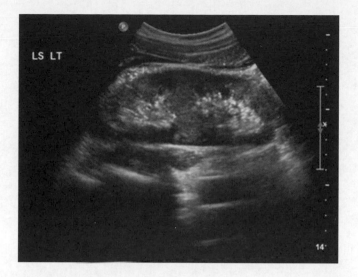

2. What anatomic variation of the kidney are the arrows pointing to?

_____

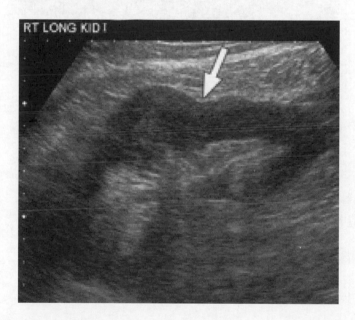

3. Identify the anatomic variant demonstrated in this image.

_____

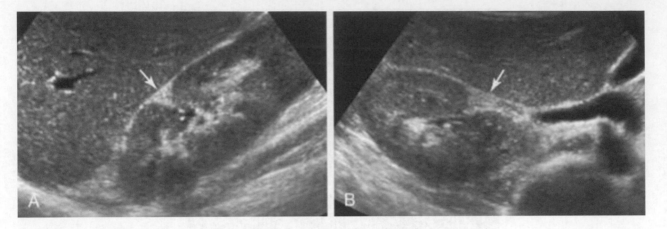

4. Name the structure that the arrow is pointing to along the anterior wall of the kidney.

_____

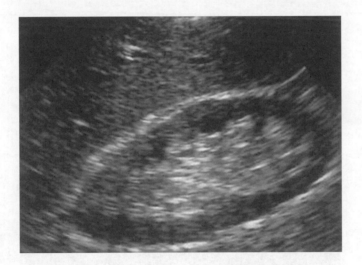

5. Describe the sonographic finding in this longitudinal image of the kidney.

_____

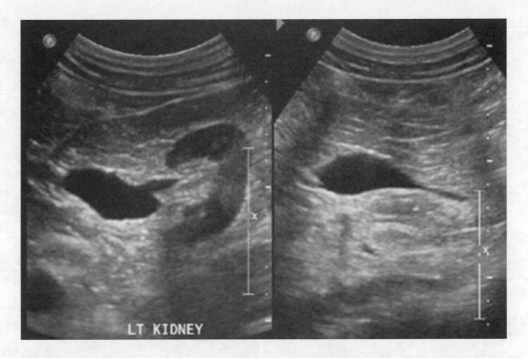

6. What pathology is demonstrated on these longitudinal scans of both kidneys of a young adult male?

_____

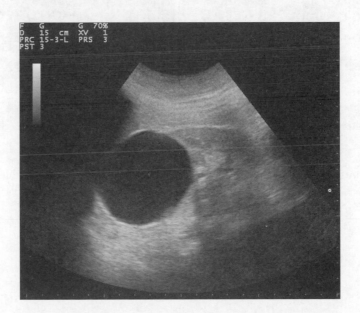

7. A 66-year-old male presents with an incidental finding on his abdominal ultrasound. What pathology do the images demonstrate?

_____

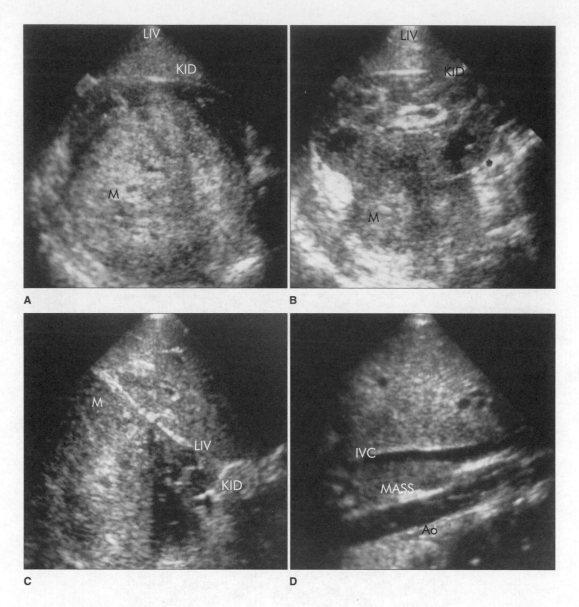

A

B

C

D

8. A 14-month-old child presents with a palpable right-sided mass, decreased appetite, and lethargy. What is the sonographic finding?

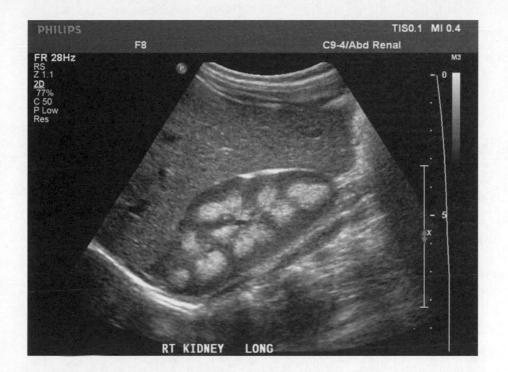

9. A 6-year-old male presents with chronic urinary tract infections. What is the ultrasound finding?

_____

16 The Retroperitoneum

KEY TERMS

Exercise 1

Match the following anatomy and physiology terms with their definitions.

_____ 1. adrenocorticotropic hormone (ACTH)

_____ 2. cortex

_____ 3. false pelvis

_____ 4. hyperplasia

_____ 5. medulla

A. Outer parenchyma of the adrenal gland that secretes steroid hormones commonly called corticoids
B. Portion of the pelvic cavity that is above the pelvic brim, bounded posteriorly by the lumbar vertebrae, laterally by the iliac fossae and iliacus muscles, and anteriorly by the lower anterior abdominal wall
C. Central tissue of the adrenal gland that secretes epinephrine and norepinephrine
D. Hormone secreted by the pituitary gland
E. An increase in the number of cells of a body part that results from an increased rate of cellular division

Exercise 2

Match the following pathology terms to their definitions.

_____ 1. adenoma

_____ 2. Addison's disease

_____ 3. Cushing's syndrome

_____ 4. lymphoma

_____ 5. neuroectodermal tissue

_____ 6. neuroblastoma

_____ 7. pheochromocytoma

_____ 8. lymphadenopathy

A. Condition caused by hyposecretion of hormones from the adrenal cortex
B. Malignant adrenal mass that is seen in pediatric patients
C. Early embryonic tissue that will eventually develop into the brain and spinal cord
D. Smooth, round, homogeneous benign tumor of the adrenal cortex associated with Cushing's syndrome
E. Malignancy that primarily affects the lymph nodes, spleen, or liver
F. Condition caused by hypersecretion of hormones from the adrenal cortex
G. Any disorder characterized by enlargement of the lymph nodes or lymph vessels
H. Benign adrenal tumor that secretes hormones that produce hypertension

Exercise 3

Label the following illustrations.

A. Identify the structures on this diagram.

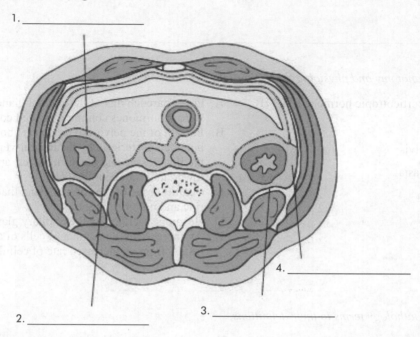

1. _____

2. _____

3. _____

4. _____

B. The right crus of the diaphragm passes posterior to the inferior vena cava.

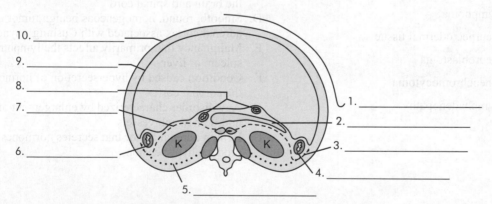

10. _____

9. _____

8. _____

7. _____

6. _____

5. _____

1. _____

2. _____

3. _____

4. _____

Exercise 4

Fill in the blank(s) with the word(s) that best completes the statements or provide a short answer about the anatomy of the retroperitoneum.

1. The retroperitoneal space is subdivided into three spaces: the anterior_____ space, the

   _____ space, and the posterior _____ space.

2. The _____ space surrounds the kidney, adrenal, and perirenal fat.

3. The anterior _____ space includes the duodenum, pancreas, and ascending and transverse colon.

4. The posterior _____ space includes the iliopsoas muscle, ureter, and branches of the inferior vena cava and their lymphatics.

5. The right adrenal is more _____ to the kidney, whereas the left adrenal is more

   _____ to the kidney.

6. The right renal artery crosses _____ to the crus and _____ to the inferior vena cava at the level of the right kidney.

Exercise 5

Fill in the blank(s) with the word(s) that best completes the statements about the physiology of the retroperitoneum.

1. Hypofunction of the adrenal cortex in humans is called _____ disease.

2. The principal mineralocorticoid is _____.

3. _____ play a principal role in carbohydrate metabolism.

4. The primary glucocorticoids are _____ and hydrocortisone.

5. Adrenal tumors in women can promote secondary _____ characteristics.

6. Epinephrine and norepinephrine are amines, sometimes referred to as _____, that elevate the blood pressure.

SONOGRAPHIC EVALUATION

Exercise 6

Fill in the blank(s) with the word(s) that best completes the statements or provide a short answer about the sonographic evaluation of the retroperitoneum.

1. Select the sonographic findings for the para-aortic lymph nodes.

   a. ____ lymph nodes measure 1 to 2 mm

   b. ____ lymph nodes are hypoechoic

   c. ____ lymph nodes are round

   d. ____ lymph nodes measure 1 to 3 cm

   e. ____ lymph nodes are found along the circulatory system

2. Select how to distinguish enlarged lymph nodes from bowel.

   a. ____ lymph nodes remain unchanged in shape with compression

   b. ____ lymph nodes present with peristaltic patterns

   c. ____ lymph nodes change in shape with compression

3. The clinical symptoms of pheochromocytoma include intermittent _____, severe headaches, heart palpitations, and excess perspiration.

4. A _____ is a walled-off collection of extravasated urine that develops spontaneously after trauma, surgery, or a subacute or chronic urinary obstruction.

Exercise 7

Provide a short answer for each question after evaluating the images.

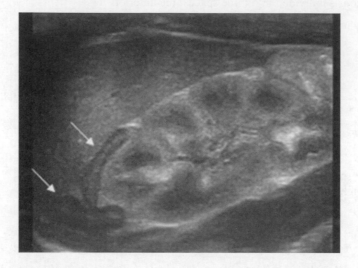

1. The arrows point to what anatomical structure?

_____

_____

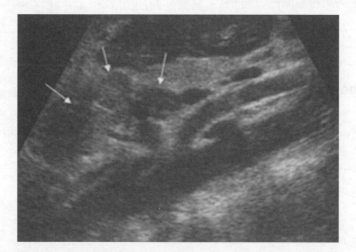

2. What are the arrows pointing to in this patient with abdominal tenderness?

_____

_____

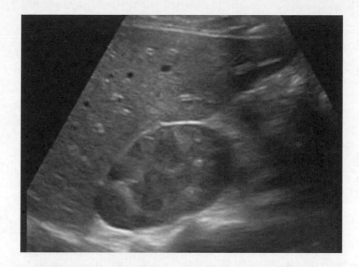

3. What is the abnormality on this right upper quadrant sonogram?

_____

_____

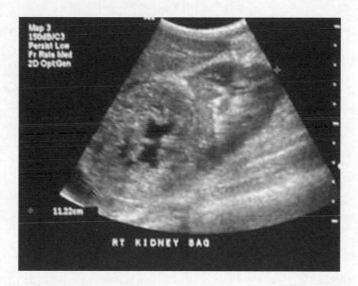

4. This two-year-old patient presents with an abdominal mass. Identify the anomaly shown in the sonograms.

_____

_____

KEY TERMS

Exercise 1

Match the following ultrasound terms to their definitions.

_____ 1. acoustic emission

_____ 2. contrast-enhanced sonography

_____ 3. tissue-specific ultrasound contrast agent

_____ 4. first-generation agents

_____ 5. gray-scale harmonic imaging

_____ 6. harmonic imaging

_____ 7. induced acoustic emission

_____ 8. intravenous injection

_____ 9. mechanical index

_____ 10. second-generation agents

_____ 11. molecular imaging agents

_____ 12. ultrasound contrast agents

_____ 13. vascular ultrasound contrast agents

A. Index that defines the low acoustic output power that can be used to minimize the destruction of microbubbles by energy in the acoustic field

B. Agents containing room air

C. After the injection of the tissue-specific UCA Sonazoid, the reflectivity of the contrast-containing tissue increases; when the right level of acoustic energy is applied to tissue, the contrast microbubbles eventually rupture, resulting in random Doppler shifts; these shifts appear as a transient mosaic of colors on the color Doppler display; masses that have destroyed or replaced normal Kupffer cells will be displayed as color-free areas

D. Agent used to reduce or eliminate some of the current limitations of ultrasound imaging and Doppler blood flow detection color flow imaging

E. Type of ultrasound contrast agent whose microbubbles are contained in the body's vascular spaces

F. Agents include Optison, Definity, Imagent, Levovist, and SonoVue

G. Allows detection of contrast-enhanced blood flow and organs with gray-scale ultrasound

H. Agents that can be administered intravenously to evaluate blood vessels, blood flow, and solid organs

I. Occurs when an appropriate level of acoustic energy is applied to the tissue; the microbubbles first oscillate and then rupture

J. Hypodermic injection into a vein for the purpose of injecting a contrast medium

K. In this mode, the ultrasound system is configured to receive only echoes at the second harmonic frequency, which is twice the transmit frequency

L. Agents containing heavy gases

M. Type of contrast agent whose microbubbles are removed from the blood and are taken up by specific tissues in the body

Exercise 2

Identify the abbreviations related to the use of contrast agents for ultrasound.

1. AE _____

2. CES _____

3. CFI _____

4. GSHI _____

5. HI _____

6. IAE _____

7. MI _____

8. PDI _____

9. UCA _____

Exercise 3

Answer the following review questions regarding ultrasound contrast agents.

1. Most of the research and development of ultrasound contrast agents has centered on creating agents that can:
   a. enhance the detection of stationary blood.
   b. be administered by intraarterial injection.
   c. be administered intravenously.
   d. enhance the detection of tumors in solid organs.
   e. be used for therapeutic applications.

2. Vascular ultrasound contrast agents enhance Doppler flow signals by:
   a. increasing the velocity of blood flow.
   b. adding more and better acoustic scatterers to the bloodstream.
   c. increasing the number of red blood cells in the vessel being evaluated.
   d. decreasing the speed of sound through tissue.
   e. a and b above.

3. For a vascular ultrasound contrast agent to be clinically useful, it should:
   a. be nontoxic.
   b. have microbubbles that are small enough to traverse the pulmonary capillary beds.
   c. be stable enough to provide multiple recirculations.
   d. be high in viscosity.
   e. a, b, and c above.

4. What type of substance does the microbubble of a "first-generation" ultrasound contrast agent contain?
   a. a heavy gas, such as a perfluorocarbon
   b. a fluid that has low solubility in blood
   c. room air
   d. a fluid that has acoustic properties that are drastically different from human blood
   e. albumin

5. Depending on the clinical application, vascular ultrasound contrast agents may be administered via:
   a. intravenous bolus injection.
   b. oral ingestion.
   c. intravenous infusion.
   d. all of the above.
   e. a and c above.

6. The microbubbles of tissue-specific ultrasound contrast agents:
   a. are significantly larger than red blood cells.
   b. are significantly larger than liver cells (hepatocytes).
   c. are taken up by or have an affinity toward specific tissue.
   d. are toxic to the targeted tissue.
   e. decrease the echogenicity of targeted tissue.

7. When in harmonic imaging mode, the ultrasound system is configured to receive:
   a. only echoes that are at one half the frequency of the transmitted frequency.
   b. only echoes that are high in amplitude.
   c. only echoes arising from contrast microbubbles.
   d. only echoes at the second harmonic frequency, which is twice the transmit frequency.
   e. only echoes arising from stationary tissue.

8. When insonating microbubble-based ultrasound contrast agents, the energy present within the acoustic field:
   a. has no effect on the microbubbles.
   b. can have a detrimental effect on the contrast microbubbles.
   c. usually increases the microbubble size.
   d. usually results in the creation of more microbubbles.
   e. c and d above.

9. Ultrasound contrast agents have shown the potential to improve the accuracy of hepatic sonography, including:
   a. enhanced detection of hepatic masses.
   b. enhanced characterization of hepatic masses.
   c. improved detection of intrahepatic and extrahepatic blood flow.
   d. a and c above.
   e. a, b, and c above.

10. Vascular ultrasound contrast agents can be useful in the evaluation of patients with suspected renal artery stenosis because they:
    a. increase the ability to visualize blood flow using color flow imaging.
    b. increase the velocity of blood flow to the kidneys.
    c. improve the intensity of spectral Doppler flow signals.
    d. a and c above.
    e. all of the above.

CLINICAL APPLICATIONS

Exercise 4

Fill in the blank(s) with the word(s) that best completes the statements or provide a short answer about the clinical applications of contrast agents in ultrasound.

1. Vascular or blood pool ultrasound contrast agents enhance Doppler (color and spectral) flow signals by adding

   more and better acoustic _____ to the bloodstream.

2. Some vascular agents also improve gray-scale ultrasound visualization of flowing blood and demonstrate changes

   to the _____ - _____ echogenicity of tissue.

3. Agents containing room air are commonly referred to as _____ generation contrast agents,

   whereas agents containing heavy gases are referred to as _____ generation agents.

4. The rupture of the _____ results in random Doppler shifts appearing as a transient mosaic of colors on a color Doppler display.

5. Currently, tissue-specific agents that are taken up by the _____ system appear to be most useful in the assessment of patients with suspected liver abnormalities.

6. In harmonic imaging mode, the ultrasound system is configured to receive only echoes at the

   _____ harmonic frequency, which is twice the transmit frequency.

Chapter **17** Abdominal Applications of Ultrasound Contrast Agents

7. When using a microbubble-based ultrasound contrast agent, the microbubbles _____ (that is, they get larger and smaller) when subjected to the acoustic energy present in the ultrasound field with gray-scale ultrasound.

8. In the harmonic imaging mode, the echoes from the oscillating microbubbles have a higher

_____ - to- _____ ratio than would be provided by using conventional US so that regions with microbubbles are more easily appreciated visually.

9. Wide-band gray-scale harmonic imaging provides a way to better differentiate areas with and without contrast and

has the potential to demonstrate real-time gray-scale blood pool imaging, or _____ imaging.

10. Although ultrasound is usually sensitive for the detection of medium to large hepatic lesions, it is limited in its

ability to detect _____, isoechoic, or peripherally located lesions, particularly in obese patients or patients with diffuse liver disease.

11. Hepatic ultrasound blood flow studies are limited by _____ -velocity blood flow (e.g., in cases of portal hypertension) or for the detection of flow in the intrahepatic artery branches.

18 Ultrasound-Guided Interventional Techniques

KEY TERMS

Exercise 1

Match the following terms with their definitions.

_____ 1. free-hand technique

_____ 2. coagulopathy

_____ 3. hypovolemia

_____ 4. international normalized ratio

_____ 5. pneumothorax

_____ 6. prostate-specific antigen

_____ 7. hypotension

_____ 8. partial thromboplastin time (PTT)

_____ 9. thoracentesis

_____ 10. vasovagal

A. Defect in blood-clotting mechanisms
B. Surgical puncture of the chest wall for removal of fluids; usually done by using a large-bore needle
C. Decreased systolic and diastolic blood pressure below normal
D. Laboratory test that can be used to evaluate the effects of heparin, aspirin, and antihistamines on the blood-clotting process by detecting clotting abnormalities of the intrinsic and common pathways
E. Method of performing an ultrasound-guided procedure without the use of a needle guide on the transducer
F. Concerning the action of stimuli from the vagus nerve on blood vessels; vasovagal syncope is a brief loss of consciousness caused by a sudden drop in heart rate and blood pressure, which reduces blood flow to the brain
G. Collection of air or gas in the pleural cavity
H. Diminished blood volume
I. Laboratory test that measures levels of this antigen in the body, elevated levels of which could indicate prostate cancer
J. Method developed to standardize prothrombin time (PT) results among laboratories by accounting for the different thromboplastin reagents used to determine PT

Exercise 2

Identify the abbreviations related to ultrasound-guided interventional techniques.

1. AFP _____

2. FNA _____

3. INR _____

4. PSA _____

5. PT _____

6. PTT _____

ULTRASOUND-GUIDED PROCEDURES

Exercise 3

Fill in the blank(s) with the word(s) that best completes the statements or provide a short answer about the ultrasound-guided procedures.

1. The most common indication for a biopsy is to confirm _____ in a mass.

2. Which laboratory test is used to evaluate the effects of heparin, aspirin, and antihistamines on the blood-clotting process? _____

3. Biopsies are used to confirm if a mass is _____,_____, or _____.

4. A(n) _____ biopsy uses an automated, spring-loaded device, termed a biopsy gun, to provide a core of tissue for histologic analysis.

5. FNA uses a(n) _____ needle to obtain cells from a mass.

6. One method of ultrasound-guided intervention is called the _____ hand technique and is performed without the use of a needle guide on the transducer.

7. The patient must be informed of the potential _____, alternate methods of obtaining the same information, and what would be the course of the disease if the biopsy were not performed and the correct treatment could not be planned.

8. The national patient safety standards (www.jcaho.org) mandate that a "timeout" be performed before beginning any procedure. Explain what a "timeout" is and what its purpose is.

_____

_____

_____

9. Complications from an ultrasound-guided biopsy are usually minor and may include _____,
_____ reactions, and _____.

10. It is important to determine how much the mass moves with _____ and also how well and how long the patient can hold his or her breath.

11. Describe how to see the needle tip in ultrasound.

_____

_____

12. Typically the _____ pole of the kidney is biopsied to prevent possible lacerations of the main renal vessels and ureter.

13. Patients may be marked for a thoracentesis or have the procedure under sonographic guidance. Patients should be scanned in the _____ position that the procedure will be performed in, which is usually in an upright position, through the back.

KEY TERMS

Exercise 1

Match the following abdominal ultrasound terms with their definitions.

_____ 1. focused assessment with sonography for trauma

_____ 2. hemoperitoneum

_____ 3. incarcerated hernia

_____ 4. intravenous urography

_____ 5. peritoneal lavage

_____ 6. pseudodissection

_____ 7. reducible hernia

_____ 8. strangulated hernia

A. Collection of bloody fluid in the abdomen or pelvis secondary to trauma or surgical procedure

B. Capable of being replaced in a normal position; the visceral contents can be returned to normal intraabdominal location

C. Invasive procedure that is used to sample the intraperitoneal space for evidence of damage to viscera and blood vessels

D. Limited examination of the abdomen or pelvis to evaluate free fluid or pericardial fluid

E. An incarcerated hernia with vascular compromise

F. Procedure used in radiography wherein contrast is administered intravenously to help the technician visualize the urinary system

G. Condition seen in a patient with aortic dissection

H. Imprisonment or confinement of a part of the bowel; the visceral contents cannot be reduced

ANATOMY AND PHYSIOLOGY

Exercise 2

Label the following illustrations.

A. Transverse view of the perihepatic space and Morison's pouch

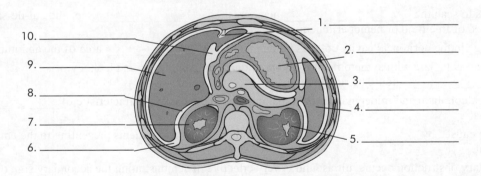

10. _____
9. _____
8. _____
7. _____
6. _____

1. _____
2. _____
3. _____
4. _____
5. _____

B. Transverse view of the perisplenic area and the splenorenal ligament.

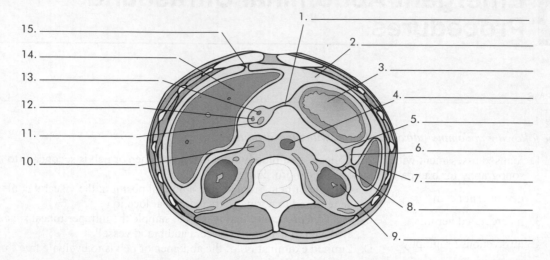

15. _____

14. _____

13. _____

12. _____

11. _____

10. _____

1. _____

2. _____

3. _____

4. _____

5. _____

6. _____

7. _____

8. _____

9. _____

EMERGENT ABDOMINAL ULTRASOUND PROCEDURES

Exercise 3

Fill in the blank(s) with the word(s) that best completes the statements or provide a short answer about emergent abdominal ultrasound procedures.

1. Peritoneal lavage is usually used as a diagnostic technique in certain cases of _____ abdominal trauma.

2. Peritoneal lavage carries a risk of organ injury and decreases the specificity of subsequent ultrasonography or computed tomography (CT) because of the introduction of _____ fluid and air.

3. The _____ scan in the emergency department is a limited examination of the abdomen or pelvis to evaluate free fluid or pericardial fluid.

4. In the context of traumatic injury, free fluid is usually a result of _____ and contributes to the assessment of the circulation.

5. The goal is to scan the _____ quadrants, _____ sac, and cul-de-sac for the presence of free fluid or hemoperitoneum.

6. Hemorrhage in the peritoneal cavity collects in the most _____ area of the abdomen.

7. If the patient is female with symptoms of right upper quadrant pain, fever, and leukocytosis, _____ should be ruled out.

8. History of alcoholism and midepigastric pain that radiates to the back is characteristic of _____ pancreatitis.

9. Flank pain caused by _____ is a common problem in patients presenting to the emergency department.

10. When urinary obstruction occurs, ultrasound is very effective in demonstrating the secondary sign of _____.

11. With the bladder distended, the color Doppler is an excellent tool to image the presence of ureteral jets into the bladder; the transducer should be angled in a(n) _____ presentation through the distended urinary bladder.

12. The pulse repetition frequency should be _____ to assess the low velocity of the ureteral jet flow.

13. Most aortic dissections are located in the _____ aorta.

14. _____ hypertension is nearly always associated with aortic dissection.

15. The most typical presentation of an aortic dissection is that of a sudden onset of severe, tearing _____ pain radiating to the arms, neck, or back.

16. The patient should be instructed to perform a(n) _____ maneuver to determine the site of wall defect and confirm the presence of the protruding hernia.

124

Provide a short answer for each question after evaluating the images.

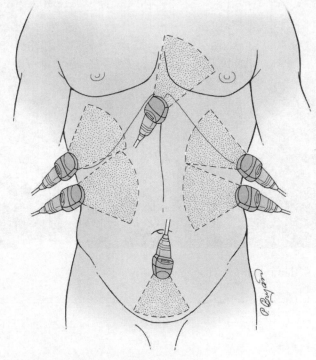

1. These images represent what type of ultrasound examination?

_____

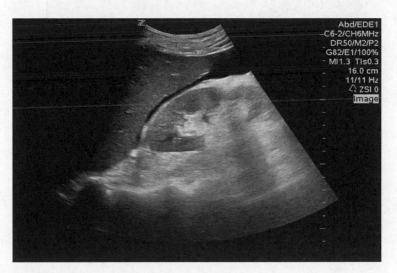

2. A trauma patient demonstrated fluid in what space?

_____

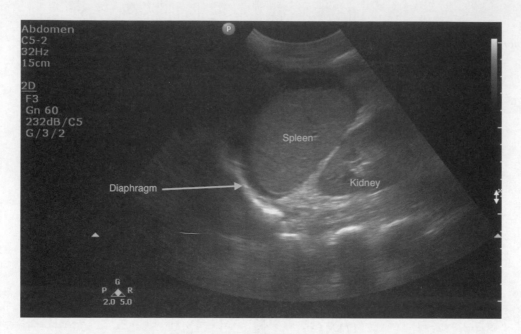

3. This sagittal image of the LUQ demonstrates what abnormality?

_____

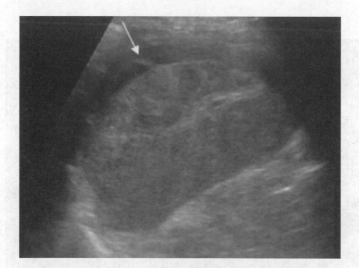

4. Trauma following a football injury to the LUQ demonstrates what abnormality?

_____

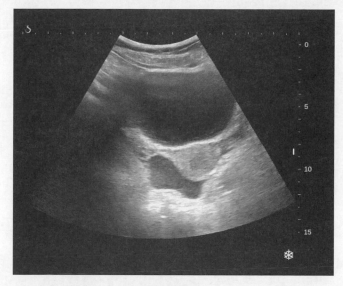

5. Transverse image of the pelvis demonstrates what abnormality?

_____

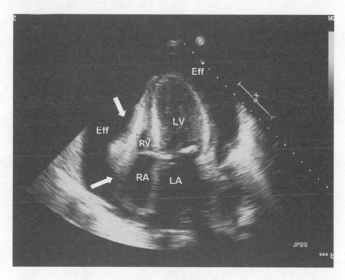

6. What is the significant finding in this patient with pericardial tamponade?

_____

20 Sonographic Techniques in the Transplant Patients

KEY TERMS

Exercise 1

Match the following abdominal ultrasound terms with their definitions.

_____ 1. Model for End-Stage Liver Disease (MELD)

_____ 2. Organ Procurement and Transplantation Network (OPTN)

_____ 3. Pediatric End-Stage Liver

_____ 4. PTLF

_____ 5. Renal autotransplantation-

_____ 6. SPK

_____ 7. United Network for Organ Sharing (UNOS)

A. The patient's own kidney is removed from the retroperitoneum, and reimplanted into the iliac fossa

B. Maintains a centralized computer networking system for all organ procurement organizations and transplant centers while seeking to be fair and effective in selecting transplant candidates.

C. Simultaneous pancreas-kidney transplant

D. Initially used to predict death within three months in patients who had a transjugular intrahepatic portosystemic shunt (TIPS) performed. The MELD score is a mathematical calculation based on lab values of bilirubin (measurement of bile pigment), creatinine (kidney function), and International Nationalized Ratio (INR) (blood clotting ability).

E. Organ allocation process

F. For children under 12 years of age

G. Post-transplant lymphoproliferative disorder

Exercise 2 Transplantation

Fill in the blank(s) with the word(s) that best completes the statements about transplantation.

1. Acute _____ failure is sudden and most commonly caused from a drug-induced injury such as an acetaminophen overdose.

2. The most common reason for transplantation in the United States is cirrhosis due to chronic _____, followed by _____ abuse.

3. The most common primary malignant tumor in the liver is _____ carcinoma.

4. The most common cause for requiring a renal transplant is _____ end-stage renal disease or renal failure.

5. High blood _____ can lead to many complications such as amputations, heart disease, stroke, vascular disease, blindness, nerve damage, or kidney damage.

Exercise 3 Evaluation of the Liver Allograft

Fill in the blanks that best completes the statements about the evaluation of the Liver Allograft.

1. The spectral waveform of the PV has _____ flow with minimal respiratory changes.

2. Postoperative edema can create _____ blood flow velocities within the HAs or venous system.

3. The most common cause for liver transplant failure is _____.

4. Intrahepatic _____ are localized fluid collections of necrotic inflammatory tissue that contains purulent material and an infectious organism.

5. Thrombosis and _____ are the most common events to occur at the anastomosis sites due to size discrepancy between the native and transplant vessels or suprahepatic caval kinking.

6. The most common cause for hepatic artery stenosis is postoperative _____.

7. The most common vascular complication of liver transplantation is _____ artery thrombosis.

8. _____complications taken as a whole are the second most common cause of allograft dysfunction following rejection.

9. The most common biliary complication is _____, usually caused from a stricture at the anastomosis but may also be secondary to choledocholithiasis.

10. _____ are clear, serous fluid collections that are usually found within the first few days after transplantation.

11. The most common complication of venovenous bypass during liver transplantation is a _____ _____.

12. Bile leaks seeps into the peritoneal cavity and may form a contained perihepatic collection, or _____.

13. Portal venous _____ is a common finding on ultrasound during the early postoperative period following transplantation.

Exercise 4 Renal Transplant

Fill in the blanks that best completes the statements about the evaluation of the Renal Allograft.

1. For all spectral Doppler, the angle should be _____with the vessel that is sampled and less than 60 degrees to ensure accurate velocity measurements.

2. Postoperative edema can create _____blood flow velocities within the RA or RV and the arcuate arteries can have an elevated RI as well demonstrating little or no diastolic flow.

3. What is the most common complication of renal biopsy? _____

4. Any peri-transplant fluid collection should be considered infected in the _____ patient.

5. The most common site of obstruction is at the site of ureteral implantation into the _____.

6. Renal transplant recipients are at a higher risk for developing urinary _____.

7. Slow flow, extrinsic compression, or a narrowing at the anastomosis may be a precursor to develop _____.

8. _____ renal vein thrombosis is an urgent finding and the patient should undergo thrombectomy to avoid allograft loss.

9. Renal artery _____is one of the most common vascular complications and usually occurs within the first year following transplantation.

10. A _____ is a focal disruption of the artery with no direct communication with a vein and can occur in any vessel.

11. The most common peri-transplant fluid collection is a _____.

Exercise 5 Pancreatic Transplant

Fill in the blanks that best completes the statements about the evaluation of the Pancreatic Transplant.

1. The tranplanted pancreas will appear different than the native organ and typically it has a _____ appearance and the borders can be difficult to visualize at times.

2. _____ is the second most common complication following transplantation.

3. _____ thrombosis is the second most common cause of allograft failure and is typically seen within the first 6 weeks following transplantation.

4. On ultrasound, _____ appears as a round cystic structure and demonstrates disorganized "yin-yang" color flow within.

5. _____ collections are the most common complication following pancreatic transplantation, with the most common being a hematoma.

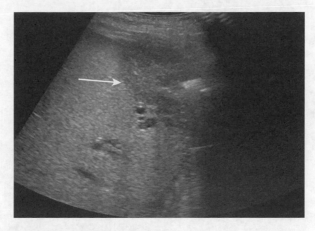

1. Describe your finding in this post-liver transplant patient.

_____

_____

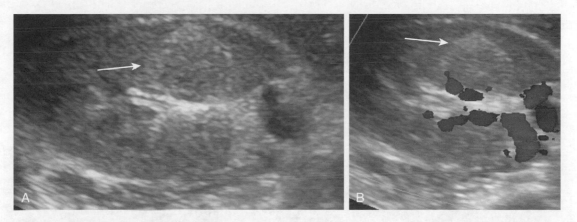

2. Describe your finding in this patient post-renal biopsy.

_____

_____

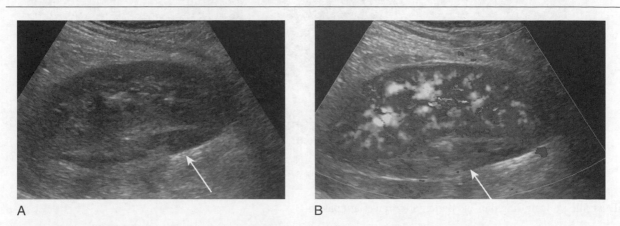

3. Describe your finding in this renal transplant patient.

_____

_____

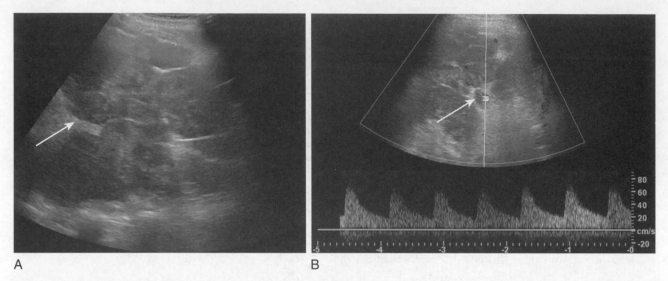

A

B

4. Describe your finding in this recent patient with a renal transplant.

_____

_____

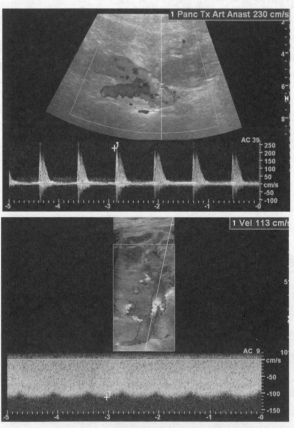

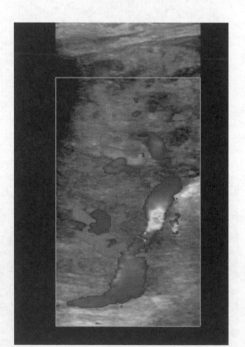

5. Describe your findings in this pancreatic transplant patient.

_____

_____

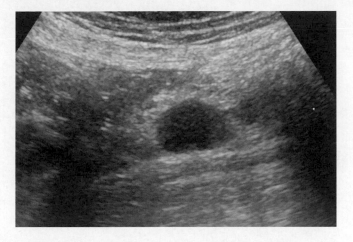 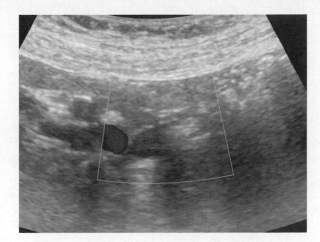

6. Describe your findings in this pancreatic transplant patient.

_____

_____

21 The Breast

KEY TERMS

Exercise 1

Match the following anatomy terms with their definitions.

_____ 1. Cooper's ligaments

_____ 2. mammary layer

_____ 3. retromammary layer

_____ 4. subcutaneous layer

_____ 5. tail of Spence

_____ 6. terminal ductal lobular unit (TDLU)

A. Connective tissue septa that connect perpendicularly to the breast lobules and extend out to the skin

B. Most superficial of the three layers of the breast identified on breast ultrasound

C. Middle layer of the breast tissue that contains the ductal, glandular, and stromal portions of the breast

D. Smallest functional portion of the breast involving the terminal duct and its associated lobule containing at least one acinus

E. Deepest of the three layers of the breast noted on breast ultrasound

F. Normal extension of breast tissue into the axillary region

Exercise 2: Crossword

Use the definitions below to solve the puzzle.

Across

1. This node represents the first lymph node along the axillary node chain.
2. Glandular (milk-producing) component of the breast lobule.
3. Armpit
4. Echo texture that is more echogenic than the surrounding tissue.
5. Differentiated apocrine sweat gland with a functional purpose of secreting milk during lactation.

Down

6. Finger-like extension of a malignan ttumor.
7. Echo texture that resembles the surrounding tissue.
8. Fluid-filled mass
9. The pigmented skin surrounding the breast nipple
10. Overgrowth of stromal and epithelial elements of the acini within terminal ductal lobular unit
11. Can be felt on clinical exam

Match the following pathology terms with their definitions.

_____ 1. apocrine metaplasia

_____ 2. atypical ductal hyperplasia

_____ 3. atypical hyperplasia

_____ 4. atypical lobular hyperplasia

_____ 5. epithelial hyperplasia

_____ 6. fibroadenoma

_____ 7. fibrocystic condition

_____ 8. Paget's disease

_____ 9. peau d'orange

_____ 10. infiltrating ductal carcinoma

_____ 11. infiltrating lobular carcinoma

_____ 12. lobular carcinoma in situ

_____ 13. lobular neoplasia

_____ 14. multicentric breast cancer

_____ 15. multifocal breast cancer

_____ 16. breast cancer

_____ 17. gynecomastia

A. Descriptive term for skin thickening of a breast that resembles the skin of an orange

B. Abnormal proliferation of cells with atypical features involving the TDLU, with an increased likelihood of evolving into breast cancer

C. Neither considered a true cancer nor treated as such

D. Most common benign solid tumor of the breast, consisting primarily of fibrous and epithelial tissue elements

E. Hypertrophy of residual ductal elements that persist behind the nipple in the male

F. Term preferred by many authors to replace LCIS and atypical hyperplasia

G. Involves two main types of cells (ductal and lobular)

H. Cancer of the lobular epithelium of the breast, arises at the level of the TDLU

I. Breast cancer occurring in more than one site within the same quadrant of the same ductal system of the breast

J. Condition that represents different, essentially normal, tissue processes within the breast that in some patients become exaggerated to the point of raising concern for breast cancer

K. The pathologist recognizes some, but not all, of the features of ductal carcinoma in situ

L. Breast cancer occurring in different quadrants of the breast at least 5 cm apart

M. Shows some, but not all, of the features of lobular carcinoma in situ

N. Surface erosion of the nipple characterized by redness with flaking and crusting caused by direct invasion of the skin of the nipple by underlying breast cancer

O. Form of fibrocystic change in which the epithelial cells of the acini undergo alteration

P. Cancer of the ductal epithelium; most common general category of breast cancer, accounting for approximately 85% of all breast cancers

Q. Proliferation (hyperplasia) of epithelial cells lining the terminal duct-lobular unit

Exercise 4

Label the following illustrations.

A. Breast anatomy.

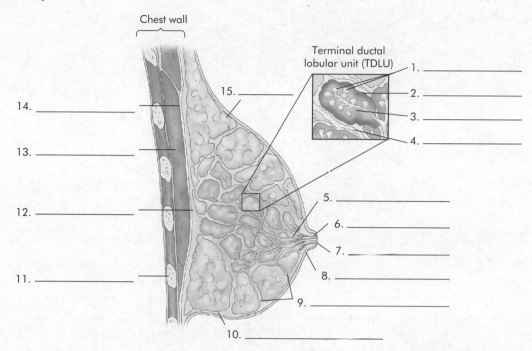

B. Lymphatic drainage of the breast.

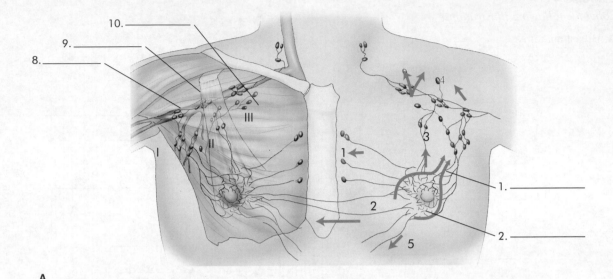

10.
9.
8.

III

II

I

1
2
5

4
3
1.
2.

A

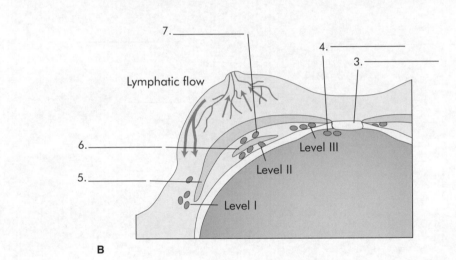

7.

Lymphatic flow

4.
3.

6.

Level III

5.

Level II

Level I

B

Exercise 5

Fill in the blank(s) with the word(s) that best completes the statements or provide a short answer about the anatomy and sonographic appearance of the breast.

1. The breast is a modified _____ gland located in the superficial fascia of the anterior chest wall.

2. Sonographically the breast is divided into three layers located between the skin and the pectoralis major muscle on the anterior chest wall. These layers are the _____ layer, the _____ layer, and the _____ layer.

3. Fat is the least _____ tissue within the breast.

4. The fatty tissue appears _____, whereas the ducts, glands, and supporting ligaments appear echogenic.

5. The _____ quadrant of the breast contains the highest concentration of lobes.

6. Each lobule contains _____ (milk-producing glands) that are clustered on the terminal ends of the ducts like grapes on a vine.

7. The _____ major muscle lies posterior to the retromammary layer.

8. The _____ tissue can situate itself in and among the areas of glandular tissue, and in some scanning planes it can mimic isoechoic or hypoechoic masses.

9. Lymphatic drainage from all parts of the breast generally flows to the _____ lymph nodes.

Exercise 6

Fill in the blank(s) with the word(s) that best completes the statements or provide a short answer about the physiology of the breast.

1. The primary function of the breast is _____ transport.

2. The _____ system is critical in the transport of fluids within the breast.

3. An important function during the reproductive years is for the breast to make _____ from nutrients and water taken from the bloodstream.

4. Milk is produced within the _____ and carried to the nipple by the ducts.

5. During this time of development, the ductal system proliferates under the influence of _____.

6. During pregnancy, acinar development is accelerated to enable milk production by estrogen, _____, and prolactin.

7. The hormone produced by the pituitary gland that stimulates the acini to produce and excrete milk is called _____.

SONOGRAPHIC EVALUATION

Exercise 7

Fill in the blank(s) with the word(s) that best completes the statements or provide a short answer about the sonographic evaluation of the breast.

1. Ultrasound may be used for screening purposes in young breasts that are _____ and difficult to penetrate by mammography, to evaluate palpable masses that are not visible on a mammogram, and to image the deep juxtathoracic tissues not normally visible by mammography.

2. Pertinent clinical information that should be provided by the referring physician includes size and location of the lump, when it was noticed, and its relation to the _____.

3. Breast cancer is usually lobular or _____ in shape, uneven in surface contour (sometimes gritty in texture), and fixed or poorly movable.

4. Most breast masses that arise during the adolescent years are _____.

5. A(n) _____ implant rupture occurs when there is a breach of the membrane surrounding an implant, but the silicone that leaks out is still confined within the fibrous scar tissue that forms a "capsule" around the implant.

6. As the implant collapses and the membrane folds inward, a series of discontinuous echogenic lines parallel to the face of the transducer may be seen and are referred to as the "stepladder sign" or "_____ sign."

7. _____ tend to grow within the ducts and will often follow the ductal system in a radial plane, toward the convergence at the nipple.

8. A rounded or oval shape is usually associated with _____ lesions, whereas sharp, angular margins are associated with _____ lesions.

9. The normal tissue planes of the breast are _____ oriented.

10. Benign lesions tend to grow within the normal tissue planes, and their long axis lies _____ to the chest wall.

11. Malignant lesions are able to grow through the connective tissue and may have a(n) _____ orientation when imaging the breast from anterior to posterior.

12. Malignant masses will often demonstrate increased _____ within the lesion and often have a feeder vessel, which can be identified with careful evaluation.

PATHOLOGY

Exercise 8

Fill in the blank(s) with the word(s) that best completes the statements about the abnormalities of the breast.

1. Lesions more common to younger women are _____ disease and fibroadenomas.

2. Older or postmenopausal women are more likely to have _____ papillomas, duct ectasia, and cancer.

3. Skin dimpling or ulceration and nipple retraction nearly always result from _____.

4. Benign tumors are rubbery, _____, and well delineated (as seen in a fibroadenoma), whereas malignant tumors are often stone hard and irregular with a gritty feel.

5. Clinical signs and symptoms of _____ disease include the lumps and pain that the patient feels that fluctuate with every monthly cycle. In most cases both breasts are equally involved.

6. If the tumor is _____, it continues to grow in one area, compressing and distorting the surrounding architecture.

7. Most cancer originates in the _____ ductal lobular units, whereas a smaller percentage originates in the glandular tissue.

8. Carcinomas that do not normally spread outside of the duct or lobule are called noninvasive, noninfiltrating, or _____ cancers, whereas cancers that spread into nearby tissue are said to be invasive or infiltrating.

Provide a short answer for each question after evaluating the images.

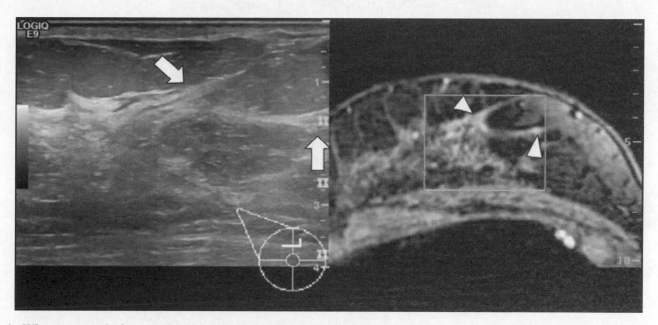

1. What structure is the arrow pointing to on this breast ultrasound?

_____

_____

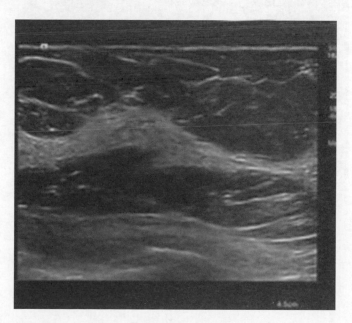

2. What classification would you give to this breast image?

_____

_____

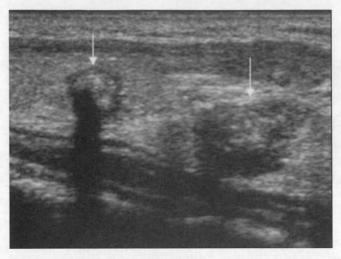

3. The arrows point to what abnormal structures in the breast?

_____

_____

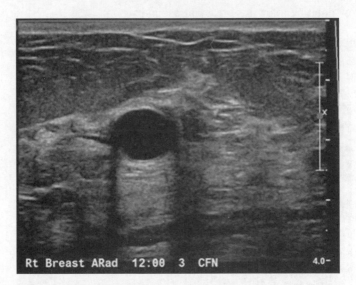

4. This image is representative of what abnormality in the breast?

_____

_____

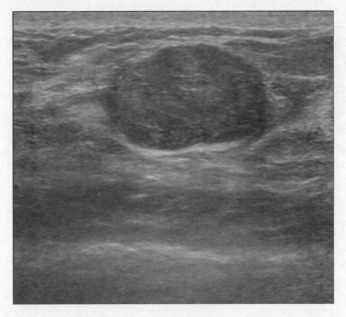

5. This image is representative of what abnormality in this young patient?

_____

_____

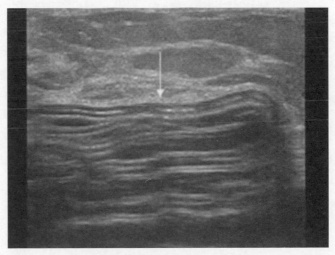

6. What abnormality is this arrow pointing to in a patient with breast implants?

_____

_____

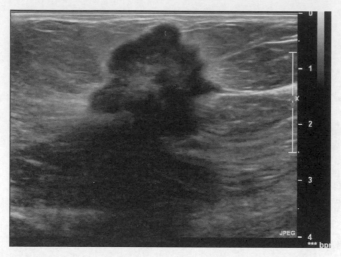

7. Would you suspect benign or malignant disease to be present in this patient?

_____

_____

22 The Thyroid and Parathyroid Glands

KEY TERMS

Exercise 1

Match the following terms related to normal and abnormal anatomy and physiology with their definitions.

_____ 1. calcitonin

_____ 2. euthyroid

_____ 3. hyperthyroidism

_____ 4. hypophosphatasia

_____ 5. hypothyroidism

_____ 6. isthmus

_____ 7. longus colli muscles

_____ 8. parathyroid hormone

_____ 9. pyramidal lobe

_____ 10. serum calcium

_____ 11. sternocleidomastoid muscles

_____ 12. strap muscles

_____ 13. thyroid-stimulating hormone

A. Group of three muscles (sternothyroid, sternohyoid, and omohyoid) that lies anterior to the thyroid
B. Undersecretion of thyroid hormones
C. Thyroid hormone important for maintaining a dense, strong bone matrix and regulating the blood calcium level
D. Low phosphate level associated with hyperparathyroidism
E. Laboratory value that is elevated with hyperparathyroidism
F. Hormone secreted by the pituitary gland that stimulates the thyroid gland to secrete thyroxine and triiodothyronine
G. Wedge-shaped muscle posterior to the thyroid lobes
H. Hormone secreted by parathyroid glands that regulates serum calcium levels
I. Refers to a normal functioning thyroid gland
J. Small piece of thyroid tissue that connects the right and left lobes of the gland
K. Large muscles anterolateral to the thyroid
L. Oversecretion of thyroid hormones
M. Present in small percentage of patients; extends superiorly from the isthmus

Exercise 2

Match the following terms related to parathyroid pathology and miscellaneous neck masses with their definitions.

_____ 1. brachial cleft cyst

_____ 2. fine-needle aspiration

_____ 3. hyperparathyroidism

_____ 4. lymphadenopathy

_____ 5. parathyroid hyperplasia

_____ 6. primary hyperparathyroidism

_____ 7. secondary hyperparathyroidism

_____ 8. thyroglossal duct cysts

A. Disorder characterized by a localized or generalized enlargement of the lymph nodes or lymph vessels
B. Remnant of embryonic development that appears as a cyst in the neck
C. Disorder associated with elevated serum calcium level, usually caused by a benign parathyroid adenoma
D. Oversecretion of parathyroid hormone, usually from a parathyroid adenoma
E. Congenital anomalies that present in the midline of the neck anterior to the trachea
F. Enlargement of the multiple parathyroid glands
G. Enlargement of parathyroid glands in patients with renal failure or vitamin D deficiency
H. Use of a fine-gauge needle to obtain cells from a mass

Exercise 3

Match the following terms related to thyroid pathology with their definitions.

_____ 1. adenoma

_____ 2. anaplastic carcinoma

_____ 3. follicular carcinoma

_____ 4. goiter

_____ 5. Graves' disease

_____ 6. Hashimoto's thyroiditis

_____ 7. medullary carcinoma

_____ 8. microcalcification

_____ 9. multinodular goiter

_____ 10. nodular hyperplasia

_____ 11. papillary carcinoma

_____ 12. subacute (de Quervain's) thyroiditis

_____ 13. thyroiditis

A. Degenerative nodules within the thyroid

B. Inflammation of the thyroid

C. Viral infection of the thyroid that causes inflammation

D. Autoimmune disorder characterized by a diffuse toxic goiter, bulging eyes, and cutaneous manifestations

E. Nodular enlargement of the thyroid associated with hyperthyroidism

F. Benign thyroid neoplasm characterized by complete fibrous encapsulation

G. Most common form of thyroid malignancy

H. Rare, undifferentiated carcinoma occurring in middle age

I. Chronic inflammation of the thyroid gland caused by the formation of antibodies against normal thyroid tissue

J. Occurs as a solitary malignant mass within the thyroid gland

K. Enlargement of the thyroid gland that can be focal or diffuse; multiple nodules may be present

L. Neoplastic growth that accounts for 10% of thyroid malignancies

M. Tiny echogenic foci within a nodule that may or may not shadow

ANATOMY AND PHYSIOLOGY

Exercise 4

Label the following illustrations.

A. Anterior view of the thyroid and parathyroid glands.

B. Cross section of the thyroid region.

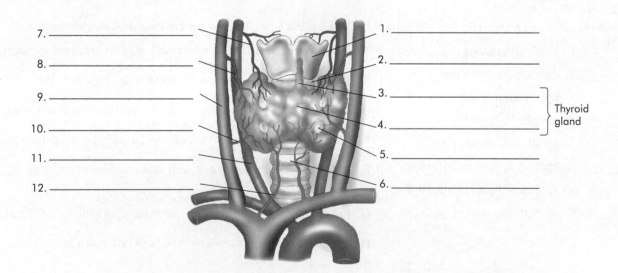

7. _____
8. _____
9. _____
10. _____
11. _____
12. _____

1. _____
2. _____
3. _____ ⎤
4. _____ ⎬ Thyroid gland
5. _____ ⎦
6. _____

1. _____

15. _____

14. _____

13. _____

12. _____

11. _____

10. _____

2. _____ ⎤
                      ⎬ Strap
3. _____ ⎭ muscles

4. _____

5. _____

6. _____

7. _____

8. _____

9. _____

THE THYROID AND PARATHYROID GLANDS

Exercise 5

Fill in the blank(s) with the word(s) that best completes the statements about the thyroid and parathyroid glands.

1. The thyroid straddles the trachea anteriorly, whereas the paired lobes extend on either side bounded laterally by the _____ arteries and _____ veins.

2. Along the anterior surface of the thyroid gland lie the _____ muscles, including the sternothyroid, omohyoid, sternohyoid, and sternocleidomastoid muscles.

3. The parathyroid glands are normally located on the _____ surface of the thyroid gland.

4. The parathyroid glands are the _____ organs in the body.

5. The parathyroid glands produce _____ and monitor the serum calcium feedback mechanism.

6. When the serum calcium level _____, the parathyroid glands are stimulated to release PTH.

7. PTH acts on bone, _____, and intestine to enhance calcium absorption.

8. Primary hyperparathyroidism is characterized by _____, hypercalciuria, and low serum levels of phosphate.

9. Primary hyperparathyroidism occurs when increased amounts of PTH are produced by a(n) _____, primary hyperplasia, or, rarely, carcinoma located in the parathyroid gland.

Exercise 6

Fill in the blank(s) with the word(s) that best completes the statements about the thyroid and parathyroid glands.

1. The thyroid gland is the part of the endocrine system that maintains body growth, development, and _____ through the synthesis, storage, and secretion of thyroid hormones.

2. These hormones include triiodothyronine (T3), thyroxine (T4), and _____.

3. The mechanism for producing thyroid hormones is _____ metabolism.

4. The secretion of TSH is regulated by thyrotropin-releasing factor, which is produced by the _____.

5. Low intake of iodine (goiter) in the body may cause either _____, or the inability of the thyroid to produce the proper amount of thyroid hormone, or a problem in the pituitary gland that does not control the thyroid production.

6. The function of the thyroid gland is evaluated by _____ medicine.

7. An enlargement of the thyroid gland is a(n) _____, which is often visible on the anterior neck.

8. One of the most common forms of thyroid disease is _____ goiter .

9. _____ disease is characterized by these findings: hypermetabolism, diffuse toxic goiter, exophthalmos (inflammatory infiltration of the orbital tissue resulting in proptosis, or bulging of the eyes), and cutaneous manifestations (thickening of the dermis of the pretibial areas and the dorsum of the feet).

10. A benign thyroid neoplasm characterized by complete fibrous encapsulation is a(n)_____.

11. The most common of the thyroid malignancies is _____ cancer of the thyroid and is the preponderant cause of thyroid cancer in children.

12. The normal thyroid gland has a fine _____ echotexture that is more echogenic than the surrounding muscle structure.

13. The _____ muscle is posterior and lateral to each thyroid lobe and appears as a hypoechoic triangular structure adjacent to the cervical vertebrae.

PATHOLOGY

Exercise 7

Provide a short answer for each question after evaluating the images.

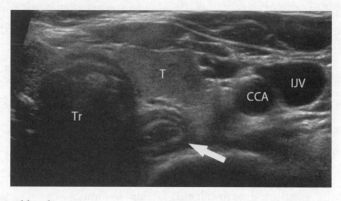

1. Identify the structure denoted by the arrow.

_____

_____

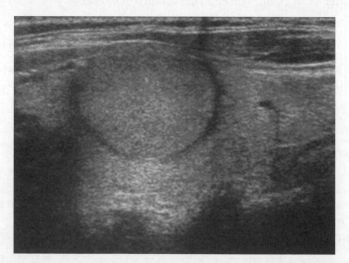

2. A young woman presented with a palpable mass in her neck. What is the sonographic finding that defines this as a thyroid nodule?

_____

_____

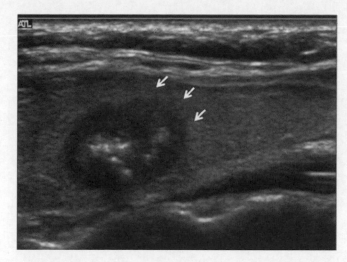

3. An female patient appeared with a mass in her neck. Would you consider this lesion to be malignant or benign?

_____

_____

23 The Scrotum

KEY TERMS

Exercise 1

Match the following anatomy terms with their definitions.

_____ 1. cremasteric muscle

_____ 2. ejaculatory ducts

_____ 3. epididymis

_____ 4. mediastinum testis

_____ 5. pampiniform plexus

_____ 6. pudendal artery

_____ 7. scrotum

_____ 8. seminal vesicles

_____ 9. septa testis

_____ 10. spermatic cord

_____ 11. testicle

_____ 12. testicular artery

_____ 13. tunica albuginea

_____ 14. tunica vaginalis

_____ 15. urethra

_____ 16. vas deferens

_____ 17. verumontanum

A. Connect the seminal vesicle and the vas deferens to the urethra at the verumontanum

B. Reservoirs for sperm located posterior to the bladder

C. Plexus of veins in the spermatic cord that drain into the right and left testicular veins

D. Junction of the ejaculatory ducts with the urethra

E. Male gonad that produces hormones that induce masculine features and spermatozoa

F. An extension of the internal oblique muscle that descends to the testis with the spermatic cord

G. Membrane consisting of a visceral layer and a parietal layer lining the inner wall of the scrotum

H. Partially supply the scrotal wall and epididymis and occasionally the lower pole of the testis

I. Tube that connects the epididymis to the seminal vesicle

J. Anatomic structure formed by the network of ducts leaving the mediastinum testis that combine into a single, convoluted epididymal tubule

K. Artery arising from the aorta just distal to each renal artery

L. Central linear structure formed by the convergence of multiple, thin septations within the testicle, which are invaginations of the tunica albuginea

M. Small membranous canal that extends from the bladder to the end of the penis

N. Multiple septa formed from the tunica albuginea that course toward the mediastinum testis and separate the testicle into lobules

O. Inner fibrous membrane surrounding the testicle

P. Structure made up of vas deferens, testicular artery, cremasteric artery, and pampiniform plexus that suspends the testis in the scrotum

Q. Sac containing the testes and epididymis

Exercise 2

Match the following vascular supply terms with their definitions.

_____ 1. centripetal artery

_____ 2. cremasteric artery

_____ 3. deferential artery

_____ 4. recurrent rami

_____ 5. testicular vein

A. Small artery arising from the inferior epigastric artery, which supplies the peritesticular tissue, including the cremasteric muscle

B. Formed by the pampiniform plexus.

C. Arises from the vesicle artery and supplies the vas deferens and epididymis

D. Terminal intratesticular arteries arising from the capsular arteries

E. Terminal ends of the centripetal arteries that curve backward toward the capsule

Exercise 3

Match the following pathology terms with their definitions.

_____ 1. cryptorchidism

_____ 2. epididymal cyst

_____ 3. epididymitis

_____ 4. hematocele

A. Dilated veins in the pampiniform plexus caused by obstruction of the venous return from the testicle

B. Cyst filled with clear, serous fluid located in the epididymis

C. Fluid formed between the visceral and parietal layers of the tunica vaginalis

D. Cyst in the vas deferens containing sperm

151

_____ 5. hydrocele	E.	Inflammation of the epididymis
_____ 6. pyocele	F.	Testicles remain within the abdomen or groin and fail to descend into the scrotal sac
_____ 7. rete testis	G.	Pus located between the visceral and parietal layers of the tunica vaginalis
_____ 8. spermatocele	H.	Network of the channels formed by the convergence of the straight seminiferous tubules in the mediastinum testis
_____ 9. varicocele	I.	Blood located between the visceral and parietal layers of the tunica vaginalis

ANATOMY AND PHYSIOLOGY

Exercise 4

Fill in the blank(s) with the word(s) that best completes the statements about the anatomy and physiology of the scrotum.

1. The testes are symmetric, oval-shaped glands residing in the _____.

2. The largest part of the epididymis is the _____, measuring 6 to 15 mm in width.

3. The ductus epididymis becomes the _____ and continues in the spermatic cord.

4. The testis is completely covered by a dense, fibrous tissue termed the _____.

5. The _____ supports the ducts coursing within the testis.

6. The space between the layers of the tunica vaginalis is where _____ can form.

7. Venous drainage of the scrotum occurs through the veins of the _____ plexus.

PATHOLOGY

Exercise 5

Fill in the blank(s) with the word(s) that best completes the statements or provide a short answer about the pathologic conditions of the scrotum.

1. The most important goal of the ultrasound examination in testicular trauma is to determine if _____ has occurred.

2. An acute hematocele is _____ with numerous, highly visible echoes that can be seen to float or move in real time.

3. The most common cause of acute scrotal pain in adults is _____ infection of the epididymis and testis.

4. With epididymitis, Doppler waveforms demonstrate _____ velocities in both systole and diastole. A low resistance waveform pattern is present.

5. _____ of the spermatic cord occurs as a result of abnormal mobility of the testis within the scrotum.

6. The bell _____ anomaly occurs when the tunica vaginalis completely surrounds the testis, epididymis, and distal spermatic cord, allowing them to move and rotate freely within the scrotum.

7. Torsion is the most common cause of acute scrotal pain in _____.

8. A(n) _____ of perfusion in the symptomatic testis with normal perfusion demonstrated in the asymptomatic side is considered to be diagnostic of torsion.

9. Extratesticular cysts are found in the tunica _____ or epididymis.

10. _____ are usually caused by incompetent venous valves within the spermatic vein.

11. A(n) _____ contains serous fluid and is the most common cause of painless scrotal swelling.

Exercise 6

Provide a short answer for each question after evaluating the images.

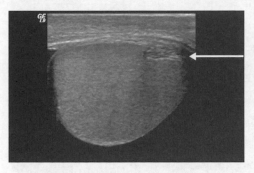

1. What anatomic structure does the arrow point to?

_____

_____

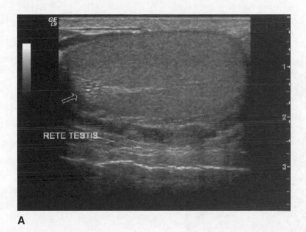

A

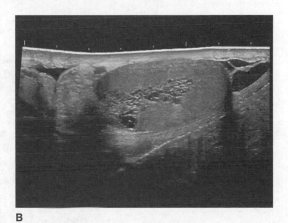

B

2. Identify the abnormality in these images of the testes.

_____

_____

153

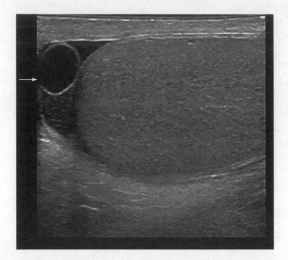

3. What is the arrow pointing to?

_____

_____

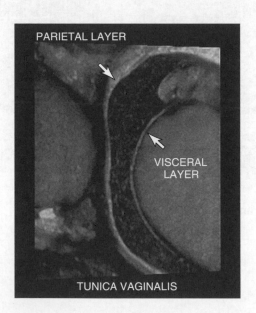

4. Describe the sonographic findings on this image of the tunica vaginalis.

_____

_____

24 The Musculoskeletal System

Exercise 1

Match the following anatomy terms with their definitions.

_____ 1. aponeurosis

_____ 2. bursa

_____ 3. epineurium

_____ 4. fasciculi

_____ 5. ligament

_____ 6. muscle

_____ 7. myelin

_____ 8. pennate

_____ 9. perineurium

_____ 10. synovial sheath

_____ 11. tendon

_____ 12. volar

A. Type of tissue consisting of contractile cells or fibers that affects movement of an organ or part of the body
B. Covering of a nerve that consists of connective tissue
C. Membrane surrounding a joint, tendon, or bursa that secretes a viscous fluid called synovia
D. Connective tissue that surrounds muscle
E. Bandlike flat tendons connecting the process of the scapula
F. Fibrous band of tissue connecting bone or cartilage to bone that aids in stabilizing a joint
G. Fibrous tissue connecting muscle to bone
H. Saclike structure containing thick fluid that surrounds areas subject to friction, such as the interface between bone and tendon
I. Substance forming the sheath of Schwann cells
J. The anterior portion of the body when in the anatomic position
K. Small bundle of muscles, nerves, and tendons
L. A feather-like pattern of muscle growth

Exercise 2

Match the following artifact, sonography, and pathology terms with their definitions.

_____ 1. acromioclavicular joint

_____ 2. anisotropy

_____ 3. nerve

_____ 4. comet tail artifact

_____ 5. dorsiflexion

_____ 6. Guyon's canal or tunnel

_____ 7. plantar flexion

_____ 8. refractile shadowing

_____ 9. seroma

_____ 10. tendinitis

A. Conduit for impulses sent to and from the muscles and the central nervous system
B. Fibrous tunnel that contains the ulnar artery and vein, ulnar nerve, and some fatty tissue
C. Accumulation of serous fluid within tissue
D. The joint found in the shoulder that connects the clavicle to the acromion process of the scapula
E. Pointing of the toes toward the plantar surface of the foot
F. The quality of comprising varying values of a given property when measured in different directions
G. The bending of the sound beam at the edge of a circular structure that results in the absence of posterior echoes
H. Upward movement of the hand and foot
I. Inflammation of the tendon
J. Posterior linear equidistant artifact created when sound reverberates between two strong reflectors, such as air bubbles, metal, and glass

155

Exercise 3

Label the following illustrations.

1. Different types of muscle.

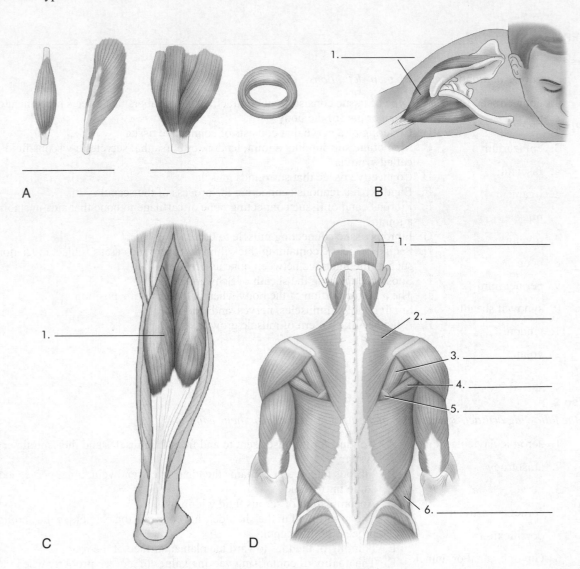

A _____   _____

_____   _____

B

C

D

1. _____

1. _____

2. _____

3. _____

4. _____

5. _____

6. _____

2. The subscapularis, biceps tendon, and the acromioclavicular joint image.

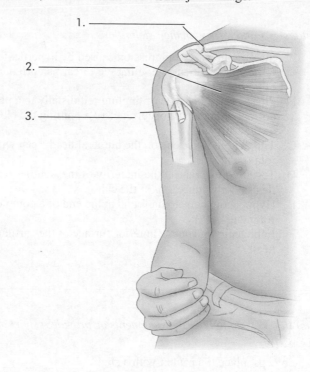

1. _____

2. _____

3. _____

Exercise 4

Fill in the blank(s) with the word(s) that best completes the statements about the anatomy of the musculoskeletal system.

1. Skeletal muscle contains long organized units called muscle _____.

2. The characteristic long fibers are under voluntary control, allowing us to contract a(n) _____ and move a joint.

3. A(n) _____ muscle has a division of several feather-like sections in one muscle, and the _____ is the convergence of fibers to a central tendon.

4. The attachment of the muscle that occurs at the proximal and distal portion of the bundle is called a(n) _____.

5. Tendons occur with or without a(n) _____ sheath.

6. The sheath surrounding a tendon has two layers. The fluid separates the layers in this part of the body: _____, _____, _____, and _____.

7. Short bands of tough fibers that connect bones to other bones are _____.

8. The saclike structure surrounding joints and tendons that contains a viscous fluid is the _____.

9. The knee joint has _____ bursa.

10. A loose areolar connective tissue that fills the fascial compartment of the tendon lacking a synovial sheath is a(n) _____.

11. The dense _____ is another layer of connective tissue that closely adjoins the tendon.

12. Interwoven and interconnected collagen fibers found in the tendon run in a(n) _____ path.

13. The proximal portion of the muscle is considered the _____, whereas the _____ is the distal end.

14. The normal nerve has a(n) _____ appearance when compared with muscle, but it is _____ to tendons.

15. The minute amount of viscous fluid contained within the bursa helps reduce _____ between the moving parts of the joint.

16. A Baker's cyst is an example of a(n) _____ bursa in the medial popliteal fossa.

Exercise 5

Match the following musculoskeletal signs and tests with their definitions.

1. ____ cartilage interface sign

2. ____ clapper-in-the-bell sign

3. ____ naked tuberosity sign

4. ____ Phalen's sign

5. ____ Thompson's test

6. ____ Tinel's sign

A. Increase in wrist compression caused by hyperflexion of the wrist for 60 seconds; patient is holding the forearms upright and pressing the ventral side of the hands together

B. Pins and needles type of tingling felt distally to a percussion site and either a normal or abnormal occurrence (e.g., hitting the elbow creates a tingling in the distal arm)

C. The deltoid muscle is on the humeral head; seen with a full-thickness tear of the rotator cuff

D. Test used to evaluate the integrity of the Achilles tendon that involves plantar flexion with squeezing of the calf

E. Hypoechoic hematoma found at the end of a completely retracted muscle fragment

F. Echogenic line on the anterior surface of the cartilage surrounding the humeral head

SONOGRAPHIC EVALUATION

Exercise 6

Fill in the blank(s) with the word(s) that best completes the statements or provide a short answer about the sonographic evaluation of the musculoskeletal system.

1. To begin the examination of the biceps, place the patient with a slight _____ rotation of the shoulder.

2. When facing the patient and imaging the right shoulder, the lateral anatomy displays on the _____ side of the image and the medial anatomy on the _____ side of the screen.

3. The groove located between the greater and lesser tuberosities, coupled with the overlying transverse ligament, maintains the _____ tendon location.

4. Using the biceps tendon as a landmark, angle the transducer _____ to locate the subscapularis tendon.

5. The bandlike tendon that has a medium level echotexture is the _____ tendon and originates from the greater tuberosity of the humerus.

6. A good landmark to help find the anteriorly located infraspinatus tendon is the posterior _____.

7. Fluid imaged _____ to the infraspinatus tendon indicates bursal fluid, whereas _____ fluid indicates joint effusion.

8. The carpal tunnel is located between the _____ bones and the _____ retinaculum on the palmar side of the wrist.

9. The ulnar artery and veins indicate the medial border of the carpal tunnel, whereas the most lateral structure is the _____ artery and veins.

10. The tendon that connects the gastrocnemius and soleus muscles to the calcaneus is the _____ tendon.

11. The _____ thickness tear involves either the bursal or articular cuff surface or the intrasubstance material.

12. The presence of large amounts of fluid in the subacromial-subdeltoid bursa raises the chance of a nonvisualized _____ tear.

13. The normal tendon cannot be compressed; however, the injured tendon _____ as the torn edges move apart.

14. Joint effusion around the biceps tendon combined with subacromial-subdeltoid bursitis results in the _____ sign.

15. Acute tendinitis involves not only the tendon but the surrounding _____ sheath.

16. The normal synovial sheath appears as a hypoechoic _____ around the tendon.

17. The abrupt stretching of the muscle beyond the maximum length results in a(n) _____ tear.

18. External force resulting in a crush injury is considered a(n) _____ tear.

PATHOLOGY

Exercise 7

Provide a short answer for each question after evaluating the images.

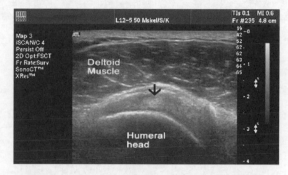

1. The arrow is pointing to which mildly hyperechoic structure in the shoulder?

_____

_____

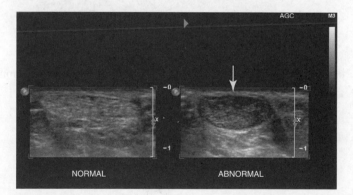

2. What abnormality does this comparison of the normal with the injured tendon reveal?

_____

_____

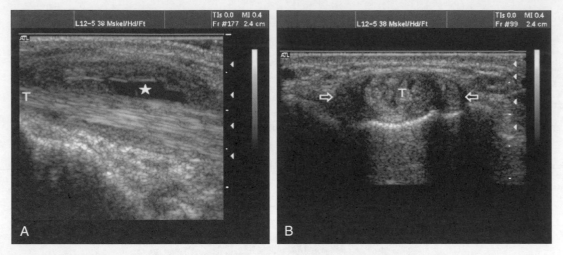

3. De Quervain's tendinitis is identified in this patient. What are the sonographic findings?

_____

_____

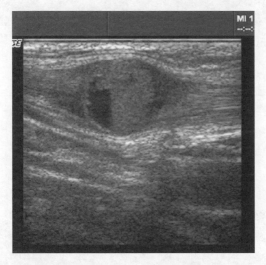

4. A soccer player experienced intense pain in his calf after a sudden blow in a championship game. What are the sonographic findings?

_____

_____

Chapter **24** **The Musculoskeletal System**

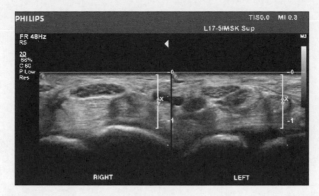

5. This sonographic image demonstrates an abnormality that may be seen in carpal tunnel syndrome. What is the abnormality?

_____

_____

25 Neonatal and Pediatric Abdomen

Exercise 1

Match the following key terms with their definitions.

_____ 1. acholic

_____ 2. appendicolith

_____ 3. atretic

_____ 4. Beckwith-Wiedemann syndrome

_____ 5. biliary atresia

_____ 6. choledochal cyst

_____ 7. hemihypertrophy

_____ 8. hypertrophic pyloric stenosis

_____ 9. intussusception

_____ 10. neuroblastoma

_____ 11. projectile vomiting

_____ 12. pyloric canal

_____ 13. target (donut) sign

_____ 14. Wilms' tumor

A. Congenital absence or closure of a normal body opening or tubular structure

B. Excessive development of one side or one half of the body or an organ

C. Frequently associated with sectional areas of the gastrointestinal tract; the muscle is hyperechoic, and the inner core is hypoechoic

D. Congenital cystic malformation of the common bile duct

E. Fecalith or calcification located within the appendix

F. Occurs when bowel prolapses into distal bowel and is propelled in an antegrade fashion

G. Autosomal recessive condition characterized by macroglossia, exophthalmos, and gigantism, often accompanied by visceromegaly and dysplasia of the renal medulla

H. Describes the absence of bile secretion or failure of bile to enter the alimentary tract

I. Located between the stomach and duodenum

J. Thickened muscle in the pylorus that prevents food from entering the duodenum

K. Closure or absence of some or all of the major bile ducts

L. Rapidly developing tumor of the kidney that usually occurs in children

M. Malignant hemorrhagic tumor composed principally of cells resembling neuroblasts that give rise to cells of the sympathetic system

N. Sign of pyloric stenosis in the neonatal period

THE PEDIATRIC ABDOMEN

Exercise 2

Fill in the blank(s) with the word(s) that best completes the statements or provide a short answer about the pediatric abdomen.

1. The right hepatic lobe should not extend more than _____ cm below the costal margin in the young infant.

2. The common bile duct should measure less than _____ mm in neonates, less than _____ mm in infants up to 1 year old, less than _____ mm in older children, and less than _____ mm in adolescents and adults.

3. The length of the gallbladder should not exceed the length of the _____.

4. The three most common causes for jaundice in the neonate are _____, _____, and

_____.

5. An abnormal cystic dilation of the biliary tree that most frequently affects the common bile duct is a(n)

_____.

6. When a choledochal cyst is present, there is usually fusiform dilatation of the common bile duct with associated

_____ ductal dilation.

7. The most common benign vascular liver tumor of early childhood is infantile hepatic _____.

8. The most common sonographic appearance of hemangioendothelioma is that of multiple hypoechoic lesions and

_____.

9. The most common primary malignant disease of the liver is _____ and occurs most frequently in children under 5 years of age.

10. The _____ is located between the stomach and duodenum.

11. Hypertrophic pyloric stenosis occurs most commonly in _____ infants between 2 and 6 weeks of age.

12. As the pyloric muscle thickens and elongates, the stomach outlet obstruction increases, and vomiting is more

constant and _____.

13. A muscle thickness of _____ mm or greater on the long-axis view, a channel length of 17 mm or greater, and pyloric muscle length of 20 mm or greater are reliable indicators of HPS.

14. In infants and young children, the progression of acute appendicitis to _____ is more rapid than in older children.

15. With ultrasound the acutely inflamed appendix is _____.

16. _____ produced by overlying transducer pressure is an additional finding consistent with appendicitis.

17. The most common acute abdominal disorder in early childhood is _____.

18. The presence of alternating hypoechoic and hyperechoic rings surrounding an echogenic center as seen in a

short-axis view of the involved area is known as the _____ sign.

Exercise 3

Provide a short answer for each question after evaluating the images.

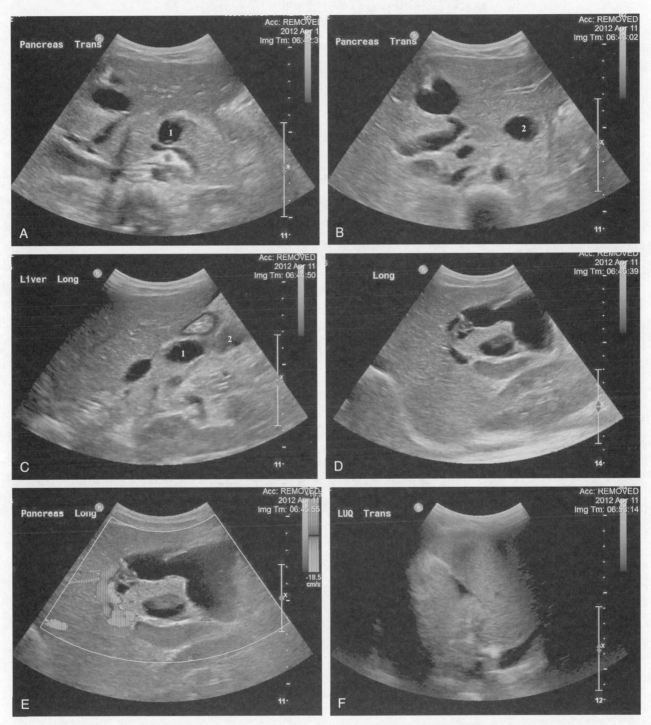

1. An 11-year-old child presented with increasing abdominal pain several days after blunt trauma to the abdomen from striking the handlebars on her bike.

_____

_____

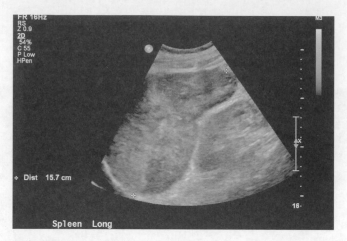

Spleen Long

2. Describe this image obtained from a 17-year-old male with leukemia.

_____

_____

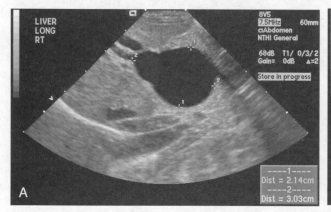

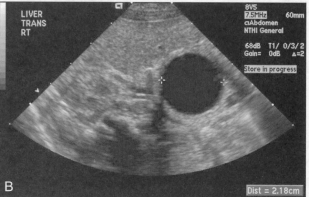

3. A 5-day-old infant with a history of a palpable abdominal mass. What are the sonographic findings?

_____

_____

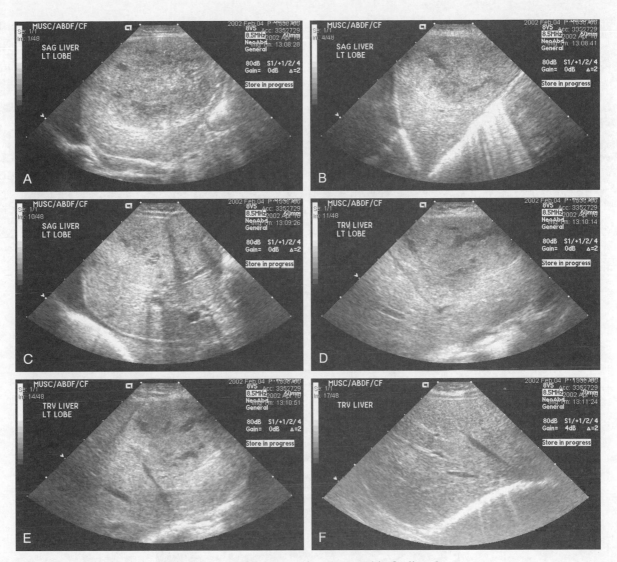

4. A neonate presented with an abdominal mass. What are the sonographic findings?

_____

_____

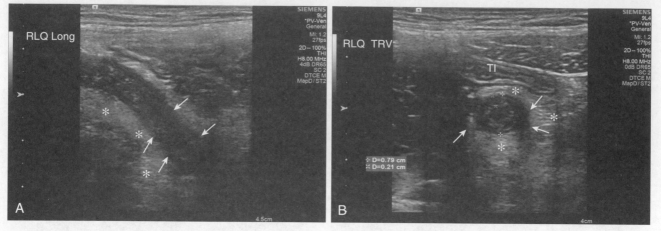

5. A child presented with nausea and vomiting, fever, and intense left lower quadrant pain. What is the sonographic finding?

_____

_____

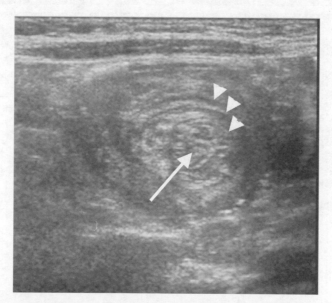

6. An infant presented with fever and peritoneal signs. What is the sonographic finding?

_____

_____

26 Neonatal and Pediatric Adrenal and Urinary System

KEY TERMS

Exercise 1

Match the following terms related to neonatal and pediatric kidneys with their definitions.

_____ 1. adrenal hemorrhage

_____ 2. arcuate arteries

_____ 3. autosomal dominant polycystic kidney disease (ADPKD)

_____ 4. autosomal recessive polycystic kidney disease (ARPKD)

_____ 5. congenital mesoblastic nephroma

_____ 6. cortex

_____ 7. ectasia

_____ 8. ectopic ureterocele

_____ 9. hydronephrosis

_____ 10. medullary pyramids

_____ 11. multicystic dysplastic kidney (MCDK)

_____ 12. nephroblastomatosis

_____ 13. neuroblastoma

_____ 14. polycystic renal disease

_____ 15. posterior urethral valves

_____ 16. Potter facies

_____ 17. prune-belly syndrome

_____ 18. pulmonary hypoplasia

_____ 19. renal vein thrombosis

_____ 20. ureteropelvic junction obstruction

_____ 21. VACTERL

_____ 22. VATER

_____ 23. Wilms' tumor (nephroblastoma)

A. Malignant adrenal mass seen in pediatric patients; hemorrhaging tumor consisting primarily of cells resembling neuroblasts
B. Dilation of the renal collecting system
C. Large and hypoechoic in the neonate
D. Poorly functioning enlarged kidneys
E. Most common benign renal tumor of the neonate and infant
F. Underdevelopment of the lung tissue that occurs in utero secondary to oligohydramnios
G. Classification of cystic renal disease
H. Abnormal persistence of fetal renal blastoma
I. Most common neonatal obstruction of the urinary tract; results from intrinsic narrowing or extrinsic vascular compression
J. Lie at the base of the medullary pyramids and appear as echogenic structures
K. Congenital polycystic kidney disease that usually presents during middle age; the severity of the disease varies widely
L. Adds cardiac and limb anomalies to the VATER syndrome
M. Most common malignant tumor in the neonate and infant
N. Dilation of any tubular vessel
O. Kidney becomes enlarged and edematous as a result of obstruction of the renal vein
P. Ectopic insertion and cystic dilation of distal ureter of duplicated renal collecting system
Q. Most common cause of bladder outlet obstruction in the male neonate
R. Occurs when the fetus is stressed during a difficult delivery or a hypoxic insult
S. Vertebral, anal, tracheoesophageal fistula and renal anomalies
T. Most common cause of renal cystic disease in the neonate; multiple cystic masses within the kidney; may have contralateral ureteral pelvic junction obstruction
U. Dilation of the fetal abdomen secondary to severe bilateral hydronephrosis and fetal ascites; fetus also has oligohydramnios and pulmonary hypoplasia
V. Outer rim of the kidney; in the neonate it has an echogenicity similar to that of the normal liver parenchyma
W. Rare, congenital polycystic renal disease; typically occurs with diffuse enlargement, sacculations, and cystic diverticula of the medullary portions of the kidneys

Exercise 2

Fill in the blank(s) with the word(s) that best completes the statements about the neonatal and pediatric kidneys and adrenal glands.

1. In the second trimester, the kidney develops from small _____ composed of a central large pyramid with a thin peripheral rim of cortex.

2. As the renunculi fuse progressively, their adjoining cortices form a(n) _____.

3. The former renunculi are at that point called _____.

4. The renal cortex continues to grow throughout childhood, whereas the renal _____ become smaller in size.

5. The larger amount of cortical _____ is not present in the neonate and pediatric patient, which allows clear distinction of the corticomedullary junction.

6. The medullary _____ are large and hypoechoic and should not be mistaken for dilated calyces or cysts.

7. The surrounding cortex is quite thin, with echogenicity essentially similar to or slightly greater than that of normal _____ parenchyma.

8. The _____ vessels are seen as intense specular echoes at the corticomedullary junction.

9. At the site of the fetal lobulation, a parenchymal triangular defect may be identified in the anterosuperior

   or inferoposterior aspect of the kidney, known as a(n) _____ parenchymal defect.

10. Each adrenal gland lies immediately _____ to the upper pole of the kidney.

PATHOLOGY

Exercise 3

Fill in the blank(s) with the word(s) that best completes the statements about the pathology of the neonatal and pediatric kidney and adrenal gland.

1. The dilatation of the urinary collecting system is known as _____.

2. The most common type of obstruction of the upper urinary tract is _____; it most often results from intrinsic narrowing or extrinsic vascular compression at the level of the ureteropelvic junction.

3. The obstruction produces _____ (proximal or distal) dilatation of the collecting system; the ureter is normal in caliber.

4. The most common cause of bladder outlet obstruction in the male neonate is _____ urethral valves.

5. Urinary _____ or a perirenal urinoma can result from high-pressure vesicoureteral reflux rupturing

   a calyceal fornix or tearing the renal parenchyma.

6. The ectopic _____ is seen as a fluid mass within the urinary bladder and is located inferomedially to the ureteral insertion of the lower pole ureter.

7. The triad of hypoplasia, or deficiency, of the abdominal musculature, cryptorchidism, and urinary tract anomalies

   is known as the _____ syndrome.

8. The most common cause of renal cystic disease presenting in the neonate is _____ dysplastic kidney, and when hydronephrosis is excluded, it is the most common cause of an abdominal mass in the newborn.

9. Sonographically, the classic appearance of MCDK is of a unilateral mass resembling a bunch of grapes, which

   represents a cluster of discrete _____ cysts, the largest of which are peripheral.

10. The kidneys are hyperechoic and greatly enlarged with a hypoechogenic outer rim, which represents the cortex

    compressed by the expanded pyramids in autosomal _____ polycystic kidney disease.

11. The most common intra-abdominal malignant renal tumor is _____ tumor in young children.

12. A(n) _____ is a malignant tumor that arises in sympathetic chain ganglia and adrenal medulla; it may be detected on antenatal sonography or at birth.

13. About half of neuroblastoma tumors arise in the medulla of the _____ gland, although tumors have also been found in the neck, mediastinum, retroperitoneum, and pelvis.

14. Sonographically, adrenal _____ results in ovoid enlargement of the gland or a portion of the gland.

Exercise 4

Provide a short answer for each question after evaluating the images.

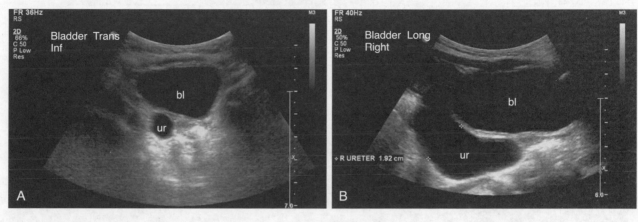

1. Describe the findings in this 28-day-old infant.

_____

_____

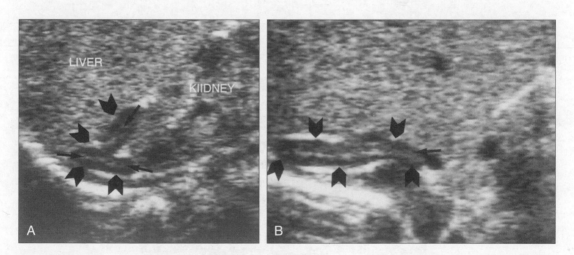

2. What anatomic structure are the arrows pointing to?

_____

_____

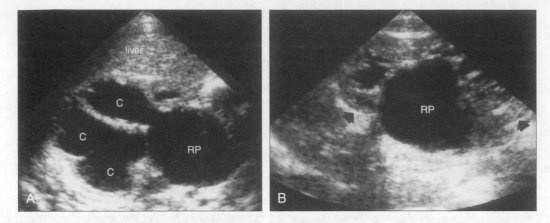

3. Identify whether this obstruction to the kidney is minor or major.

_____

_____

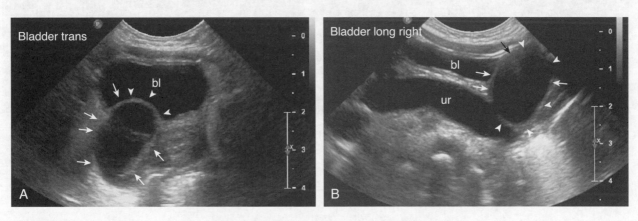

4. Identify the abnormality demonstrated in these views of the neonatal pelvis.

_____

_____

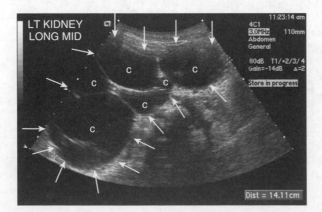

5. Does this neonate show sonographic evidence of hydronephrosis or of multicystic dysplastic kidney disease?

_____

_____

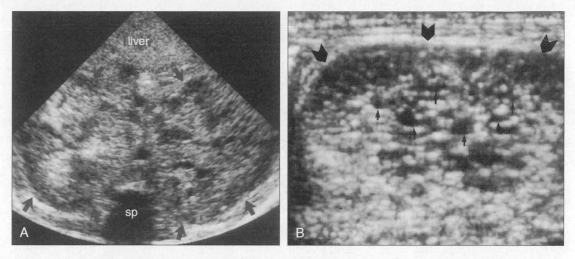

6. This neonate had abdominal distention at 1 day after birth. Describe the appearance of the kidneys.

_____

_____

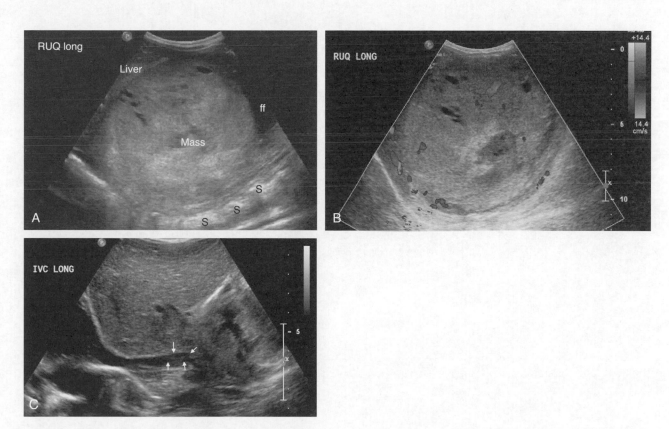

7. A 2-year-old with a palpable abdominal mass, nausea and vomiting, and appetite loss was imaged with ultrasound. Describe the sonographic findings.

_____

_____

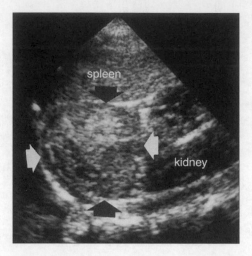

8. A 2-week-old male neonate with a history of neonatal infections, increased bilirubin, and an abdominal mass had an ultrasound. Describe the sonographic findings.

_____

_____

27 Neonatal Echoencephalography

KEY TERMS

Exercise 1

Match the following embryology and anatomy terms with their definitions.

_____ 1. neonate

_____ 2. atrium (trigone) of the lateral ventricles

_____ 3. brain stem

_____ 4. caudate nucleus

_____ 5. cavum septum pellucidum

_____ 6. cerebellum

_____ 7. cerebrum

_____ 8. choroid plexus

_____ 9. cistern

_____ 10. corpus callosum

_____ 11. falx cerebri

_____ 12. fontanelle

_____ 13. germinal matrix

_____ 14. meninges

_____ 15. sulcus

_____ 16. tentorium cerebelli

_____ 17. thalamic-caudate groove

_____ 18. thalamus

A. Echogenic cluster of cells important in the production of cerebrospinal fluid that lies along the atrium of the lateral ventricles

B. Three membranes enclosing the brain and spinal cord

C. Echogenic fibrous structure that separates the cerebral hemispheres

D. Part of the brain connecting the forebrain and spinal cord; consists of the midbrain, pons, and medulla oblongata

E. Prominent structure best seen in the midline filled with cerebrospinal fluid in the premature infant

F. The region at which the thalamus and caudate nucleus join

G. Largest part of the brain consisting of two equal hemispheres

H. Prominent group of nerve fibers that connect the right and left sides of the brain

I. Infant during the early newborn period

J. Fragile periventricular tissue that bleeds easily in the premature infant; includes the caudate nucleus

K. Area of the brain that forms the lateral borders of the anterior horns, anterior to the thalamus

L. Echogenic V-shaped "tent" structure in the posterior fossa that separates the cerebellum from the cerebrum

M. Area of the brain that lies posterior to the brain stem below the tentorium

N. Two ovoid brain structures located midbrain, situated on either side of the third ventricle superior to the brain stem

O. The ventricle is measured at this site on the axial view; anterior, occipital, and temporal horn junction

P. Groove on the surface of the brain that separates the gyri

Q. Soft space between the bones

R. Reservoir for cerebrospinal fluid

Exercise 2

Match the following terms related to pathology and sonographic evaluation with their definitions.

_____ 1. aqueductal stenosis

_____ 2. asphyxia

_____ 3. axial plane

_____ 4. Chiari malformation

_____ 5. coronal plane

_____ 6. Dandy-Walker malformation

_____ 7. extracorporeal membrane oxygenation

_____ 8. holoprosencephaly

A. Transducer is placed above the ear (above the canthomeatal line)

B. Ventriculomegaly in the neonate resulting in compression and often destruction of brain tissue

C. Abnormal development of the fourth ventricle; often accompanied by hydrocephalus

D. Severe case of inadequate oxygenation

E. Echogenic white matter necrosis best seen in the posterior aspect of the brain or adjacent to the ventricular structures

F. Congenital defect characterized by abnormal single ventricular cavity with some form of thalami fusion

G. Congenital blockage of the aqueduct connecting the third and fourth ventricles causing dilation of the third and fourth ventricles

H. Treatment for infants with severe respiratory failure who have not responded to conventional ventilatory support

175

_____ 9. hydrocephalus

_____ 10. hypoxia

_____ 11. periventricular leukomalacia

_____ 12. sagittal plane

_____ 13. subependyma

_____ 14. subependymal cyst

_____ 15. ventriculitis

I. Perpendicular to the coronal plane with the transducer in the anterior fontanelle

J. Transducer is perpendicular to the anterior fontanelle in the coronal axis of the head

K. Site of hemorrhage for the germinal matrix; fragile area beneath the ependyma that is subject to bleeding in the premature neonate

L. Congenital defect in which the cerebellum and brain stem are pulled toward the spinal cord (banana sign)

M. Decreased oxygen in the body

N. Inflammation/infection of the ventricles, which appears as echogenic linear structures along the gyri

O. Cyst that occurs at the site of a previous bleed in the germinal matrix

ANATOMY AND PHYSIOLOGY

Exercise 3

Label the following illustrations.

A. Neonatal skull showing the sutures and open anterior fontanelle.

1._____

2._____

3._____

4._____

5._____

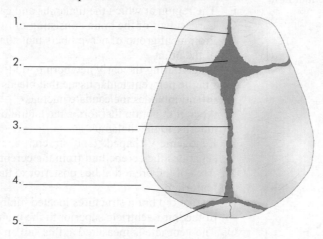

B. Sagittal view of the ventricular system.

1._____

8._____

7._____

6._____

5._____

2._____

3._____

4._____

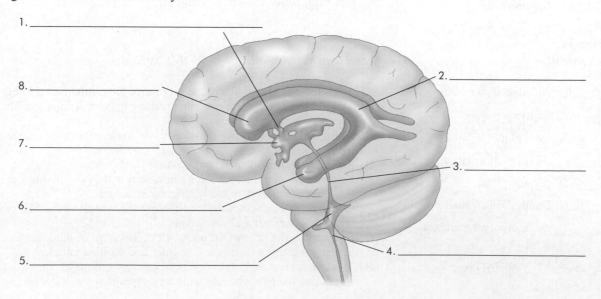

C. Sagittal view of choroid plexus and cisterns of the ventricular system.

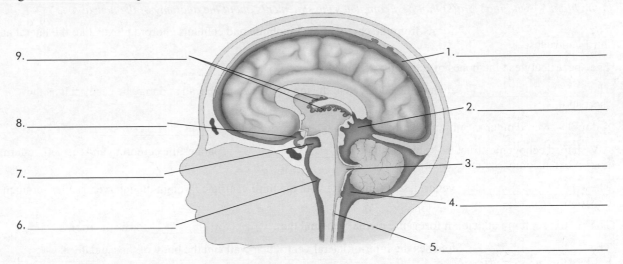

9. _____

8. _____

7. _____

6. _____

1. _____

2. _____

3. _____

4. _____

5. _____

D. Coronal view of cerebral lobes, corpus callosum, and sylvian fissure.

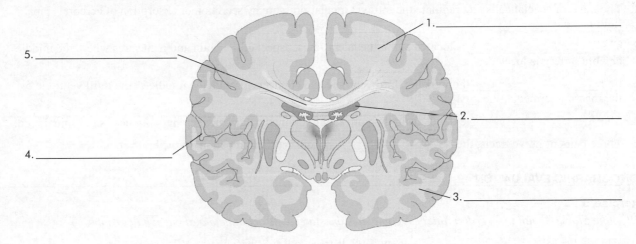

5. _____

4. _____

1. _____

2. _____

3. _____

177

Exercise 4

Fill in the blank(s) with the word(s) that best completes the statements about the anatomy of the neural axis.

1. The _____ forms from the cavity of the hindbrain and contains choroid plexus like the lateral and third ventricles.

2. The spaces between the bones of the skull are called _____.

3. The _____ fontanelle is located at the top of the neonatal head and may be easily felt as the "soft spot."

4. A double-layered outer membrane that forms the toughest barrier is the _____.

5. A V-shaped echogenic structure known as the _____ separates the cerebrum and the cerebellum; it is an extension of the falx cerebri.

6. The _____ ventricles communicate with the third ventricle through the interventricular foramen of Monro.

7. The cavum septum pellucidum forms the medial wall and the _____ forms the roof.

8. The _____ touches the inferior lateral ventricular wall and the body of the caudate _____ borders the superior wall.

9. The third and fourth ventricles are connected by the _____.

10. The lateral angles of the fourth ventricle form the foramen of _____.

11. The mass of special cells that regulate the intraventricular pressure by secretion or absorption of cerebral spinal fluid is the _____.

12. The _____ is located along the lateral-most aspect of the brain and is the area where the middle cerebral artery is located.

13. The _____ borders the third ventricle and connects through the middle of the third ventricle by the massa intermedia.

14. The _____ extends from the pons to the foramen magnum where it continues as the spinal cord.

15. Three pairs of nerve tracts, the _____, connect the cerebellum to the brain stem.

SONOGRAPHIC EVALUATION

Exercise 5

Fill in the blank(s) with the word(s) that best completes the statements about neonatal encephalography.

1. Technically a(n) _____ view is 90 degrees to Reid's baseline.

2. When the transducer is angled _____, the frontal horns of the lateral ventricles appear as slitlike hypoechoic to cystic formations.

3. As the transducer is angled _____, the ventricles acquire a comma-like shape.

4. Sonography depicts the choroid plexus as a very _____ structure inside the ventricular cavities surrounding the thalamic nuclei.

5. In premature infants, the caudate nuclei may have _____ echogenicity than the rest of the brain parenchyma.

6. The _____ ventricle appears in the midline as a small anechoic space approximately 2 to 3 mm wide, located anteriorly to the vermis.

Exercise 6

Fill in the blank(s) with the word(s) or provide a short answer that best completes the statements about the pathology of the neonatal head.

1. A congenital anomaly associated with spina bifida is a(n) _____ malformation in which the cerebellum and brain stem are pulled toward the spinal cord and secondary hydrocephalus develops.

2. Chiari malformation is frequently associated with myelomeningocele, _____, dilation of the third ventricle, and absence of the septum pellucidum.

3. _____ is characterized by a grossly abnormal brain in which there is a common large central ventricle.

4. Dandy-Walker syndrome is a congenital anomaly in which a huge _____ ventricle cyst occupies the area where the cerebellum usually lies, with secondary dilation of the third and lateral ventricles.

5. A Dandy-Walker variant is present when there is an enlarged _____ communicating with the fourth ventricle in the presence of a normal or hypoplastic cerebellar vermis.

6. Complete absence of the _____ is distinguished by narrow frontal horns, as well as marked separation of the anterior horns and bodies of the lateral ventricles associated with widening of the occipital horns and the third ventricle.

7. Any condition in which enlargement of the ventricular system is caused by an imbalance between production and reabsorption of cerebrospinal fluid (CSF) is referred to as _____.

8. The CSF pathways are open within the ventricular system in _____ hydrocephalus, but there is decreased absorption of CSF.

9. The most common cause of congenital hydrocephalus is _____.

10. The most common hemorrhagic lesions in preterm newborn infants are _____-_____ hemorrhages.

11. Subependymal hemorrhages (SEHs) are caused by capillary bleeding in the _____.

12. Studies from the anterior fontanelle may not detect small IVHs, because intraventricular blood tends to "settle out" in the _____ horns.

13. Intraparenchymal hemorrhages appear as very _____ zones in the white matter adjacent to the lateral ventricles.

14. _____ can result from a variety of insults including respiratory failure, congenital heart disease, and sepsis.

15. White matter ischemia leads to white matter volume loss or _____ leukomalacia.

16. The chronic stage of WMN is identified with ultrasound when _____ develop in the echogenic white matter.

17. A common complication of purulent meningitis in newborn infants is _____.

18. _____ occurs when the ependyma becomes thickened and hyperechoic as a result of irritation from hemorrhage within the ventricle.

Provide a short answer for each question after evaluating the images.

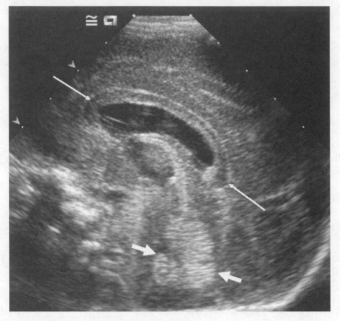

1. What structure is the arrow pointing to in this sagittal image?

_____

_____

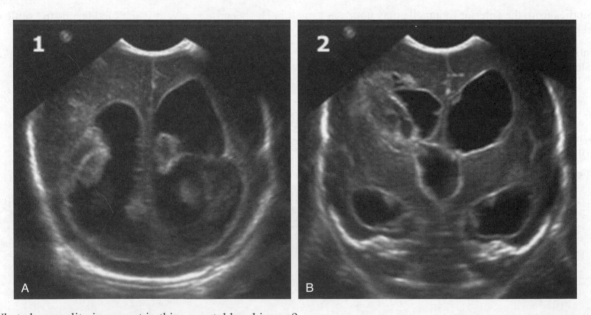

2. What abnormality is present in this neonatal head image?

_____

_____

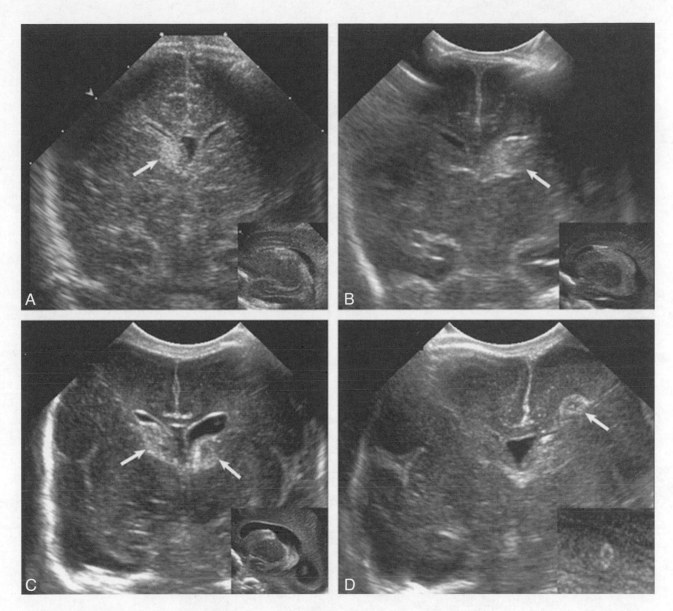

3. Describe the abnormality in this newborn infant on ECMO.

_____

_____

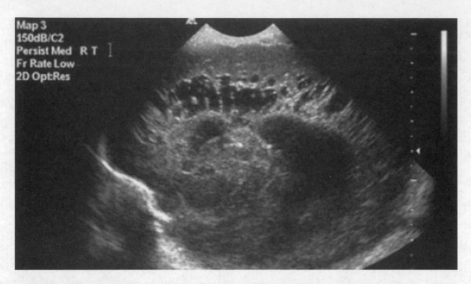

4. This sonographic image is typical of what abnormality of the premature neonatal head?

_____

_____

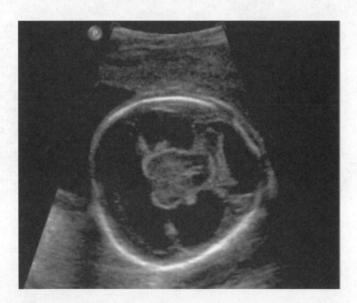

5. Identify the abnormality in this neonatal head ultrasound.

_____

_____

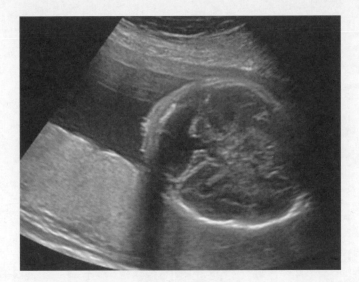

6. Identify the abnormality.

_____

_____

28 The Neonatal Hip

KEY TERMS

Exercise 1

Match the following anatomy terms with their definitions.

_____ 1. fascia lata

_____ 2. femoral triangle

_____ 3. hip joint

_____ 4. pelvic girdle

_____ 5. saphenous opening

_____ 6. sciatic nerve

A. Formed by the articulation of the head of the femur with the acetabulum of the hip bone
B. Deep fascia of the thigh
C. Largest nerve in the upper thigh
D. Formation of the hip bones by the ilium, ischium, and pubis
E. Description of a region at the front of the upper thigh, just below the inguinal ligament
F. Gap in the fascia lata, which is found 4 cm inferior and lateral to the pubic tubercle

Exercise 2

Match the following sonographic evaluation and pathology terms with their definitions.

_____ 1. Barlow maneuver

_____ 2. developmental displacement of the hip (DDH)

_____ 3. frank dislocation

_____ 4. Galeazzi sign

_____ 5. Ortolani maneuver

_____ 6. subluxation

A. The hip is laterally and posteriorly displaced to the extent that the femoral head has no contact with the acetabulum and the normal "U" configuration cannot be obtained on ultrasound.
B. The patient lies in the supine position. The examiner's hand is placed around the hip to be examined with the fingers over the femoral head. The hip is flexed 90 degrees, and the thigh is abducted.
C. On physical exam, the knee is lower in position on the affected side of the neonate with DDH when the patient is supine and the knees are flexed.
D. The patient lies in the supine position with the hip flexed 90 degrees and adducted. Downward and outward pressure is applied. If the hip is dislocated, the examiner will feel the femoral head move out of the acetabulum.
E. This occurs when the femoral head moves posteriorly and remains in contact with the posterior aspect of the acetabulum.
F. This abnormal condition of the hip results in congenital hip dysplasia; includes dysplastic, subluxated, dislocatable, and dislocated hips.

Exercise 3

Label the following illustrations.

A. Coronal section of the right hip joint and articular surfaces of the right hip joint.

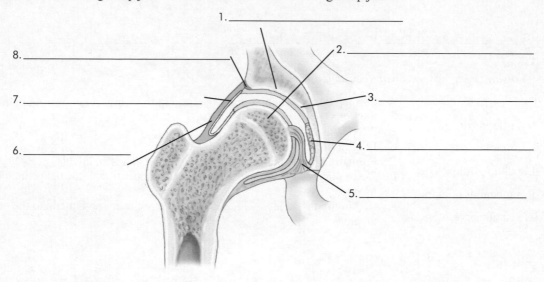

B. Coronal section of the right hip joint and arterial supply of the head of the femur.

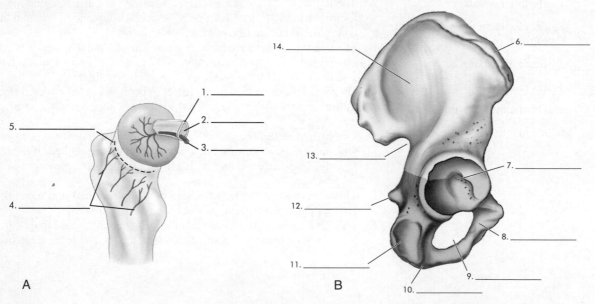

A

B

Exercise 4

Fill in the blank(s) with the word(s) that best completes the statements about the anatomy of the neonatal hip.

1. The _____ joints unite the two hip bones with the sacral part of the vertebral column.

2. The hip bones are the fusion of three separate bones, the _____, the _____, and the _____, which together form the pelvic girdle.

3. The bone of the upper thigh is the _____.

4. The femoral artery branches into the _____ femoris artery, which is the main artery supply for the thigh muscles.

5. The largest nerve in the upper thigh is the _____ nerve.

6. The deep fascia of the thigh, the _____, forms a tough connective tissue surrounding the muscles.

7. The _____ triangle is formed by the inguinal ligament, the adductor longus (medially), and the sartorius (laterally).

8. The contents of the femoral triangle include the femoral canal, the femoral _____ and _____, and the femoral nerve.

9. The femoral vein and artery and the femoral canal are enclosed in a connective tissue sleeve called the femoral _____.

10. The contents of the femoral triangle are separated from the more deeply lying hip joint by muscles; the _____ is medial, and the _____ is lateral.

11. The articulation of the head of the femur with the acetabulum of the hip bone forms the _____.

12. The gluteus _____ muscle is the immediate cover for the upper part of the hip joint, whereas the obturator externus is found winding below it from front to back.

13. The _____ muscle is immediately posterior to the joint, and the obturator internus and the gemelli and quadratus femoris are lower down.

14. The rounded shape of the femur and the cup shape of the _____ form the "ball and socket" hip joint.

15. One of the strongest ligaments in the body is the _____ ligament; it is very important for standing and maintaining correct upright balance.

MOVEMENTS OF THE HIP

Exercise 5

Match the following terms regarding movements of the hip with their definitions.

_____ 1. flexion

_____ 2. extension

_____ 3. abduction

_____ 4. adduction

_____ 5. medial rotation

_____ 6. lateral rotation

A. To move away from the body
B. Turning inward
C. Bending forward
D. Turning outward
E. Bending backward
F. To move toward the body

Exercise 6

Fill in the blank(s) with the word(s) that best completes the statements about the movement of the hip.

1. The primary flexors of the hip are the _____ major, the _____, and the _____ femoris.

2. When the trochanter moves forward, the femur rotates _____, and when the trochanter moves backward, the femur rotates _____.

3. The medial rotators are the anterior fibers of gluteus _____ and _____.

4. The lateral rotators are the small muscles at the back of the joint: _____, _____ internus, and quadratus femoris, with assistance of the gluteus maximus.

SONOGRAPHIC EVALUATION

Exercise 7

Fill in the blank(s) with the word(s) that best completes the statements or provide a short answer about the sonographic evaluation of the neonatal hip.

1. Ossification of the femoral head begins between _____ and _____ months of age, occurs earlier in girls than boys, and is often complete by 1 year.

2. Sonography of the neonatal hip is performed with a(n)_____ transducer.

3. Sonographically, the femoral head is _____ because it is cartilaginous and contains a focal echogenic ossification nucleus.

4. The femoral head sits within the acetabulum, which is _____ and has a deep concave configuration.

5. Two-thirds of the head should be covered by the _____.

6. The _____ view is performed with the infant in the supine position from the lateral aspect of the hip joint with the plane of the transducer oriented coronally with respect to the hip joint.

7. The transducer is maintained in the lateral position while the hip is moved into a 90-degree angle of flexion in the _____ view. During this assessment, the transducer is moved in an anteroposterior direction with respect to the body to allow visualization of the entire hip.

8. A normal hip gives the appearance of a "ball on a spoon" in the midacetabulum. The _____ is the ball, the _____ forms the spoon, and the iliac line is the handle.

9. The transverse plane is rotated 90 degrees and moved posteriorly into a posterolateral position over the hip joint in the _____ view.

10. From the transverse or flexion view, the leg is brought down into a neutral position to the _____ view.

PATHOLOGY

Exercise 8

Fill in the blank(s) with the word(s) that best completes the statements or provide a short answer about the pathology of the neonatal hip.

1. _____ causes of hip dislocation can be traumatic or nontraumatic (i.e., neuromuscular diseases).

2. _____ dislocations occur in utero and are associated with neuromuscular disorders.

3. _____ of the hip includes dysplastic, subluxated, dislocatable, and dislocated hips.

Provide a short answer for each question after evaluating the images.

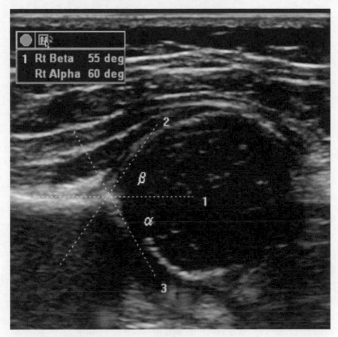

1. Is this neonatal hip image normal or abnormal ?

_____

_____

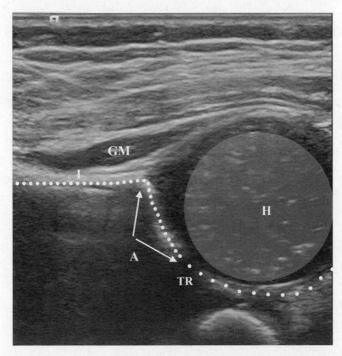

2. Name the normal "_____" appearance seen in this coronal/flexion view.

_____

_____

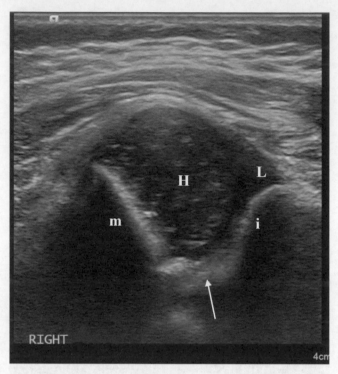

3. This transverse view without any added stress is the normal "_____" shape.

_____

_____

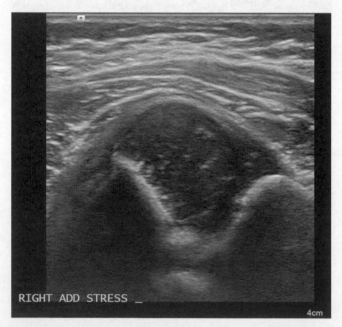

4. With stress added in the transverse view, this demonstrates the "_____" shape.

_____

_____

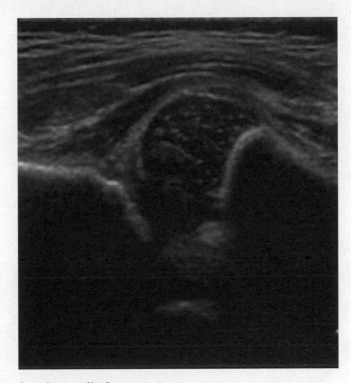

5. This image demonstrates what abnormality?

_____

_____

29 Neonatal and Infant Spine

KEY TERMS

Exercise 1

Match the following neonatal spine anatomy and pathology terms with their definitions.

_____ 1. cauda equine

_____ 2. conus medullaris

_____ 3. diastematomyelia

_____ 4. dysraphic

_____ 5. filum terminale

_____ 6. hydromyelia

_____ 7. lipoma

_____ 8. meningocele

_____ 9. myelomeningocele

_____ 10. myeloschisis

_____ 11. spina bifida aperta

_____ 12. spina bifida occulta

_____ 13. tethered spinal cord

A. Protrusion of the meninges through the gap in the spine, the skin covering being vestigial

B. Bundle of nerve roots from the lumbar, sacral, and coccygeal spinal nerves that descend nearly vertically from the spinal cord until they reach their respective openings in the vertebral column

C. Slender tapering terminal section of the spinal cord

D. Caudal end of the spinal cord

E. Fixed spinal cord that is in an abnormal position

F. Congenital fissure of the spinal cord, frequently associated with spina bifida cystica

G. Open (non-skin-covered lesions) neural tube defects, such as myelomeningocele and meningocele

H. Dilation of the central canal of the spinal cord

I. Describes anomalies associated with incomplete embryologic development

J. Closed (skin-covered lesions) neural tube defects, such as spinal lipoma and tethered cord

K. Cleft spinal cord resulting from failure of the neural tube to close

L. Spinal cord and nerve roots are exposed, often adhering to the fine membrane that overlies them

M. Common benign tumor composed of fat cells

Exercise 2

Label the following illustrations.

A. Basic features of the vertebrae.

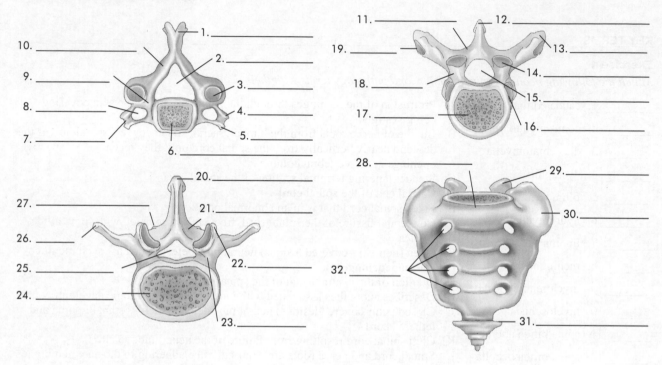

10. _____
9. _____
8. _____
7. _____
1. _____
2. _____
3. _____
4. _____
5. _____
6. _____

11. _____
19. _____
18. _____
17. _____
12. _____
13. _____
14. _____
15. _____
16. _____

20. _____
27. _____
26. _____
25. _____
24. _____
21. _____
22. _____
23. _____

28. _____
29. _____
30. _____
32. _____
31. _____

B. Longitudinal section through the sacrum.

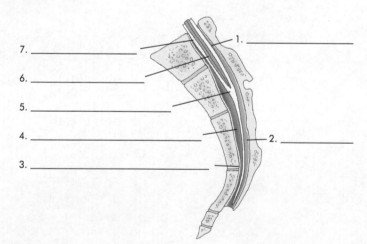

7. _____
6. _____
5. _____
4. _____
3. _____
1. _____
2. _____

C. Third lumbar vertebrae showing relationship between the intervertebral disk and cauda equina.

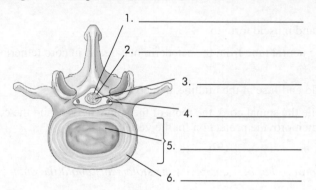

1. _____

2. _____

3. _____

4. _____

5. _____

6. _____

D. Section through the thoracic part of the spinal cord showing the anterior and posterior roots of the spinal nerves and meninges.

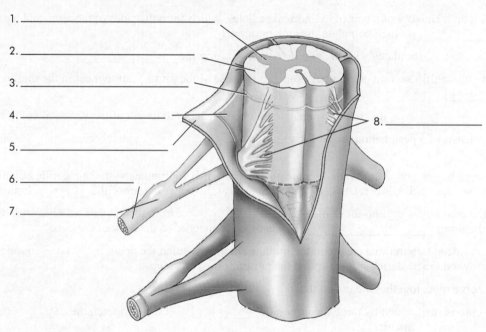

1. _____

2. _____

3. _____

4. _____

5. _____

6. _____

7. _____

8. _____

ANATOMY AND PATHOLOGY

Exercise 3

Fill in the blank(s) with the word(s) that best completes the statements about the anatomy and pathology of the neonatal spine.

1. One of the clinical signs of a spinal problem in an infant is a(n) _____ on the posterior surface of the body along the spinal canal.

2. Other suspicious findings that an abnormality may be present include a(n) _____, a raised midline area, a(n) _____ patch, or even a tail-like projection from the lower spine.

3. A dimple is suspicious if it is of greater than _____ from the anus.

4. Spinal _____ includes disorders of the spine involving absent or incomplete closure of the neural tube.

5. The defects of the spinal canal occur in the first _____ weeks of life as the fetal nervous system develops.

6. The bony spine, meninges, and muscle form the _____.

7. Incomplete separation of the neural tube from the ectoderm may result in cord tethering, _____, or a dermal sinus.

8. If the neural tube fails to fold and fuse in the midline, defects, such as _____, occur.

9. Within the vertebral cavity lie the spinal cord, the roots of the spinal nerves, and the covering _____, which provide protection for the vertebral column.

Exercise 4

Fill in the blank(s) with the word(s) that best completes the statements about the anatomy of the vertebral column and spinal cord.

1. Each vertebra consists of a rounded body _____ and a vertebral arch posteriorly.

2. The vertebrae enclose a space called the vertebral _____, through which run the spinal cord and its coverings.

3. The vertebral arch consists of a pair of cylindrical pedicles, which form the sides of the arch, and a pair of flattened _____, which complete the arch posteriorly.

4. Laterally the sacrum articulates with the two iliac bones to form the _____ joints.

5. The laminae of the fifth sacral vertebra (and sometimes those of the fourth) fail to meet in the midline, forming the sacral _____.

6. The _____ disks are responsible for one fourth of the length of the vertebral column.

7. Each disk consists of a peripheral part, the *annulus* _____, and a central part, the *nucleus* _____.

8. The spinal cord begins above at the foramen magnum, where it is continuous with the medulla oblongata of the brain. In the younger child, it is relatively longer and ends at the upper border of the _____ lumbar vertebra.

9. Inferiorly the cord tapers off into the conus _____, from the apex of which a prolongation of the pia mater, the filum _____, descends to be attached to the back of the coccyx.

10. The cord has a deep longitudinal fissure in the midline anteriorly called the anterior _____ fissure, and a shallow furrow on the posterior surface called the posterior median sulcus.

11. The lower nerve roots together are called the _____.

12. The spinal cord is surrounded by three meninges: the _____ mater, the _____ mater, and the _____ mater.

13. The most external membrane is the _____ mater and is a dense, strong, fibrous sheet that encloses the spinal cord and cauda equina.

14. The _____ mater is a delicate impermeable membrane covering the spinal cord and lying between the pia mater internally and the dura mater externally.

15. The vascular membrane that closely covers the spinal cord is the _____ mater; below it fuses with the filum terminale.

Exercise 5

Fill in the blank(s) with the word(s) that best completes the statements about the anatomy and pathology of the spinal cord.

1. The spinal cord is _____ with slightly echogenic borders and an echogenic line extending longitudinally along its midline.

2. This central echo complex represents or is close to the cord's central _____.

3. The spinal cord and roots of the cauda equina are normally observed to _____ with the frequency of the heartbeat, and there is also a superimposed motion that occurs with respirations.

4. The _____ spinal cord is a pathologic fixation of the spinal cord in an abnormal caudal location so that the cord suffers mechanical stretching, distortion, and ischemia with daily activities, growth, and development.

5. In addition to being in a more caudal location, the tethered spinal cord is often fixed _____ within the canal.

6. Lipomas are usually _____ and may present as a small or large mass.

7. A(n) _____ shows a flat nontubulated cord (neural placode) with nerve roots extending into the defect.

8. In contrast, a(n) _____ shows nothing but fluid within the sac.

9. _____ seem to have a high association with tethered spinal cord.

Exercise 6

Provide a short answer for each question after evaluating the images.

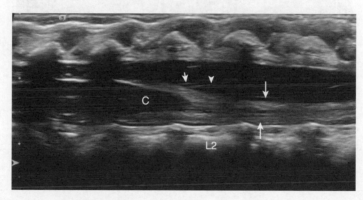

1. Identify the structure the arrows are pointing to on this image.

_____

_____

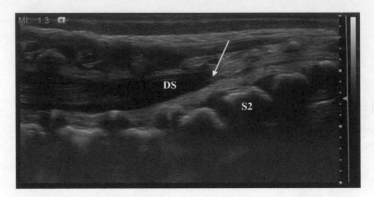

2. Identify the structures lettered on this sagittal image.

_____

_____

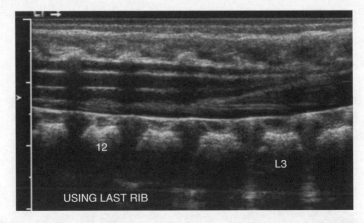

3. A neonate presented with fatty mass near the lower back with increased areas of pigmentation. Describe the sonographic finding.

_____

_____

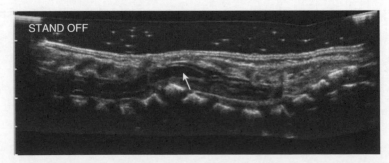

4. What abnormality of the neonatal spine is demonstrated in this image?

_____

_____

KEY TERMS

Exercise 1

Match the following heart and cardiac cycle terms with their definitions.

_____ 1. atrioventricular valves

_____ 2. endocardium

_____ 3. epicardium

_____ 4. myocardium

_____ 5. pericardium

_____ 6. semilunar valves

A. Outer layer of the heart wall
B. Inner layer of the heart wall
C. Sac surrounding the heart, reflecting off the great arteries
D. Valves located between the atria and ventricles
E. Thick, contractile middle layer of the heart
F. Valves located in the aortic or pulmonic artery

Exercise 2

Match the following electrical conduction system and auscultation terms with their definitions.

_____ 1. continuous murmur

_____ 2. depolarization

_____ 3. diastolic murmur

_____ 4. electrocardiography

_____ 5. frequency

_____ 6. intensity

_____ 7. murmur

_____ 8. repolarization

_____ 9. systolic murmur

A. The predominant frequency band of the murmur, which varies from high to low as determined by auscultation
B. Method of recording the electrical activity generated by the heart muscle
C. Heart murmur that begins with or after the time of the first heart sound and ends at or before the time of the second heart sound
D. Describes the electrical activity that triggers contraction of the heart muscle
E. A relatively prolonged series of auditory vibrations of varying intensity (loudness), frequency (pitch), quality, configuration, and duration; produced by structural changes and/or hemodynamic events in the heart or blood vessels
F. Heart murmur that begins with or after the time of the second heart sound and ends at or before the time of the first heart sound
G. Describes electrical activity just before the relaxation phase of cardiac muscle activity
H. Heart murmur that begins in systole and continues without interruption through the time of the second heart sound into all or part of diastole
I. A grading scale of 1 to 6 describes this aspect of systolic and diastolic murmurs

Exercise 3

Label the following illustrations.

A. Anterior view of the right ventricle.

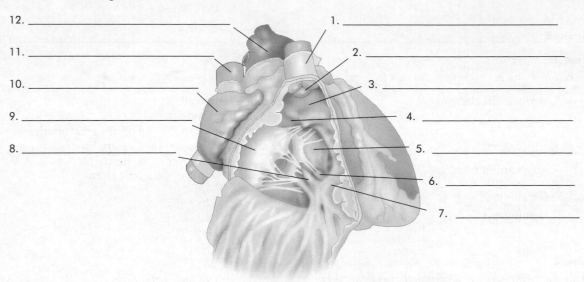

12. _____

11. _____

10. _____

9. _____

8. _____

1. _____

2. _____

3. _____

4. _____

5. _____

6. _____

7. _____

B. Right atrium viewed from the right side.

12. _____

11. _____

10. _____

9. _____

8. _____

7. _____

6. _____

1. _____

2. _____

3. _____

4. _____

5. _____

C. Tricuspid valve.

1. _____
12. _____
11. _____
10. _____
9. _____

2. _____
3. _____
4. _____
5. _____

8. _____
7. _____
6. _____

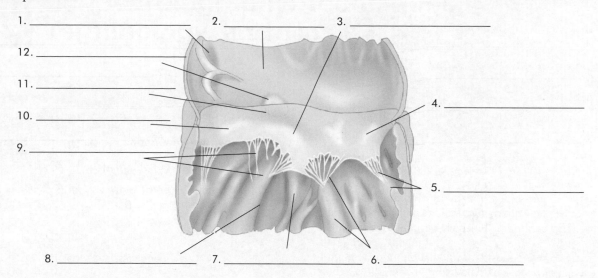

D. Posterolateral view of the left atrium and ventricle.

1. _____
12. _____
11. _____

2. _____
3. _____
4. _____
5. _____
6. _____
7. _____

10. _____

9. _____
8. _____

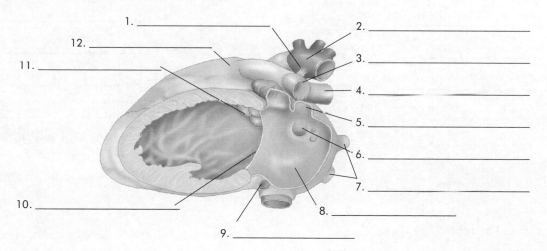

Chapter **30** **Anatomic and Physiologic Relationships Within the Thoracic Cavity**

E. Mitral valve.

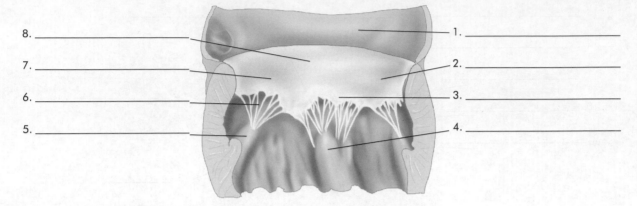

8. _____

7. _____

6. _____

5. _____

1. _____

2. _____

3. _____

4. _____

F. Aortic valve.

1. _____

2. _____

10. _____

9. _____

8. _____

3. _____

4. _____

5. _____

6. _____

7. _____

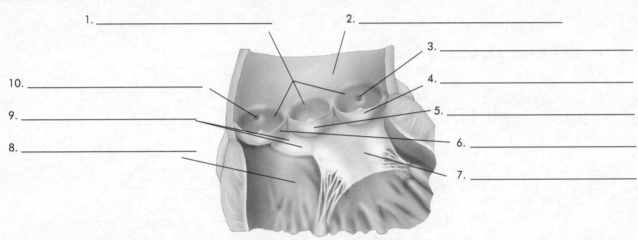

G. Aortic arch and branches.

13. _____

12. _____

11. _____

10. _____

9. _____

8. _____

1. _____

2. _____

3. _____

4. _____

5. _____

6. _____

7. _____

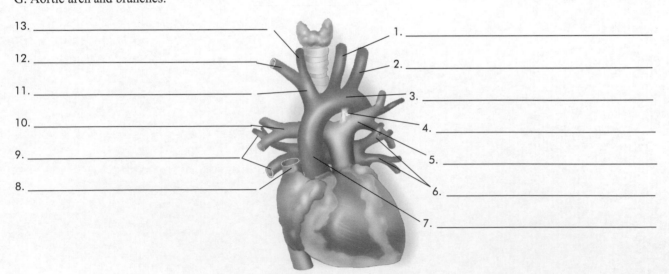

Exercise 4

Match the following landmarks of the thorax with their locations.

_____ 1. midaxillary line

_____ 2. sternal angle

_____ 3. costal margin

_____ 4. midsternal line

_____ 5. xiphoid

_____ 6. suprasternal notch

_____ 7. midclavicular line

_____ 8. xiphisternal joint

A. Lies in the median plane over the sternum
B. Superior margin of the manubrium sterni; lies opposite the lower border of the body of the second thoracic vertebra
C. Angle between the manubrium and the body of the sternum; also known as the angle of Louis
D. Junction between the xiphoid and the sternum
E. Runs vertically from a point midway between the anterior and posterior axillary folds
F. Vertical line from the midpoint of the clavicle
G. Lower boundary of the thorax, formed by the cartilages of the seventh through tenth ribs and the ends of the eleventh and twelfth cartilages
H. Lowest point of the sternum

Exercise 5

Fill in the blank(s) with the word(s) that best completes the statements about the anatomy of the cardiovascular system.

1. The cardiovascular system delivers _____ blood to tissues in the body and removes _____ products from these tissues.

2. The thoracic cavity lies within the thorax and is separated from the abdominal cavity by the _____.

3. The junction between the manubrium and the body of the sternum is a prominent ridge called the angle of _____.

4. The greater part of the thoracic cavity is occupied by two lungs that are enclosed by the _____ sac.

5. The pleural reflection between the costal and diaphragmatic portions of the parietal pleura is known as the _____ sinus.

6. The heart lies obliquely in the chest, posterior to the sternum, with the greater portion of its muscular mass lying slightly to the _____ of midline.

7. The right heart is located more _____ than its left-side chambers.

8. The right atrium is more _____ than the left atrium and lies to the right of the sternum.

9. The left atrium becomes the most _____ chamber to the left of the sternum.

10. The _____ layer lines the fibrous pericardium and is reflected around the roots of the great vessels to become continuous with the visceral layer of serous pericardium.

11. The slit between the parietal and visceral layers is the _____ cavity.

12. The intimal lining of the heart is the _____ and is continuous with the intima of the valvular structures connecting to it.

13. The muscular part of the heart is the _____.

14. The primary purpose of the atrium is to act as a _____ chamber that drives the blood into the ventricular cavity.

15. The left ventricle has the greatest muscle mass because it must pump blood to the entire body, whereas the right ventricle needs only enough pressure to pump the blood to the _____.

16. The _____ vena cava enters the upper posterior border and the _____ vena cava enters the lower posterolateral border of the right atrium.

17. The medial wall of the right atrium is formed by the _____ septum.

Chapter **30 Anatomic and Physiologic Relationships Within the Thoracic Cavity**

18. The _____ part of the membranous septum separates the right atrium and the left ventricle.

19. The inferior vena cava is guarded by a fold of tissue called the _____ valve, and the coronary sinus is guarded by the thebesian valve.

20. The _____ sinus drains the blood supply from the heart wall.

21. The valve that separates the right atrium from the right ventricle is the _____ valve.

22. The base of the right ventricle lies on the diaphragm, and the roof is occupied by the crista _____, which lies between the tricuspid and pulmonary orifices.

23. The outflow portion of the right ventricle, or _____, is smooth walled and contains few trabeculae.

24. The valve that separates the left atrium from the left ventricle is the _____ valve.

25. The functions of the _____tendinae are to prevent the opposing borders of the leaflets from inverting into the atrial cavity, to act as mainstays of the valves, and to form bands or foldlike structures that may contain muscle.

26. The smaller end of the ventricle represents the _____ of the heart, and the larger end, near the left atrium, is

called the _____ of the heart.

27. The _____ septum is located just inferior to the aortic root in the area of the left ventricular outflow tract.

28. The _____ arteries arise from the right and left coronary cusps.

Exercise 6
Fill in the blank(s) with the word(s) that best completes the statements about the cardiac cycle and conduction system of the heart.

1. The average normal heart beats in sinus rhythm at _____ beats per minute.

2. Forceful contraction of the cardiac chambers is _____, and the relaxed phase of the cycle is

_____.

3. Oxygenated blood returns from the lungs through the _____veins to enter the left atrium.

4. The _____ pressure in the ventricular cavity closes the atrioventricular valves.

5. The blood fills the sinuses of _____ and forces the cusps to close.

6. The _____ node initiates the normal cardiac impulse and is often called the pacemaker of the heart.

7. The _____ node is located in the right posterior portion of the interatrial septum.

8. Atrial contraction follows the _____ wave on ECG and generates the atrial systolic activity.

9. The impulse spreads via the Purkinje fibers to activate the ventricles, generating the _____ waves of the ECG.

10. The _____ wave represents ventricular repolarization.

11. The Frank _____ law of the heart states that the output of the heart increases in proportion to the degree of diastolic stretch of the muscle fibers.

12. The longer the initial resting length of the cardiac muscle, called _____, the greater the strength of contraction of the following beat.

13. The shortening velocity of cardiac muscle is inversely related to the _____.

Exercise 7

Fill in the blank(s) with the word(s) that best completes the statements about cardiac physiology.

1. When the blood moves in smooth layers, which slide against each other, this is known as _____ flow.

2. When blood cells move in different directions with varying velocities, this is known as _____ flow.

3. The flow dynamics depend on the fluid _____ and the momentum of molecules in the fluid.

4. The _____ flow velocity profile is such that as fluid moves through a tube, fluid layers in the center have a higher velocity than those on outer surfaces.

5. The _____ flow velocity profile states that as flow accelerates and converges, more fluid travels at velocities closer to peak velocity than layers in the center.

6. In _____, the ventricles eject blood into the aorta and pulmonary artery.

7. In _____, the ventricles fill with blood from the atria that flows to the body organs.

8. Blood flow through a constriction creates a _____ fluid pressure upstream from the constriction.

31 Hemodynamics

KEY TERMS

Exercise 1

Match the following heart and cardiac cycle terms with their definitions.

_____ 1. Afterload

_____ 2. Bernoulli Equation

_____ 3. Blood flow velocity profiles

_____ 4. Cardiac Output

_____ 5. Color Doppler

_____ 6. Continuous Wave Doppler

_____ 7. Continuity Principle

_____ 8. Doppler Effect

_____ 9. Frequency shift

_____ 10. Hemodynamics

_____ 11. Preload

_____ 12. Pressure

_____ 13. Pulsed Wave Doppler

_____ 14. Stroke Volume

_____ 15. Velocity

_____ 16. Volume

A. the product of stroke volume and heart rate

B. refers to a change in the frequency of waves (through sound, light etc.) that occurs as the source and observer change in motion relative to each other (away or toward)

C. measures the pressure gradient across the orifice using blood flow velocities. Three components are present: convective acceleration, flow acceleration, and viscous friction

D. the exertion of force upon a surface by an object, fluid, etc., it is in contact with, or the force per unit area

E. displays intracavitary blood flow in shades of red, blue, yellow, green depending on the velocity, direction, and extent of turbulence

F. refers to the aortic arterial pressure and vascular resistance the ventricle must overcome to eject blood or any resistance against which the ventricles must pump in order to eject its volume

G. transducers send and receive ultrasound pulses at timed intervals so that the location of where the sample volume is positioned can be known.

H. depends on many factors including the shape and size of the vessel or chamber it's traveling through, wall characteristics, the timing within the cardiac cycle, flow rate, and the viscosity of the blood.

I. refers to the change or shift in received sound waves from the initial transmitted sound waves or pulse

J. transducer delivers continuous pulses out and back, it constantly transmits and receives, with no specific pulse duration or sample volume area

K. the amount of space occupied by a three-dimensional object as measured in cubic units such as cm^3 or ml

L. derived from one of the fundamental laws of physics—the conservation of energy which states that energy cannot be created or destroyed, only transferred from one form to another

M. the speed with which something moves in a given direction

N. the study of the forces involved with blood flow and circulation

O. the volume of blood ejected by the ventricles with each contraction

P. the degree that the muscle fiber stretches prior to contraction (end-diastole)

Exercise 2

1.

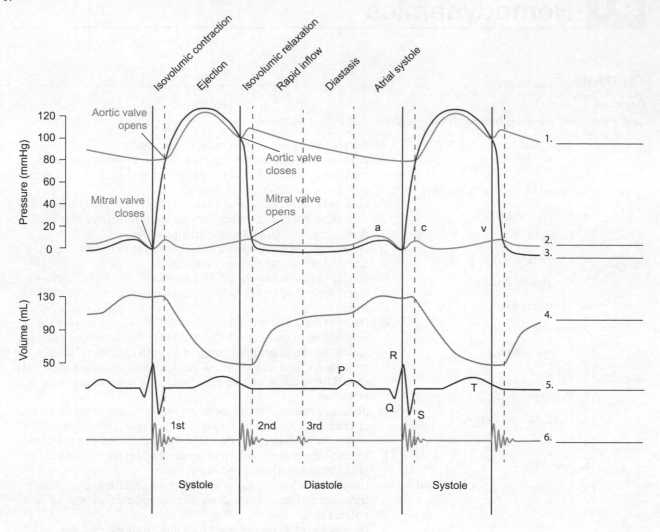

2. Fill in the correct mmHg for each structure in the box:

Right Atrium (RA) ___ mmHg	**Left Atrium** (LA) _____ mmHg
Right Ventricle (RV): _____ mmHg in systole _____ mmHg in diastole	**Left ventricle** (LV): _____ mmHg in systole _____ mmHg in diastole
Pulmonary Artery (PA) _____ mmHg in systole _____ mmHg in diastole	**Aorta** (Ao) _____ mmHg in systole _____ mmHg in diastole

3. The average CO for adults is _____ liters per minute.

4. Cardiac output has a direct effect on blood pressure; as the cardiac output _____, so does the blood pressure.

5. _____ can also be considered the diastolic filling or ventricular end-diastolic volume and pressure.

6. The flow velocities will be _____ toward the middle of the vessel or area and slowest along the walls or edges of the surface it travels through.

7. When the flow is moving away from the transducer or source, the velocity will be _____, displaying a negative shift with lower frequencies.

8. As flow moves toward the transducer or source, the velocity is _____ displaying a positive shift.

9. If flow is _____ to the transducer it will exhibit no change in frequency, giving no frequency shift.

10. One of the limitations of pulsed wave Doppler is that higher velocities will exceed the Nyquist limit and

_____ of the spectral trace will occur

11. The _____ pressure is estimated by ultrasound from the size and collapsibility of the inferior vena cava (IVC).

Exercise 3

Identify and answer the questions for the following images:

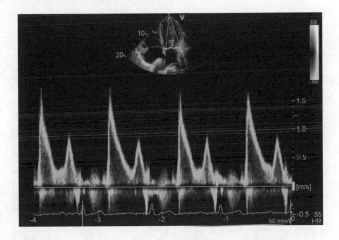

1. Which valve is demonstrated? Is the Doppler waveform Pulsed or Continuous?

_____

_____

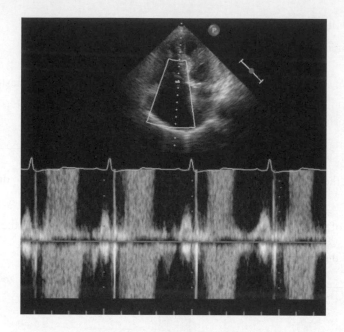

2. Describe this Doppler artifact.

_____

_____

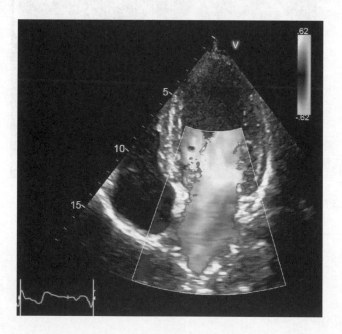

3. Is this image captured in systole or diastole?

_____

_____

32 Echocardiography: Techniques, Terminology, and Tips

KEY TERMS

Exercise 1

Match the following echocardiography terms with their definitions.

_____ 1. color flow mapping (CFM)

_____ 2. continuous wave probe

_____ 3. diastole

_____ 4. Doppler frequency

_____ 5. pulsed wave transducer

_____ 6. spectral analysis waveform

_____ 7. systole

A. Name for the change in frequency when red blood cells move from a lower-frequency sound source at rest toward a higher-frequency sound source

B. Part of the cardiac cycle in which the ventricles are filling with blood; the tricuspid and mitral valves are open during this time

C. Sound is continuously emitted from one transducer and is continuously received by a second transducer

D. Graphic display of flow velocity over time

E. Ability to display blood flow in multiple colors, depending on the velocity, direction of flow, and extent of turbulence

F. Part of the cardiac cycle in which the ventricles are pumping blood through the outflow tract into the pulmonary artery or the aorta

G. Single crystal that sends and receives sound intermittently; a pulse of sound is emitted from the transducer, which also receives the returning signal

ECHOCARDIOGRAPHY EXAMINATION

Exercise 2

Use the definitions below to complete the puzzle.

ACROSS

1. *Transducer located over the cardiac apex (at the point of maximal impulse).*
2. *Transects the heart approximately parallel to the dorsal and ventral surfaces of the body.*
3. *Transects the heart perpendicular to the dorsal and ventral surfaces of the body and perpendicular to the long axis of the heart.*
4. *Transducer placed in the suprasternal notch*

DOWN

5. *Transects the heart perpendicular to the dorsal and ventral surfaces of the body and parallel to the long axis of the heart.*
6. *Transducer placed over the area bounded superiorly by the left clavicle, medially by the sternum, and inferiorly by the apical region.*

7. *Transducer located near the body midline and beneath the costal margin.*

Exercise 3

Fill in the blank(s) with the word(s) that best completes the statements about the echocardiography examination.

1. The cardiac window is usually found between the third and _____ intercostal spaces, slightly to the left of the sternal border. The cardiac window may be considered that area on the anterior chest where the heart is just beneath the skin surface, free of lung interference.

2. Doppler echocardiography has emerged as a valuable noninvasive tool in clinical cardiology to provide

   _____ information about the function of the cardiac valves and chambers of the heart.

3. The best quality Doppler signals are obtained when the sample volume is _____ to the direction of flow.

4. Blood flow toward the transducer is displayed by a time velocity waveform above the baseline at point zero, or a

   _____ deflection.

5. The maximum frequency shift that can be measured by a pulsed Doppler system is called the

   _____ limit and is one half of the pulsed repetition frequency.

6. The _____ analysis waveform allows the operator to print a graphic display of what the audio signal is recording as it provides a representation of blood flow velocities over time.

7. The Doppler equation is based on the principle that the velocity of blood flow is _____ proportional to the Doppler frequency shift and the speed of sound in tissue and is inversely related to twice the frequency of transmitted ultrasound and the cosine of the angle of incidence between the ultrasound beam and the direction of blood flow.

Exercise 4

Identify the echocardiographic view demonstrated in each image.

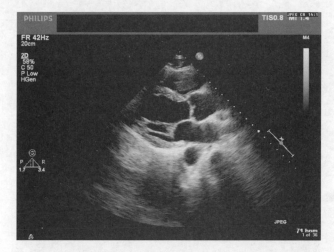

1. Name the echo view.

_____

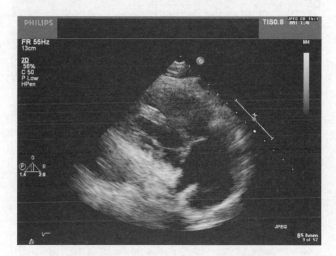

2. Name the echo view.

_____

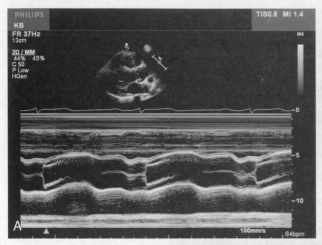
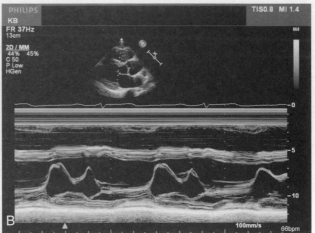
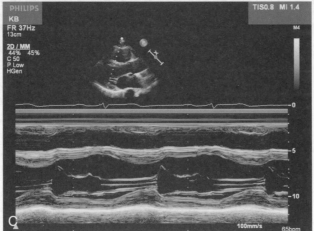

3. What is demonstrated in each M-mode image?

A._____ B _____ C _____

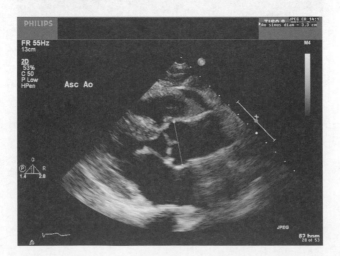

4. What is measured in this image?

_____

Chapter **32 Echocardiography: Techniques, Terminology, and Tips**

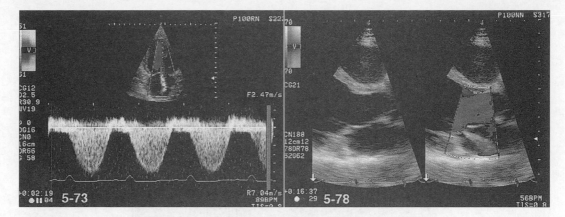

5. What pathology is demonstrated?

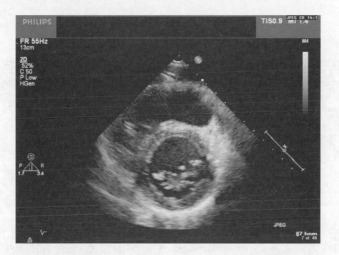

6. Name the echo view.

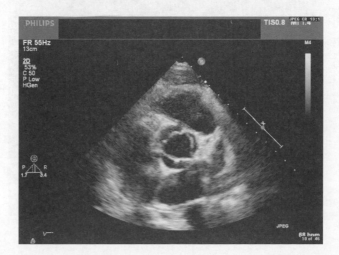

7. Name the echo view.

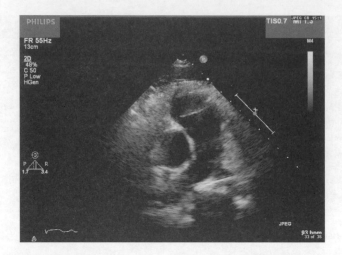

8. Name the echo view.

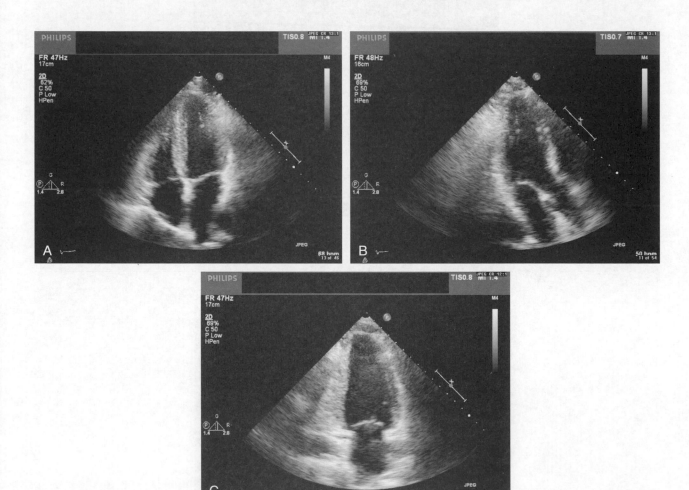

9. Name the echo view.

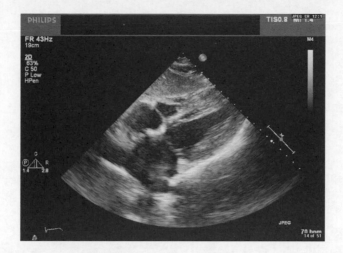

10. Name the echo view.

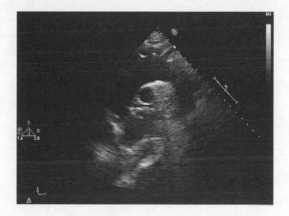

11. Name the echo view.

33 Introduction to Clinical Echocardiography: Left Side Valvular Heart Disease

EXERCISE 1

_____ 1. Aortic stenosis

_____ 2. Bicuspid aortic valve

_____ 3. Pressure Half Time (PHT)

_____ 4. Pseudoaneurysm

_____ 5. PISA

_____ 6. Mitral regurgitation

A. time it takes for the transmitral pressure gradient to decrease by half

B. Abnormal development of the cusps that results in thickened and domed leaflets.

C. Proximal isovelocity surface area (PISA) method

D. Congenital abnormality that causes two of the three aortic leaflets to fuse together, resulting in a two-leaflet valve instead of the normal three-leaflets.

E. well-defined collection of blood and connective tissue outside the vessel wall, typically results from a contained rupture of the aortic wall.

G. occurs when the mitral leaflet is thickened and deformed and unable to close properly, allowing blood to leak from the left ventricle into the left atrium during systole

EXERCISE 2

Fill in the blank(s) with the word(s) that best completes the statements regarding valvular heart disease.

1. The anterior and posterior leaflets are pliable with chordae _____ attached to the tips of the leaflets.

2. The chordae tendinae are attached to the _____ and posterior papillary muscles.

3. The atrioventricular leaflets open in _____ and close in _____.

4. Mitral regurgitation is defined as the systolic retrograde flow from the left _____ into the left

   _____.

5. The vena contracta width should be measured in the parasternal _____ axis view at the narrowest portion of the regurgitant jet, just after the orifice.

6. Analysis of the pulmonary vein flow into the left atrium with PW Doppler may show systolic flow

   _____ due to the MR jet and elevated LA pressure.

7. The two common causes of mitral stenosis are _____ fever and degenerative mitral stenosis.

8. Degenerative mitral stenosis is secondary to mitral annular _____ which is associated with advanced age, hypertension, artherosclerosis, and renal disease/ dialysis.

9. The reduced valve area in mitral stenosis leads to _____ diastolic flow into the left ventricle

   causing _____ of the left atrial pressure and pulmonary venous pressure, which leads to pulmonary edema and right-sided heart failure.

10. With _____ aortic regurgitation there is a sudden large regurgitant volume on the left ventricle causing early closure of the mitral valve.

11. The vena contracta is measured in the parasternal long axis view with the beam _____ to the jet of regurgitation at the smallest neck of the flow region at the level of the aortic valve immediately below the flow convergence region.

12. Aortic regurgitation may show flow reversal in the _____ aorta as imaged from the suprasternal notch view.

13. The _____ aortic stenosis occurs inferior to the aortic leaflets in the left ventricular outflow tract.

14. What is the most common congenital valvular aortic stenosis? _____

15. The most common cause of adult aortic stenosis is _____ and senile or degenerative disease.

16. The high flow rate (hyperdynamic status secondary to aortic insufficiency) may lead to _____ of the severity of aortic stenosis, while the low-flow rate (left ventricular dysfunction or mitral regurgitation)

    may lead to _____ of the severity of aortic stenosis.

EXERCISE 3

Fill in the blank(s) with the word(s) that best completes the statements regarding aortic abnormalities.

1. The parasternal _____ *axis* view will image the aortic sinuses of Valsalva, the sinotubular junction and ascending aorta.

2. The aortic arch is seen from the _____ notch, the descending thoracic aorta is imaged from the

   apical _____ chamber view, and the subcostal long axis view demonstrates the distal thoracic

   and proximal _____ aorta.

3. The definition of an aneurysm implies there has been _____ expansion of all three layers of the vessel wall in diameter.

4. The risk of rupture is greatest when the aneurysm exceeds _____ cm or if the aneurysm is rapidly expanding.

5. The aortic _____ is a tear in the aortic intima that leads to a false lumen with blood between the intima and media and /or adventitia.

6. The true lumen expands with _____ *(diastole/systole)* and shows normal laminar flow with color Doppler.

   The false lumen may be cresant shaped, usually _____ *(larger/smaller)* than the true lumen, with thrombosis within the lumen.

EXERCISE 4

Provide an answer to the question regarding each of the following images.

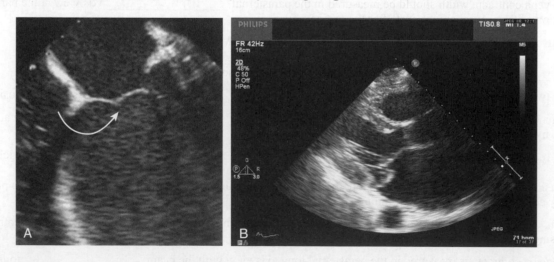

1. Which image shows "tenting" of the mitral valve?

_____

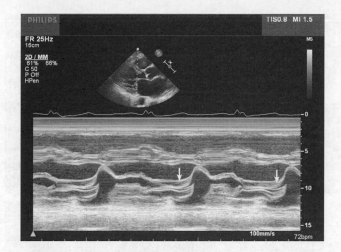

2. What structure are the arrows pointing to in this image?

_____

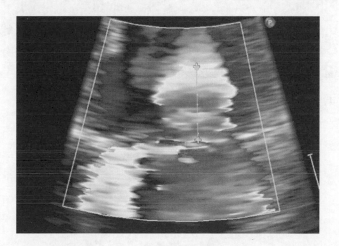

3. What measurement is this used for?

_____

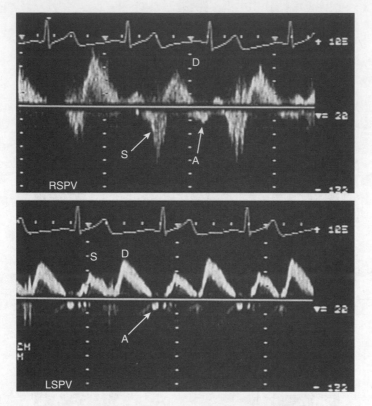

4. Describe what is happening to the systolic flow in the pulmonary vein analysis.

_____

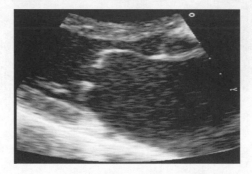

5. What does this parasternal long-axis image represent?

_____

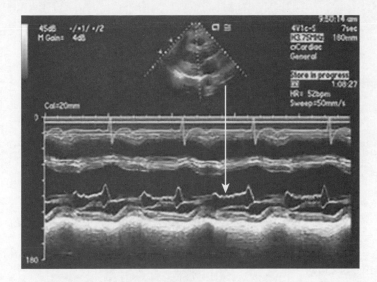

6. Describe what is happening with the anterior leaflet of the mitral valve.

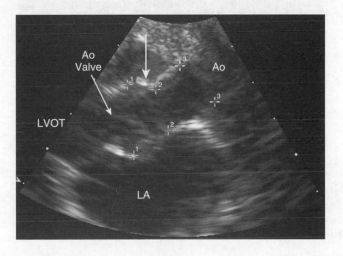

7. What is this arrow pointing to in the ascending aorta?

Chapter **33** **Introduction to Clinical Echocardiography: Left Side Valvular Heart Disease**

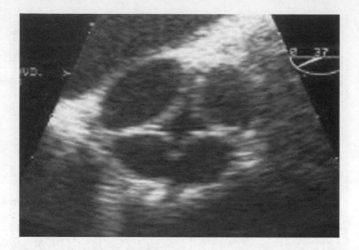

8. What type of aortic valve is shown?

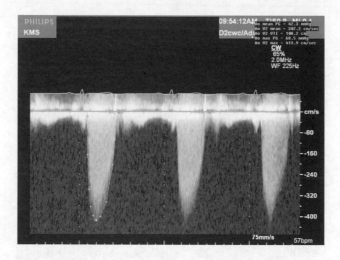

9. This is a patient with aortic valve disease. What is the aortic gradient?

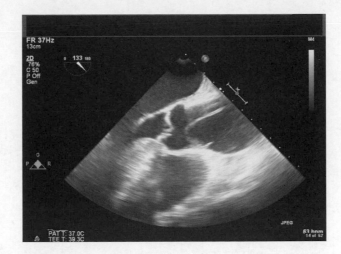

10. A patient presented in the E hypertensive with acute onset of chest pain. What do you see on the TEE image of the ascending aorta?

_____

Chapter **33** **Introduction to Clinical Echocardiography: Left Side Valvular Heart Disease**

34 Introduction to Clinical Echocardiography: Pericardial Disease, Cardiomyopathies, and Tumors

KEY TERMS

EXERCISE 1

_____ 1. Cardiac Tamponade

_____ 2. Constrictive Pericarditis

_____ 3. Dilated cardiomyopathy

_____ 4. Exudative

_____ 5. Fibrous pericardium

_____ 6. Hypertrophic cardiomyopathy

_____ 7. Lipomatous hypertrophy

_____ 8. Malignant Primary Cardiac Tumors

_____ 9. Myxoma

_____ 10. Papillary Fibroelastoma

_____ 11. Rhabdomyoma

_____ 12. Serous pericardium

_____ 13. Takotsubo Cardiomyopathy

_____ 14. Transudative

A. In chronic pericardial disease the pericardium may become thickened and inelastic, which in turn limits the ventricular filling, leading to chronic biventricular diastolic dysfunction, right-sided heart failure and low systemic output.

B. tumors include angiosarcomas, rhabdomyosarcoma, mesothelioma, fibrosarcoma, and synovial fibrosarcoma

C. accumulative fluid in a cavity

D. benign cardiac tumor is the most common tumor in children with tuberous sclerosis

E. common benign tumor of the heart

F. outer sac of the pericardium

G. inner sac of the pericardium with 2 layers: visceral and parietal

H. hypertrophied, non-dilated left ventricle in the absence of another cardiac or systemic disease capable of producing hypertrophy.

I. thickening that is seen along the superior/inferior interatrial septum

J. arises on the aortic or mitral valve tissue and is usually quite small

K. acute cardiac syndrome that is characterized by transient left ventricular regional wall motion abnormalities, chest pain and/or dyspnea, ST-segment elevations, and minor elevations in cardiac enzymes

L. This condition occurs when the intrapericardial pressure increases to the point of compromising systemic venous return to the right atrium.

M. fluid that passes through a membrane

N. characterized by the dilation and reduced contractility of the left ventricle or both the left and right ventricles.

Exercise 2

Fill in the blank(s) with the word(s) that best completes the statements regarding pericardial disease.

1. The inner layer of the pericardium is further divided into the _____ layer (epicardium) that is continuous with the pericardial surface and covers the heart and proximal great vessels and the fibrous parietal layer.

2. The visceral layer is reflected to form the _____ epicardium.

3. The effusions first accumulate _____ to the heart and as the size increases, extend laterally and then circumferentially.

4. The pericardial effusion always is found _____ to the descending aorta.

5. The pleural effusion is _____ to the descending aorta.

Exercise 3

Fill in the blank(s) with the word(s) that best completes the statements regarding cardiomyopathies.

1. The _____ cardiomyopathy is characterized by the dilation and reduced contractility of the left ventricle or both the left and right ventricles.

2. _____ of the left ventricle implies that the myocardial wall segments are extremely thick (>2 mm) with peaks and valleys.

3. The _____ properties of the left ventricle may be determined by the E/A ratio, dispersion of the E-wave velocity, color Doppler M-mode velocity of propagation, deceleration time, pulmonary vein flow, and annular Doppler tissue imaging.

4. The acute cardiac syndrome that is characterized by transient left ventricular regional wall motion abnormalities, chest pain and/or dyspnea, ST-segment elevations, and minor elevations in cardiac enzymes is called

    _____ cardiomyopathy.

5. The predominant anatomical features of _____ cardiomyopathy include a narrowed left ventricular outflow tract secondary to the asymmetric septal hypertrophy.

6. The sonographer should evaluate the presence of _____ anterior motion of the mitral leaflet to see if further flow velocity is obstructed in the LVOT.

Exercise 4

Fill in the blank(s) with the word(s) that best completes the statements regarding cardiac masses.

1. _____ is a tumor of the kidney that may travel through the renal vein into the inferior vena cava and into the right atrium.

2. _____ malignancy affects the right side of the heart, causing severe tricuspid regurgitation.

3. The more common benign tumor of the heart that is seen in the atrial cavity is a _____.

4. This benign tumor, _____, has a stippled edge with a shimmer or vibration at the tumor-blood interface that is always found downstream of the flow.

5. _____ hypertrophy is a thickening that is seen along the superior/inferior interatrial septum.

6. Predisposing conditions for left ventricular _____ include blood stasis with low velocity flow, ventricular aneurysm, dilated cardiomyopathy with "swirling" blood flow, or pseudoaneurysm.

7. Contrast injected into the heart will clearly demonstrate a _____ anechoic area if thrombus is present.

8. Patients are usually present clinically as very symptomatic with _____ _____, appearing with fever, chills, and perhaps a new cardiac murmur.

Exercise 5

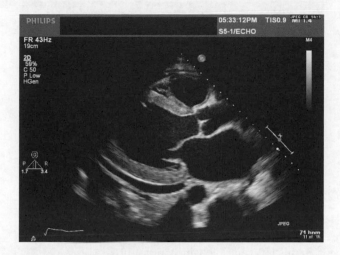

1. Does this image show a pleural effusion or pericardial effusion?

_____

_____

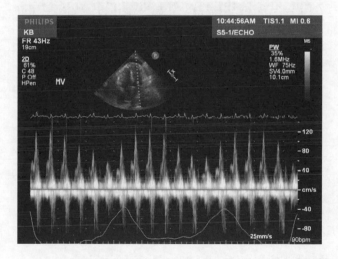

2. This M-mode through the mitral valve is suggestive of what abnormality?

_____

_____

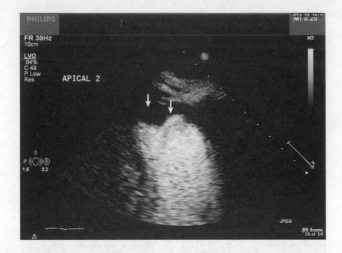

3. What are the areas pointing to in this left ventricle with contrast?

_____

_____

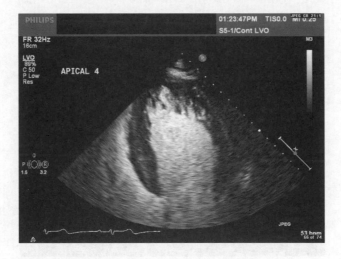

4. What does this apical four-chamber view reveal about the left ventricle?

_____

_____

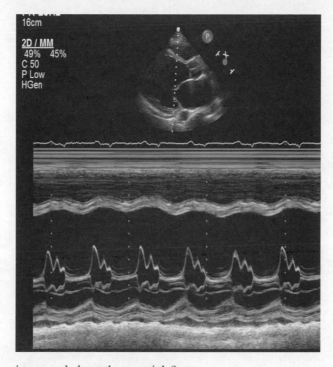

5. What does this M-mode tracing reveal about the ventricle?

_____

_____

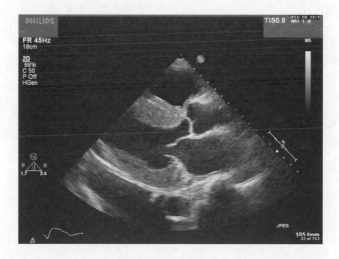

6. What does this parasternal long-axis view of the heart reveal?

_____

_____

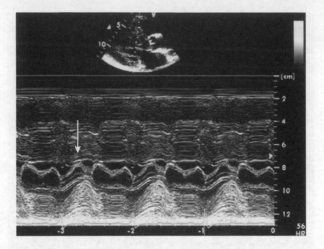

7. What are the arrows pointing to in this M-mode image?

_____

_____

35 Fetal Echo: Normal

KEY TERMS

Exercise 1

Match the following embryology of the cardiovascular system terms with their definitions.

_____ 1. atrioventricular node

_____ 2. bulbus cordis

_____ 3. foramen ovale

_____ 4. left and right atria

_____ 5. left and right ventricles

_____ 6. septum primum

_____ 7. septum secundum

_____ 8. sinoatrial node

A. Filling chambers of the heart

B. First part of the atrial septum to grow from the dorsal wall of the primitive atrium; fuses with the endocardial cushions

C. Primitive chamber that forms the right ventricle

D. Pumping chambers of the heart

E. Area of cardiac muscle that receives and conducts the cardiac impulse

F. Forms in the wall of the sinus venosus near its opening into the right atrium

G. Also termed *fossa ovale*; opening between the free edge of the septum secundum and the dorsal wall of the atrium

H. Grows into the atrium to the right of the septum primum

Exercise 2

Match the following fetal circulation terms with their definitions.

_____ 1. bicuspid aortic valve

_____ 2. ductus arteriosus

_____ 3. fossa ovale

_____ 4. inferior vena cava

_____ 5. main pulmonary artery

_____ 6. mitral valve

_____ 7. patent ductus arteriosus

_____ 8. pulmonary veins

_____ 9. right ventricle

_____ 10. superior vena cava

_____ 11. tricuspid valve

A. Vessel receiving venous return from the head and upper extremities into the upper posterior medial wall of the right atrium

B. Four veins that bring blood from the lungs back into the posterior wall of the left atrium

C. Pumping chamber of the heart that sends blood into the pulmonary artery

D. Also termed *foramen ovale*; opening between the free edge of the septum secundum and the dorsal wall of the atrium

E. Atrioventricular valve between the left atrium and the left ventricle

F. Two leaflets instead of the normal three leaflets with asymmetrical cusps

G. Atrioventricular valve found between the right atrium and the right ventricle

H. Venous return into the right atrium of the heart along the posterior lateral wall

I. Open communication between the pulmonary artery and the descending aorta that does not constrict after birth

J. Communication between the pulmonary artery and the descending aorta that closes after birth

K. Main artery that carries blood from the right ventricle to the lungs

Exercise 3

Label the following illustrations.

A. The heart during the fourth week of development.

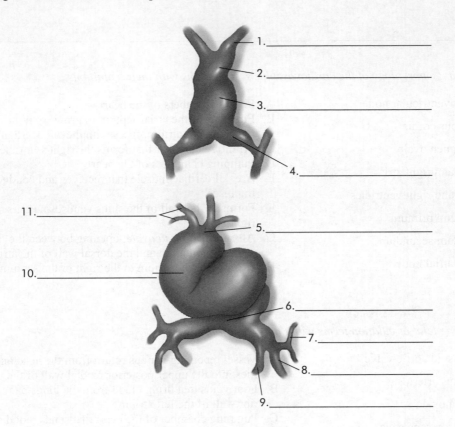

1._____

2._____

3._____

4._____

11._____

5._____

10._____

6._____

7._____

8._____

9._____

B. Partitioning of the primitive atrioventricular canal, atrium, and ventricle in the developing heart.

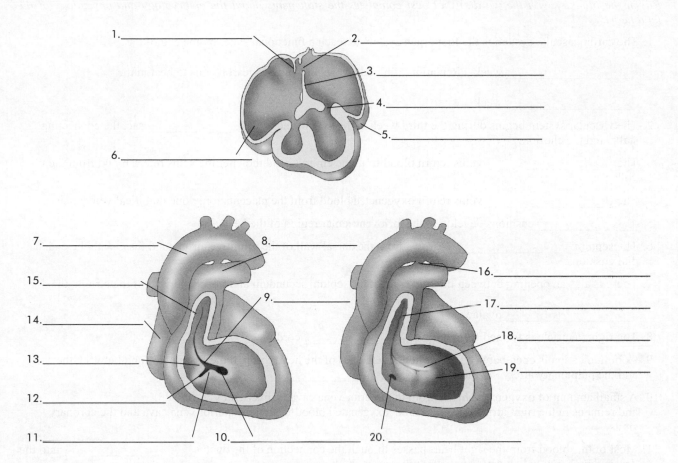

1._____   2._____
                            3._____
                            4._____
6._____   5._____

7._____   8._____
15._____
14._____   9._____
13._____   16._____
12._____   17._____
11._____   10._____ 18._____
                                                        19._____
                            20._____

C. Fetal circulation.

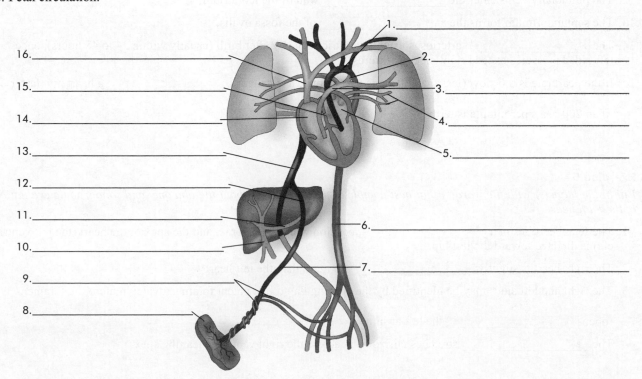

16._____   1._____
15._____   2._____
14._____   3._____
13._____   4._____
12._____   5._____
11._____
10._____   6._____
9._____   7._____
8._____

Exercise 4

Fill in the blank(s) with the word(s) that best completes the statements about the embryology and physiology of the fetal heart.

1. The cardiovascular system is the first organ system to reach a functional state; by the end of the

   _____ week, circulation of blood has begun, and the heart begins to beat in the

   _____ week.

2. The vascular system begins during the third week in the wall of the _____ sac, the connecting stalk, and the chorion.

3. The _____ veins return blood from the embryo, and the vitelline veins return blood from the yolk sac.

4. The _____ veins return oxygenated blood from the placenta; only one umbilical vein persists.

5. _____ cushions develop in the atrioventricular region of the heart.

6. The septum _____ grows from the dorsal wall of the primitive atrium and fuses with the endocardial cushions.

7. There is also an opening between the free edge of the septum secundum and the dorsal wall of the atrium, the

   _____ ovalae.

8. The right ventricle is formed from the _____ cordis.

9. Communication is open between the right and left sides of the heart through the fossa ovale and between the aorta and the pulmonary artery via the _____ _____.

10. A small amount of oxygenated blood from the inferior vena cava is diverted by the crista _____ and remains in the right atrium to mix with deoxygenated blood from the superior vena cava and the coronary sinus.

11. Most of this blood from the right heart passes through the connection of the ductus _____ into the descending aorta; only a very small amount goes to the lungs.

12. The pulmonary veins enter the _____ wall of the left atrium.

13. The septum primum forms the _____ of the fossa ovalis.

14. The _____ arteriosus usually constricts shortly after birth (usually within 24 to 48 hours), once left-sided pressures exceed right-sided pressures.

15. If the heart rate is too slow (less than 60 beats per minute), it is called _____; a heart rate faster

    than 200 beats per minute is termed _____.

Exercise 5

Fill in the blank(s) with the word(s) that best completes the statements about the anatomy and sonographic evaluation of the fetal heart.

1. The fetal heart lies in a _____ position within the thorax, and the apex of the heart (the left ventricle) is directed toward the left hip.

2. The right heart is slightly _____ in utero than the left heart.

3. The right and left sides may be identified by the opening flap of the patent foramen ovale; in utero the foramen

   opens _____ the left atrium.

4. The _____ stretches horizontally across the right ventricle near the apex.

236

5. Normally the tricuspid valve is located just slightly _____ to the mitral valve.

6. The right and left ventricular width measurements are performed in the four-chamber view at the level of the

_____ annulus.

7. The pulmonary artery normally is _____ and to the _____ of the aorta.

8. The _____ membranous septum is best seen on the apical four-chamber view at the level of the atrioventricular valves, whereas the _____ may be seen on the long-axis view.

9. On the long-axis view, the continuity of the right side of the _____ with the

_____ wall of the aortic root is important to rule out the presence of a membranous ventricular septal defect (VSD), conal truncal abnormality (such as truncus arteriosus), endocardial cushion defect, or tetralogy of Fallot.

10. Normally the three aortic cusps open in _____ to the full extent of the aortic root and close in

midposition in _____.

11. On the short-axis view, normally the right ventricular outflow tract and the pulmonary artery "drape"

_____ to the circular aorta.

12. The three head and neck branch arteries (_____, _____, and _____) may be seen to arise from the perfect curve of the aortic arch as they ascend into the fetal head.

13. A second "arch-type" pattern (which appears as large as the aorta) is shown as the transducer is angled inferior

from the aortic arch. This represents the _____ _____ _____, a communication between the pulmonary artery and the aorta.

Exercise 6
Provide a short answer for each question after evaluating the images.

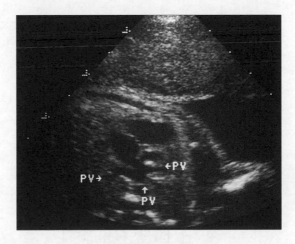

1. Which pulmonary vein is **not** shown?

_____

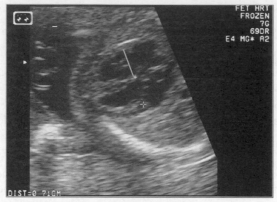

2. The left ventricle should be measured at the level of which structure?

_____

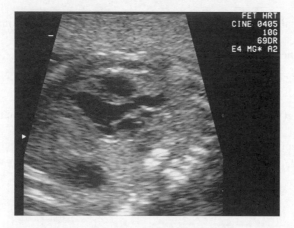

3. This image shows the mitral valve in which stage of the cardiac cycle?

_____

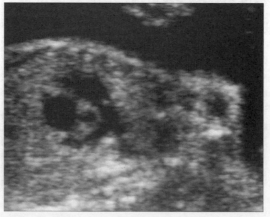

4. What important relationship does this image show?

_____

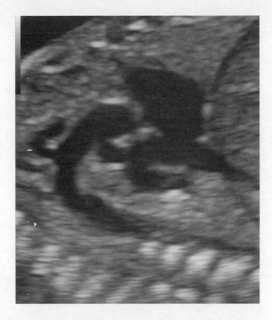

5. Does this image show the ductus arteriosus or the aortic arch?

_____

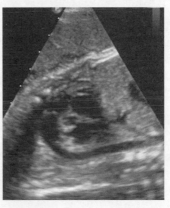

6. What anatomic structure does this image show?

_____

36 Fetal Echocardiography: Congenital Heart Disease

KEY TERMS

Exercise 1

Match the terms related to cardiac malposition, cardiac enlargement, and septal defects with their definitions.

_____ 1. atrial septal defect

_____ 2. atrioventricular septal defect (AVSD)

_____ 3. bicuspid aortic valve

_____ 4. cardiomyopathy

_____ 5. dextrocardia

_____ 6. dextroposition

_____ 7. levocardia

_____ 8. levoposition

_____ 9. mesocardia

_____ 10. myocarditis

_____ 11. partial anomalous pulmonary venous return

_____ 12. pericardial effusion

_____ 13. ventricular septal defect

A. Disease of the myocardial muscle layer of the heart that causes the heart to dilate secondary to regurgitation; also affects cardiac function

B. The heart is in the right chest with the apex pointed to the right of the thorax

C. Atypical location of the heart in the middle of the chest with the cardiac apex pointing toward the midline of the chest

D. Condition in which the pulmonary veins do not all enter the left atrial cavity

E. Normal position of the heart in the left chest with the cardiac apex pointed to the left

F. Congenital abnormality that causes two of the three aortic leaflets to fuse together, resulting in a two-leaflet valve, instead of the normal three-leaflet valve; usually the cusps are asymmetrical in size and position; may be the cause of adult aortic stenosis and/or insufficiency

G. Cardiac disease process of necrosis and destruction of myocardial cells that involves an inflammatory infiltrate

H. Condition in which the heart is located in the right side of the chest with the cardiac apex pointing medially or to the left

I. Condition in which the heart is displaced farther toward the left chest, usually in association with a space-occupying lesion

J. Defect that provides communication between the left atrium and the right atrium that continues after birth

K. Defect in the ventricular septum that provides communication between the right and left chambers of the heart; most common congenital lesion in the heart

L. Abnormal collection of fluid surrounding the epicardial layer of the heart

M. Failure of the endocardial cushion to fuse; this defect of the central heart provides communication between the ventricles, between the atria, or between the atria and ventricles

Exercise 2

Match the terms related to right and left ventricular inflow and outflow disturbances with their definitions.

_____ 1. aortic stenosis

_____ 2. Ebstein's anomaly of the tricuspid valve

_____ 3. hypoplastic left heart syndrome

_____ 4. hypoplastic right heart syndrome

_____ 5. tetralogy of Fallot

_____ 6. mitral atresia

_____ 7. mitral regurgitation

_____ 8. pulmonary stenosis

_____ 9. subpulmonic stenosis

_____ 10. supravalvular pulmonic stenosis

_____ 11. tricuspid atresia

A. Most common form of cyanotic heart disease characterized by a high, membranous ventricular septal defect; large, anteriorly placed aorta; pulmonary stenosis; and right ventricular hypertrophy

B. Abnormal pulmonary valve characterized by thickened, domed leaflets that restrict the amount of blood flowing from the right ventricle to the pulmonary artery to the lungs

C. Abnormal development of the mitral leaflet (valve between the left atrium and the left ventricle); may lead to development of hypoplastic left ventricle; also called congenital mitral stenosis

D. Abnormal narrowing in the main pulmonary artery superior to the valve opening

E. Abnormal displacement of the septal leaflet of the tricuspid valve toward the apex of the right ventricle; the right ventricle above this leaflet becomes the "atrialized" chamber

F. Underdevelopment of the tricuspid valve; usually associated with hypoplasia of the right ventricle and pulmonary stenosis

G. Underdevelopment of the right ventricular outflow tract secondary to pulmonary stenosis; tricuspid atresia is often found

H. Abnormal development of the cusps of the aortic valve, which results in thickened and domed leaflets

I. Underdevelopment of the left ventricle with aortic and/or mitral atresia; left ventricle is extremely thickened compared with the right ventricle

J. Occurs when the mitral leaflet is deformed and is unable to close properly, allowing blood to leak from the left ventricle into the left atrium during systole

K. Occurs when a membrane or muscle bundle obstructs the outflow tract into the pulmonary artery

Exercise 3

Match the following terms related to great vessel abnormalities, complex cardiac abnormalities, and dysrhythmias with their definitions.

_____ 1. atrioventricular block

_____ 2. coarctation of the aorta

_____ 3. corrected transposition of the great arteries

_____ 4. cor triatriatum

_____ 5. ductal constriction

_____ 6. premature atrial contractions (PACs) and premature ventricular contractions (PVCs)

_____ 7. single ventricle

_____ 8. supraventricular tachyarrhythmias

_____ 9. total anomalous pulmonary venous return

_____ 10. transposition of the great arteries

_____ 11. truncus arteriosus

A. Benign condition that arises from the electrical impulses generated outside the cardiac pacemaker (sinus node); immature development of the electrical pacing system causes irregular heartbeats scattered throughout the cardiac cycle

B. Right atrium and left atrium are connected to the morphologic left and right ventricles, respectively, and the great arteries are transposed

C. Congenital heart lesion in which only one great artery arises from the base of the heart; the pulmonary trunk, systemic arteries, and coronary arteries arise from this single great artery

D. Congenital anomaly in which there are two atria but only one ventricular chamber, which receives both mitral and tricuspid valves

E. Block of the transmission of electrical impulses from the atria to the ventricles

F. Condition in which the pulmonary veins do not return at all into the left atrial cavity; the veins may return into the right atrial cavity or into a chamber posterior to the left atrial cavity

G. Occurs when flow is diverted from the ductus secondary to tricuspid or pulmonary atresia or secondary to maternal medications given to stop early contractions

H. Occurs when the left atrial cavity is partitioned into two compartments; pulmonary veins drain into an accessory left atrial chamber proximal to the true left atrium

I. Abnormal condition that exists when the aorta is connected to the right ventricle and the pulmonary artery is connected to the left ventricle; the atrioventricular valves are normally attached and related

J. Abnormal cardiac rhythm above 200 beats per minute with a conduction rate of 1:1

K. Narrowing of the aortic arch (discrete, long segment, or tubular); occurs most commonly as a shelflike protrusion in the isthmus of the arch or at the site of the ductal insertion near the left subclavian artery

CONGENITAL HEART DISEASE

Exercise 4

Fill in the blank(s) with the word(s) that best completes the statements about congenital heart disease.

1. The most common type of congenital heart disease is the _____ _____

   _____, followed by atrial septal defects and then pulmonary stenosis.

2. The _____ _____ defect is the defect in the central atrial septum near the foramen ovale; it is the most difficult to see in utero because the flap of the foramen ovale is mobile at this period of development.

3. The _____ _____ defect is usually associated with the chromosome abnormality of trisomy 21; it often will consist of a cleft mitral valve and abnormalities of the atrioventricular septum.

4. The flap of the foramen ovale should not be so large as to touch the lateral wall of the atrium; when this redundancy of the foramen occurs, the sinoatrial node may become agitated in the right atrium and cause fetal

   _____.

5. Ventricular septal defects may close with the formation of _____ tissue that is commonly found along the right side of the septal defect.

6. Failure of the endocardial cushion to fuse is termed _____ atrioventricular septal defect.

7. The most primitive form of endocardial cushion defect is called _____ atrioventricular septal defect. This defect has a single, undivided, free-floating leaflet stretching across both ventricles.

8. Findings in tricuspid atresia include a large dilated _____ ventricular cavity with a small, underdeveloped _____ ventricular cavity.

9. The portion of the right ventricle underlying the adherent tricuspid valvular tissue is quite thin and functions as a receiving chamber analogous to the right atrium. This is referred to as the _____ chamber.

10. The right heart is underdeveloped because of obstruction of the right ventricular outflow tract secondary to

   _____ _____.

11. A large septal defect with mild to moderate pulmonary stenosis is classified as _____ disease, and a large septal defect with severe pulmonary stenosis is considered _____ disease ("blue baby" at birth).

12. If the override is greater than 50%, the condition is called a _____ _____

   _____ ventricle. (Both great vessels arise from the right heart.)

13. In pulmonic stenosis, the abnormal pulmonic cusps become thickened and _____ during diastole.

14. In a _____ _____ valve, the raphe between cusp tissues has not separated; thus, the leaflet opens asymmetrically and may show "doming" on the parasternal long-axis view.

15. _____ _____ _____ occurs when a membrane covers the left ventricular outflow tract.

16. _____ _____ heart syndrome is characterized by a small, hypertrophied left ventricle with aortic and/or mitral dysplasia or atresia.

17. _____ of the _____ _____ is an abnormal condition that exists when the aorta is connected to the right ventricle and the pulmonary artery is connected to the left ventricle. The atrioventricular valves are normally attached and related.

18. _____ _____ shows an abnormal, large, single great vessel arising from the ventricles. Usually an infundibular ventricular septal defect is present. Significant septal override occurs.

19. In the normal fetus, the ductus arteriosus transmits about 55% to 60% of combined ventricular output from the

   _____ artery to the aorta.

20. _____ tumors tend to be multiple and involve the septum. These tumors are associated with tuberous sclerosis (50% to 86%).

21. _____ _____ occurs when the left atrial cavity is partitioned into two compartments. This anomaly is characterized by drainage of the pulmonary veins into an accessory left atrial chamber that lies proximal to the true left atrium.

22. An enlarged _____ system can serve an important function as a conveyor of inferior vena caval blood to the right atrium even though the inferior vena cava itself communicates with the left atrium.

23. In total _____ _____ _____ _____, the venous return may occur totally into the right atrium or into a "common chamber" posterior to the left atrium, into the superior or inferior vena cava, or into the left subclavian vein, azygos vein, or portal vein.

FETAL CARDIAC RHYTHM

Exercise 5

Fill in the blank(s) with the word(s) that best completes the statements about fetal cardiac rhythm.

1. _____ atrial and ventricular contractions arise from electrical impulses generated outside the cardiac pacemaker (sinus node).

2. To adequately assess fetal rhythm, ventricular and atrial rates must be analyzed _____.

3. _____ _____ include abnormal rhythms above 200 beats per minute with a conduction ratio of 1:1.

4. In atrial flutter, the _____ rate is recorded at 300 to 460 beats per minute with a normal ventricular rate.

5. _____ _____ shows the atria to have a rate of more than 400 beats per minute with a ventricular rate of 120 to 200 beats per minute.

6. With supraventricular tachycardia, the fetus develops _____ filling of the ventricles, decreased cardiac output, and right ventricular volume overload leading to subsequent congestive heart failure.

7. When transmission of the electrical impulse from the atria to the ventricles is blocked, the condition is called

   _____ _____.

8. In _____ heart block, atrial and ventricular rates are independent of each other, and the atrial rate is slower.

Exercise 6

Provide a short answer for each question after evaluating the images.

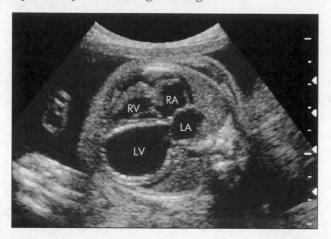

1. From this image, identify and answer the following questions:

   a. Where is the fetal spine? (Use a clock identification.)

   b. Describe the left ventricle.

   c. What is the ratio of the cardiac circumference to the thoracic circumference?

   d. What would you expect the contractility to be?

a. _____

b. _____

c. _____

d. _____

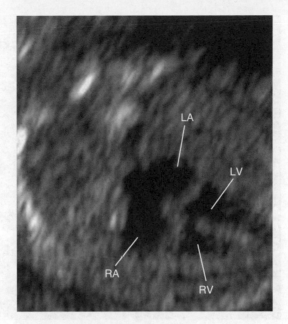

2. What fetal defect does this four-chamber view demonstrate?

_____

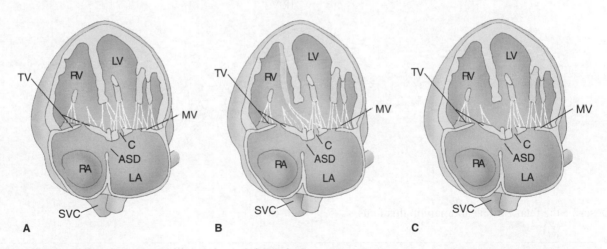

A　　　　　　　　　　**B**　　　　　　　　　　**C**

3. Describe the differences among illustrations *A* through *C*.

_____

_____

_____

　　　　Chapter **36** **Fetal Echocardiography: Congenital Heart Disease**

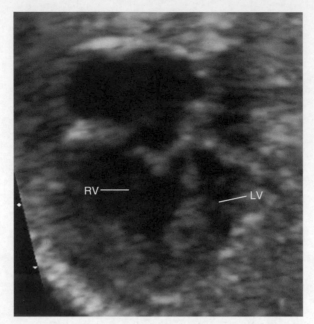

4. Identify the fetal cardiac anomaly in this image.

_____

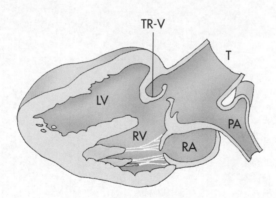

5. Describe the fetal cardiac anomaly in this fetus.

_____

_____

_____

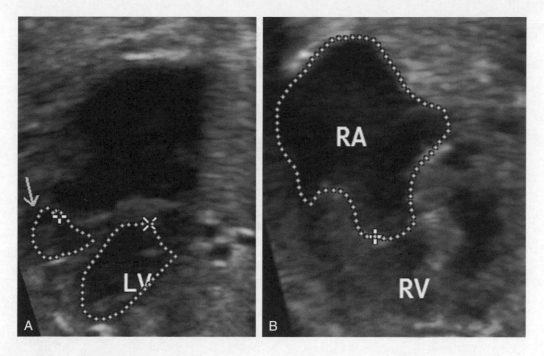

6. Identify the abnormality in this fetus.

_____

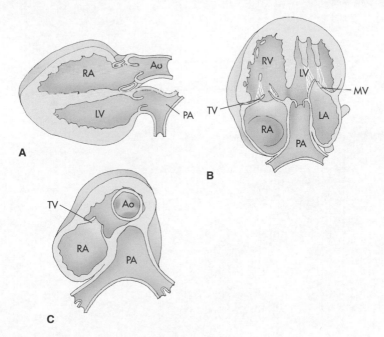

7. Describe the cardiac anomaly represented by this illustration.

_____

_____

_____

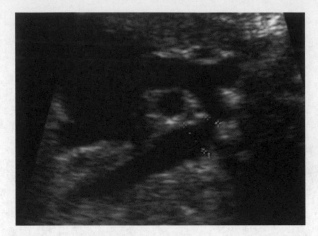

8. Identify the anomaly that is demonstrated in this fetal heart.

_____

_____

37 Extracranial Cerebrovascular Evaluation

Exercise 1

Match the following extracranial terms with their definitions.

_____ 1. amaurosis fugax

_____ 2. aphasia

_____ 3. ataxia

_____ 4. bruit

_____ 5. collateral pathway

_____ 6. common carotid artery (CCA)

_____ 7. cerebrovascular accident

_____ 8. diplopia

_____ 9. dysarthria

_____ 10. dysphagia

_____ 11. external carotid artery (ECA)

_____ 12. hemiparesis

_____ 13. internal carotid artery (ICA)

_____ 14. reversible ischemic neurologic deficit

_____ 15. transient ischemic attack

_____ 16. vertebral artery

_____ 17. vertigo

A. Difficulty with speech caused by impairment of the tongue or muscles essential to speech

B. Arises from the aortic arch on the left side and from the innominate artery on the right side

C. Noise caused by tissue vibration produced by turbulence that causes flow disturbance

D. Inability to swallow or difficulty in swallowing

E. Impaired ability to coordinate movement, especially disturbances in gait

F. Sensation of having objects move about the person or sensation of moving around in space

G. Larger of the two terminal branches that arise from the common carotid artery

H. Large branches of the subclavian artery that merge to form the basilar artery

I. Transient partial or complete loss of vision in one eye

J. Cerebral infarct that lasts longer than 24 hours but less than 72 hours

K. Unilateral partial or complete paralysis

L. Develops because of vessel obstruction; smaller side branches of the vessel provide alternative flow pathways

M. Inability to communicate by speech or writing

N. Abnormal condition of the brain characterized by occlusion by an embolus, thrombus, cerebrovascular hemorrhage, or vasospasm that results in ischemia of brain tissues normally perfused by the damaged vessels

O. Smaller of the two terminal branches of the common carotid artery

P. Episode of cerebrovascular insufficiency, usually associated with partial occlusion of a cerebral artery by an atherosclerotic plaque or an embolus

Q. Double vision

Exercise 2

Label the following illustrations.

A. Anatomy of the extracranial carotid system.

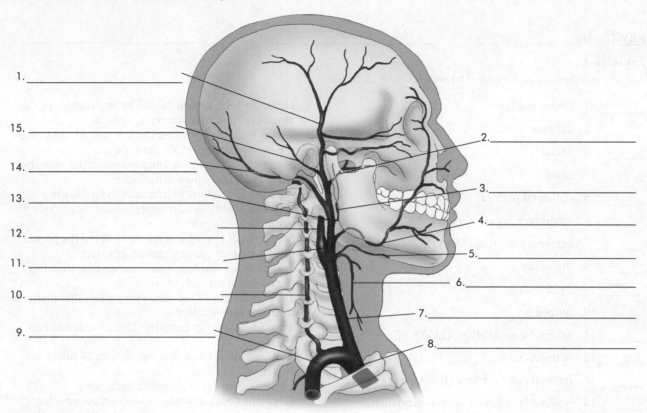

1. _____

15. _____

14. _____

13. _____

12. _____

11. _____

10. _____

9. _____

2. _____

3. _____

4. _____

5. _____

6. _____

7. _____

8. _____

Exercise 3

Fill in the blank(s) with the word(s) that best completes the statements or provide a short answer about the anatomy of extracranial cerebrovascular imaging.

1. The ascending aorta originates from the _____ ventricle of the heart.

2. Three main arteries arise from the superior convexity of the arch in its normal configuration: the

   _____ trunk (innominate artery) is the first branch; the _____

   common carotid artery the second; and the left _____ artery the third branch in approximately 70% of cases.

3. The right CCA and the right subclavian artery are divided by the _____ artery, which gives rise to the right vertebral artery.

4. Each CCA ascends through the superior mediastinum anterolaterally in the neck and lies _____ to the jugular vein.

5. The left common carotid is usually _____ than the right, because it originates from the aortic arch.

6. The termination of the CCA is the carotid _____, which is the origin of the ICA and the ECA.

7. The ECA originates at the midcervical level and is usually the _____ of the two terminal branches of the CCA.

8. The larger of the CCA terminal branches is usually the _____.

9. In most individuals, the ICA lies _____ to the ECA and courses medially as it ascends in the neck.

10. The vertebral arteries are large branches of the _____ arteries.

11. The _____ segment of the vertebral artery courses superiorly and medially from its subclavicular origin to enter the transverse foramen of the sixth cervical vertebra.

STROKE

Exercise 4

Fill in the blank(s) with the word(s) that best completes the statements or provide a short answer about stroke risk factors, warning signs, and symptoms.

1. A stroke or "brain attack" is caused by a(n) _____ of blood flow to the brain (ischemic stroke) or by a ruptured intracranial blood vessel (intracranial hemorrhage).

2. Approximately 80% of all known strokes are _____, and the remaining 20% are hemorrhagic.

3. Symptoms of weakness or numbness of a leg or arm on one side of the body indicate disease in the

_____ carotid system.

CAROTID DUPLEX IMAGING

Exercise 5

Fill in the blank(s) with the word(s) that best completes the statements about the technical aspects of carotid duplex imaging.

1. Arm pressures are recorded, and a difference of _____ mmHg pressure between arms suggests a proximal stenosis and/or occlusion of the subclavian or innominate artery on the side of the lower pressure.

2. In the normal setting, the CCA spectral waveform will demonstrate a _____ resistance pattern (end diastole above the zero baseline) because blood travels from the CCA to the brain via the ICA.

3. The CCA Doppler signal will display a _____ Doppler shift throughout the cardiac cycle.

4. The ICA demonstrates blood flow velocity that is _____ and _____ the zero baseline throughout the cardiac cycle.

5. The normal color pattern of the ICA will have _____ color throughout the cardiac cycle because the ICA has diastolic blood flow caused by the low peripheral resistance of the brain.

6. The ECA demonstrates a more _____ Doppler signal (minimum diastolic flow) because it supplies blood to the skin and the muscular bed of the scalp and face.

7. The ECA usually has a _____ slope to peak systole and blood flow velocity at or very close to zero in late diastole.

8. The vertebral arteries are located by angling the transducer slightly _____ from a longitudinal view of the middle or proximal CCA.

Exercise 6

Fill in the blank(s) with the word(s) that best completes the statements or provide a short answer about the interpretation of carotid duplex imaging.

1. The _____ velocity obtained from an ICA stenosis is used to classify the degree of narrowing.

2. A _____ _____ is present if reversal of vertebral artery blood flow direction occurs secondary to a significant obstruction proximal to the origin of the vertebral artery in the ipsilateral subclavian or innominate artery.

3. Evaluation of normal subclavian arteries produces _____ high-resistance Doppler signals.

4. Carotid duplex imaging performed after carotid endarterectomy may reveal residual or _____ stenosis in the ipsilateral ICA and disease progression in the contralateral ICA.

PATHOLOGY

Exercise 7

Fill in the blank(s) with the word(s) that best completes the statements or provide a short answer about the pathology of the extracranial vessels.

1. The echogenicity of plaque is usually described as _____ if it demonstrates a uniform level of

   echogenicity and texture throughout the plaque, and as _____ if the plaque has mixed areas

   of echogenicity and textures.

2. A _____ plaque is usually visualized with an accompanying acoustic shadow that obscures imaging information deep to it.

3. When describing whether the ICA is occluded, the color PRF should be _____ to document the presence of any slow-moving blood flow, and the color gain should be increased to enhance any blood flow that may be present.

4. The ICA should be sampled at _____ sites with Doppler.

5. A nonatherosclerotic disease that usually affects the media of the arterial wall is _____.

Exercise 8

Provide a short answer for each question after evaluating the images.

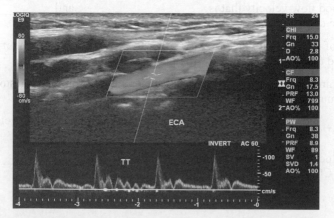

1. How can the sonographer be certain the vessel is the external carotid artery?

_____

2. Does the vertebral artery demonstrate high resistance or low resistance?

_____

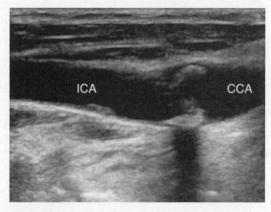

3. What does this image of the carotid artery demonstrate?

_____

_____

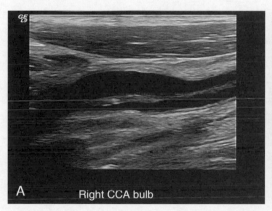 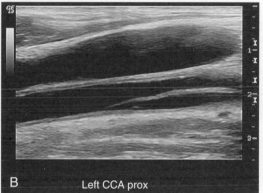

4. What does this image show of the carotid artery in a 39-year-old patient with stroke like symptoms?

_____

_____

_____

Chapter **37** **Extracranial Cerebrovascular Evaluation**

38 Intracranial Cerebrovascular Evaluation

KEY TERMS

Exercise 1

Match the following intracranial anatomic terms with their definitions.

_____ 1. anterior cerebral artery (ACA)

_____ 2. anterior communicating artery (ACoA)

_____ 3. basilar artery (BA)

_____ 4. circle of Willis

_____ 5. internal carotid artery (ICA)

_____ 6. middle cerebral artery (MCA)

_____ 7. posterior cerebral artery (PCA)

_____ 8. posterior communicating artery (PCoA)

_____ 9. vertebral artery

A. A polygon vascular ring at the base of the brain
B. A short vessel that connects the anterior cerebral arteries at the interhemispheric fissure
C. Courses posteriorly and medially from the internal carotid artery to join the posterior cerebral artery
D. Branch of the subclavian artery
E. Smaller of the two terminal branches of the internal carotid artery
F. Originates from the terminal basilar artery and courses anteriorly and laterally
G. Formed by the union of the two vertebral arteries
H. Arises from the common carotid artery to supply the anterior brain and meninges
I. Large terminal branch of the internal carotid artery

Exercise 2

Match the following intracranial terms with their definition.

_____ 1. cerebral vasospasm

_____ 2. mean velocity

_____ 3. ophthalmic artery

_____ 4. subclavian steal syndrome

_____ 5. submandibular window

_____ 6. suboccipital window

_____ 7. transorbital window

_____ 8. transtemporal window

A. Characterized by symptoms of brain stem ischemia associated with stenosis or occlusion of the left subclavian, innominate, or right subclavian artery proximal to the origin of the vertebral artery
B. Transducer is placed on the posterior aspect of the neck inferior to the nuchal crest
C. First branch of the internal carotid artery
D. Transducer is placed on the temporal bone cephalad to the zygomatic arch anterior to the ear
E. Vasoconstriction of the arteries
F. Transducer is placed at the angle of the mandible and is angled slightly medially and cephalad toward the carotid canal
G. Transducer is placed on the closed eyelid
H. Based on the time average of the outline velocity (maximum velocity envelope)

Exercise 3

Label the following illustrations.

A. The arteries of the circle of Willis.

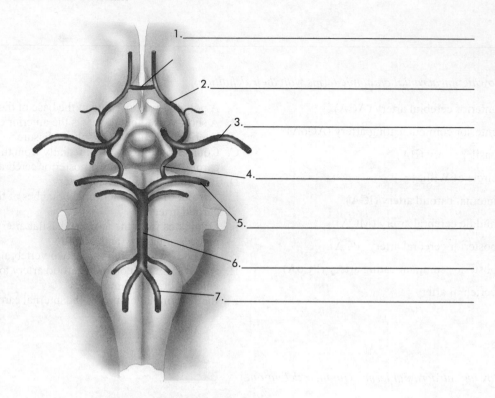

1. _____

2. _____

3. _____

4. _____

5. _____

6. _____

7. _____

B. Identify the pathway of blood in the subclavian steal.

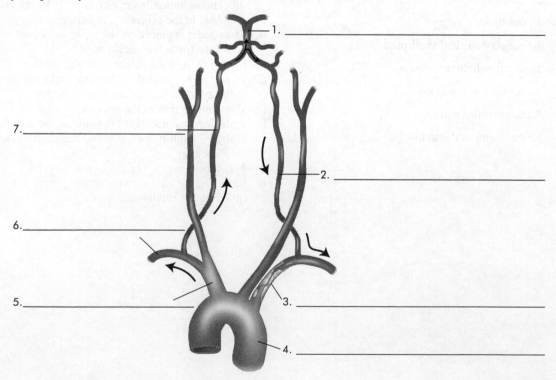

1. _____

2. _____

7. _____

6. _____

3. _____

5. _____

4. _____

Exercise 4

Fill in the blank(s) with the word(s) that best completes the statements about the anatomy of the intracranial cerebrovascular system.

1. Blood supply to the brain is provided by the _____ (anterior) and _____ (posterior) arteries.

2. The first branch of the ICA is the _____ artery, which courses anterior laterally and slightly downward through the optic foramen to supply the globe, orbit, and adjacent structures.

3. The artery that courses posteriorly and medially from the ICA to join the posterior cerebral artery is the posterior

   _____ artery.

4. The larger terminal branch of the ICA is the middle _____ artery.

5. The smaller of the two terminal branches of the ICA is the anterior _____ artery.

6. A short vessel that connects the ACAs at the interhemispheric fissure is the anterior _____ artery.

7. The large branches of the subclavian arteries are the _____ arteries.

8. The artery that is formed by the union of the two vertebral arteries and is evaluated during TCD imaging is the

   _____ artery.

9. The arteries that originate from the terminal basilar artery and course anteriorly and laterally are the

   _____ _____arteries.

10. A polygon vascular ring at the base of the brain that permits communication between the right and left cerebral hemispheres (via the ACoA) and between the anterior and posterior systems (via the PCoAs) is the

    _____ of_____.

Exercise 5

Fill in the blank(s) with the word(s) that best completes the statements about the hemodynamics of the intracranial cerebrovascular system.

1. The percentage of red blood cells by volume in whole blood and a major determinant of blood viscosity is

   _____.

2. Blood viscosity is an important factor influencing intracranial arterial blood _____ velocity.

3. A deficiency of CO_2 in the blood known as hypocapnia or _____ causes a decrease in the MCA mean velocity and an increase in the PI.

4. An excess of CO_2 in the blood referred to as hypercapnia or _____ causes an increase in MCA mean velocity and a decrease in the PI.

Exercise 6

Fill in the blank(s) with the word(s) that best completes the statements about the sonographic evaluation of intracranial evaluation.

1. The approach that is performed with the patient in the supine position with the head aligned straight with the body is

   the _____ window.

2. When the vertebrobasilar system is evaluated, the best results are obtained with the patient lying on his or her side

   with the head bowed slightly toward the chest. This is called the _____ window.

3. The large, circular, anechoic area seen from the suboccipital window is the _____

   _____, and the bright, echogenic reflection is from the occipitaol bone.

4. The _____ window evaluation provides information about the ophthalmic artery and the carotid
   siphon.

5. To evaluate the extracranial distal ICA, the transducer is placed at the angle of the mandible and is angled slightly

   medially and cephalad toward the carotid canal with the _____ window.

PATHOLOGY

Exercise 7

Fill in the blank(s) with the word(s) that best completes the statements about the pathology of the intracranial cerebrovascular system.

1. The most common cause of SAH is leakage of blood from intracranial cerebral aneurysms into the

   _____ space.

2. The hemodynamic effect of vasospasm produces a(n) _____ in blood flow velocity coupled with a
   pressure drop distal to the narrowed segment.

3. When intracranial pressure is increased or the vasomotor reserve has been exhausted, cerebral blood flow can be

   reduced to critical levels, resulting in _____ or infarction.

4. Intracranial arterial _____ cause characteristic alterations in the Doppler signal (audio and spectral waveform),
   including focal increases in velocity, local turbulence, and a poststenotic drop in velocity.

5. An artery providing collateral circulation usually demonstrates a(n) _____ blood flow velocity.

6. Brain stem ischemia associated with stenosis or occlusion of the left subclavian, innominate, or right subclavian

   artery proximal to the origin of the vertebral artery is a symptom of _____ steal syndrome.

7. The "stealing" of blood from the _____ artery, via retrograde vertebral artery flow, causes the

   patient to experience neurologic symptoms of brain stem ischemia.

8. Blood flow is normally _____ from the transducer (suboccipital approach) in the vertebrobasilar

   system. If flow is _____ the transducer in a vertebral artery and the basilar artery, there is evidence of a steal.

Provide a short answer after evaluating the image.

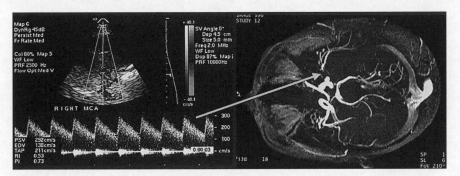

1. Describe the abnormality demonstrated on this transcranial image.

_____

_____

_____

Exercise 1

Match the following peripheral artery terms with their definitions.

_____ 1. anterior tibial artery

_____ 2. corpus cavernosum

_____ 3. axillary artery

_____ 4. brachial artery

_____ 5. claudication

_____ 6. dorsalis pedis artery

_____ 7. innominate artery

_____ 8. ischemic rest pain

_____ 9. Raynaud's phenomenon

_____ 10. popliteal artery

_____ 11. profunda femoris artery

_____ 12. pseudoaneurysm

_____ 13. radial artery

_____ 14. reactive hyperemia

_____ 15. subclavian artery

_____ 16. femoral artery

_____ 17. thoracic outlet syndrome

_____ 18. tibial-peroneal trunk

_____ 19. ulnar artery

A. Continuation of the anterior tibial artery on the top of the foot

B. Perivascular collection (hematoma) that communicates with an artery or a graft; pulsating blood is entering the collection

C. Continuation of the axillary artery

D. Posterior and lateral to the superficial femoral artery

E. Changes in arterial blood flow to the arms may be related to intermittent compression of the proximal arteries (or neural and venous structures)

F. Arterial branch that exits after the anterior tibial artery and bifurcates into the posterior tibial artery and the peroneal artery

G. Supplies the corpus cavernosum with blood

H. Begins at the opening of the adductor magnus muscle and travels behind the knee in the popliteal fossa

I. Originates at the inner border of the scalenus anterior and travels beneath the clavicle to the outer border of the first rib to become the axillary artery

J. Branch of the brachial artery that runs parallel to the radial artery in the forearm

K. Walking-induced muscular discomfort of the calf, thigh, hip, or buttock caused by ischemia

L. First branch artery from the aortic arch

M. Branch of the brachial artery that runs parallel to the ulnar artery in the forearm

N. Begins at the popliteal artery and travels down the lateral calf in the anterior compartment to the level of the ankle

O. Courses the length of the thigh through Hunter's canal and terminates at the opening of the adductor magnus muscle

P. Intermittent digital ischemia in response to cold or emotional stress (primary) or caused by vascular occlusion or stenosis to the digits (secondary)

Q. Alternative method to stress the peripheral arterial circulation

R. Continuation of the subclavian artery

S. Symptom of critical ischemia of the distal limb when the patient is at rest

Exercise 2

Label the following illustrations.

A. The arteries of the lower extremity.

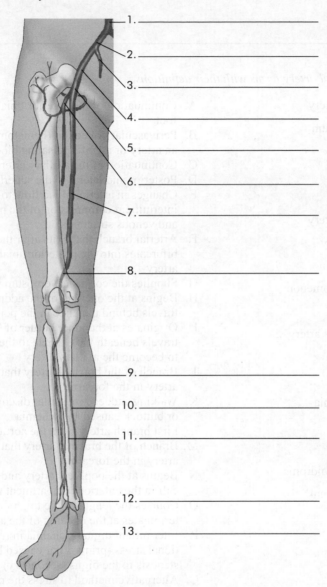

1. _____
2. _____
3. _____
4. _____
5. _____
6. _____
7. _____
8. _____
9. _____
10. _____
11. _____
12. _____
13. _____

B. The arteries of the upper extremity.

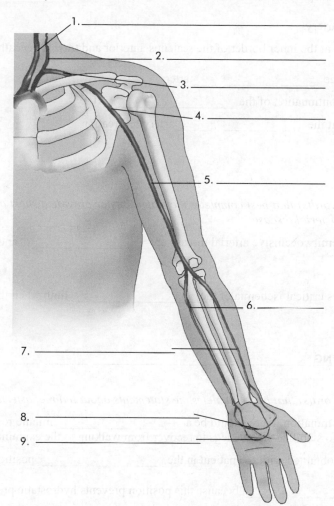

1. _____
2. _____
3. _____
4. _____
5. _____
6. _____
7. _____
8. _____
9. _____

Exercise 3

Fill in the blank(s) with the word(s) that best completes the statements about peripheral arterial anatomy.

1. The descending aorta is divided into a(n)_____ section and a(n) _____section.

2. The abdominal aorta terminates in the _____ of the right and left common iliac arteries

   (approximately at the level of the fourth lumbar vertebra).

3. The external iliac artery terminates at the inguinal ligament, where it becomes the common _____ artery.

4. The common femoral artery originates beneath the inguinal ligament and terminates by dividing into the femoral

   artery and the _____ femoris artery.

5. The popliteal artery begins at the opening of the adductor magnus muscle and travels behind the knee in the

   _____ fossa.

6. The popliteal artery terminates distally into the _____ tibial artery and the tibial

   _____ trunk.

7. A continuation of the anterior tibial artery on the top of the foot is the _____ pedis artery.

8. The artery that is located deep within the calf and travels near the medial aspect of the fibula is the

   _____ artery.

9. The artery that originates at the inner border of the scalenus anterior and travels beneath the clavicle to the outer

   border of the first rib is the _____ artery.

10. The brachial artery is a continuation of the _____ artery.

11. The radial artery begins at the _____ artery bifurcation.

Exercise 4

Fill in the blank(s) with the word(s) that best completes the statements or provide a short answer about the risk factors and symptoms of peripheral arterial disease.

1. Symptoms of lower extremity occlusive arterial disease are _____ and pain at

   _____.

2. Ischemic rest pain implies critical ischemia of the _____ limb when the patient is at rest.

INDIRECT ARTERIAL TESTING

Exercise 5

Fill in the blank(s) with the word(s) that best completes the statements about indirect arterial testing.

1. Before beginning the examination, there should be a _____ minute rest period to allow the patient's blood pressure to stabilize and the legs to recover from walking to the examination room.

2. Segmental pressures are obtained with the patient in the _____ position; the legs should be at the

   same level as the _____ because this position prevents hydrostatic pressure artifact.

3. To obtain pressures comparable with direct intra-arterial measurements, the blood pressure cuff must have a width

   _____ greater than the diameter of the limb.

4. Pressures may be falsely _____ in obese patients, and a proximal thigh pressure may be

   _____ in extremely thin patients.

5. Pulse volume recordings measure changes in _____ limb volume with each cardiac cycle.

Exercise 6

Fill in the blank(s) with the word(s) that best completes the statements or provide a short answer about arterial stress testing.

1. In a healthy individual without occlusive arterial disease, blood flow will _____ with exercise

   because of a _____ in peripheral vascular resistance.

2. Indirect arterial testing is helpful in predicting the likelihood of the _____ of skin lesions.

Exercise 7

Fill in the blank(s) with the word(s) that best completes the statements or provide a short answer about arterial duplex imaging.

1. Arterial duplex imaging provides direct anatomic and physiologic information, but it does not provide information regarding overall limb _____.

2. If a _____ -degree angle cannot be maintained, documentation of the angle used during the examination is important, especially in following the patient over time.

3. In normal vessels, the arterial Doppler signal is _____ from the abdominal aorta to the tibial arteries at the ankle.

4. The characteristic aortic waveform has a high-velocity _____ flow component during systole (ventricular contraction), followed by a brief _____ of flow in early diastole (because of peripheral resistance), and a final low-velocity forward flow phase in late diastole (elastic recoil of the vessel wall).

5. Peak systolic velocity gradually _____ from the proximal to the distal arteries.

6. A pseudoaneurysm may be unilocular or multilocular and may partially contain _____.

7. Identification of the _____ of the pseudoaneurysm is important when ultrasound-guided compression therapy is attempted and color Doppler imaging permits identification of the vessel of origin, which is important when surgical interventions are planned.

8. During _____, blood flows from the native artery into the pseudoaneurysm, and during _____, blood flow returns to the native artery.

Provide a short answer for each question after evaluating the images.

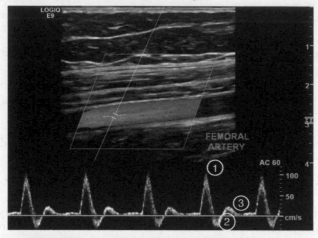

1. Describe the flow pattern in this femoral artery tracing.

_____

_____

_____

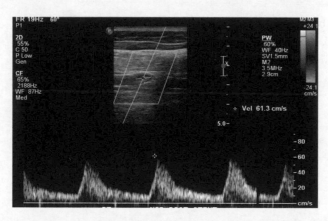

2. This patient presented with claudication. A 40-mmHg drop in pressure was noted from the upper to the lower thigh. The Doppler signal is proximal to the narrowed segment. What does this image show?

_____

_____

_____

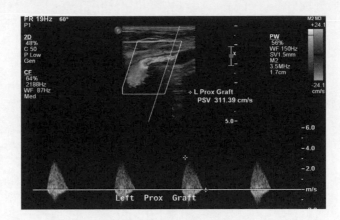

3. Describe what this waveform tells about flow in the bypass graft.

_____

_____

_____

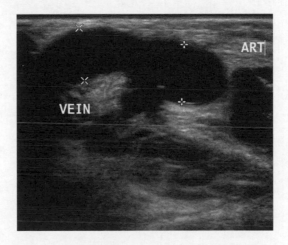

4. This image was taken along the cephalic vein and brachial artery. What vascular abnormality does it demonstrate?

_____

_____

_____

Anterior

Posterior

Uterus

Foregoing

G. Diagram of the fallopian tube.

KEY TERMS

Exercise 1

Match the following anatomy terms with their definitions.

_____ 1. anterior tibial veins

_____ 2. axillary vein

_____ 3. cephalic vein

_____ 4. common iliac vein

_____ 5. gastrocnemius veins

_____ 6. innominate veins

_____ 7. perforating veins

_____ 8. popliteal vein

_____ 9. posterior tibial veins

_____ 10. respiratory phasicity

_____ 11. subclavian vein

_____ 12. valves

_____ 13. internal iliac vein

_____ 14. external iliac vein

A. Paired veins that lie in the medial and lateral gastrocnemius muscles; terminate into the popliteal vein

B. Blood flow velocity changes with respiration

C. Connect the superficial and deep venous systems

D. Begins where the basilic vein joins the brachial vein in the upper arm and terminates beneath the clavicle at the outer border of the first rib

E. Originate from the plantar veins of the foot and drain blood from the posterior compartment of the lower leg

F. Begins on the thumb side of the dorsum of the hand and joins the axillary vein just below the clavicle

G. Folds of the intima that temporarily close to permit blood flow in one direction only

H. Right vein: courses vertically downward to join the left innominate vein below the first rib to form the superior vena cava; left vein: longer than right, courses from left chest to the right beneath the sternum to join the right vein

I. Continuation of the axillary vein joins the internal jugular vein to form the innominate vein

J. Drain blood from the dorsum of the foot and the anterior compartment of the calf

K. Originates from the confluence of the anterior tibial vein with the posterior and peroneal veins

L. Formed by the confluence of the internal and external iliac veins

M. Single vein that travels with the artery beginning at the level of the inguinal ligament

N. Single vein that travels with the iliac artery; drains the pelvis

Exercise 2

Match the following peripheral venous terms with their definitions.

_____ 1. augmentation

_____ 2. basilic vein

_____ 3. common femoral vein

_____ 4. deep femoral vein

_____ 5. greater saphenous vein

_____ 6. lesser saphenous vein

_____ 7. peroneal veins

_____ 8. posterior arch vein

_____ 9. pulmonary embolism

_____ 10. soleal sinuses

_____ 11. femoral vein

_____ 12. varicose veins

_____ 13. Baker's cyst

A. Formed by the confluence of the profunda femoris and the femoral vein; also receives the greater saphenous vein

B. Originates at the hiatus of the adductor magnus muscle in the distal thigh and ascends through the adductor (Hunter's) canal

C. Main tributary of the greater saphenous vein

D. Travels with the profunda femoris artery to unite with the superficial femoral vein to form the common femoral vein

E. Blockage of the pulmonary circulation by foreign matter

F. Blood flow velocity increases with distal limb compression or with the release of proximal limb compression

G. Dilated, elongated, tortuous superficial veins

H. Originates on the dorsum of the foot and ascends posterior to the lateral malleolus and runs along the midline of the posterior calf; terminates as it joins the popliteal vein

I. Large venous reservoirs that lie in the soleus muscle and empty into the posterior tibial or peroneal veins

J. Fluid collection that can be found in the popliteal fossa or upper posterior calf; associated with synovial fluid drainage

K. Originates on the small finger side of the dorsum of the hand and enters the brachial veins in the upper arm

L. Drain blood from the lateral compartment of the lower leg

M. Originates on the dorsum of the foot and ascends anterior to the medial malleolus and along the anteromedial side of the calf and thigh; joins the common femoral vein in the proximal thigh

Exercise 3

Label the following illustrations.

A. The deep veins of the lower extremity.

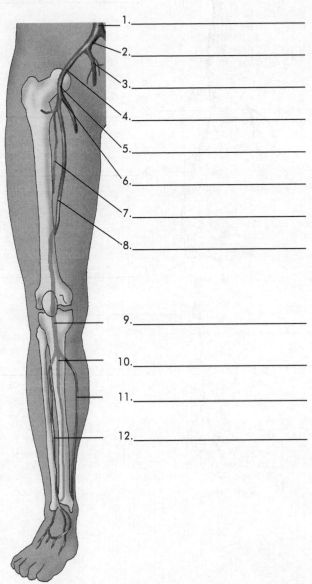

1. _____
2. _____
3. _____
4. _____
5. _____
6. _____
7. _____
8. _____

9. _____
10. _____
11. _____
12. _____

B. The greater saphenous vein.

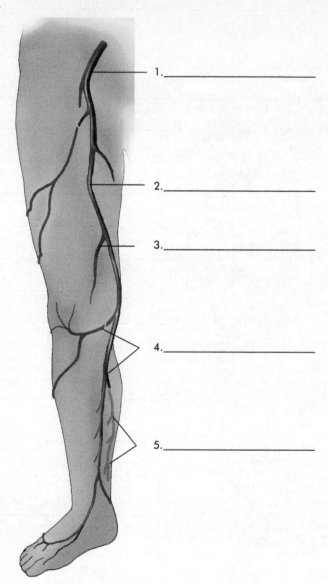

1._____

2._____

3._____

4._____

5._____

C. The lesser saphenous vein.

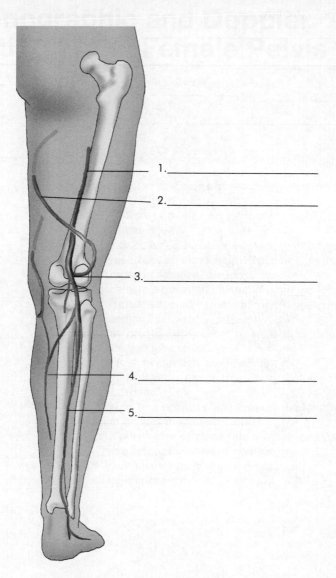

1._____

2._____

3._____

4._____

5._____

D. The deep veins of the upper extremity.

1._____

11._____

10._____

9._____

8._____

2._____

3._____

4._____

5._____

6._____

7._____

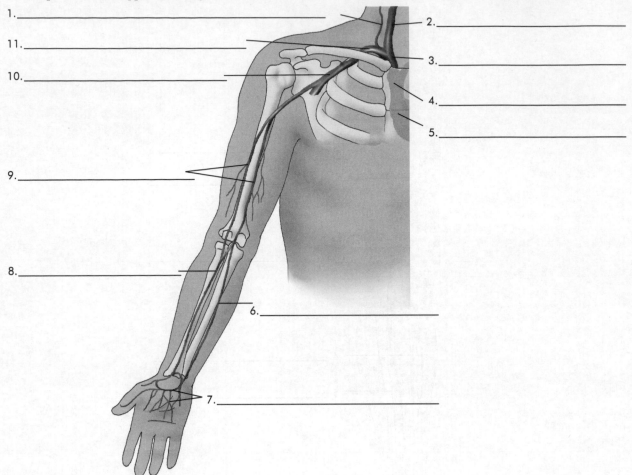

E. The superficial veins of the upper extremity.

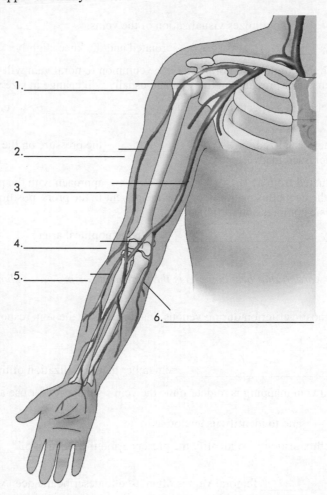

1._____

2._____

3._____

4._____

5._____

6._____

PERIPHERAL VENOUS EVALUATION

Exercise 4

Fill in the blank(s) with the word(s) that best completes the statements about the risk factors and symptoms of vascular disease.

1. A potentially lethal complication of acute DVT is _____ embolism.

2. The chronic process, post-_____syndrome, is a complication that may follow DVT.

3. Varicose veins are dilated, elongated, tortuous _____ veins.

4. Perforating veins provide a channel between the _____ and _____ veins.

5. Venous valves are important in maintaining _____ blood flow from the peripheral veins to the central veins.

Exercise 5

Fill in the blank(s) with the word(s) that best completes the statements about the technical aspects of venous duplex imaging.

1. If the patient is symptomatic, it helps to locate the _____ of pain and to measure any limb

   swelling at the _____ level.

277

2. The bed or table should be placed in reverse Trendelenburg (head elevated) position, which promotes venous

_____ and optimizes visualization of the veins.

3. The leg being evaluated is _____ rotated and the knee slightly _____.

4. In general, compared with the common femoral artery, the common femoral vein will _____ with light to moderate transducer pressure on the skin and usually will change in size with respiration.

5. If superficial thrombophlebitis is suspected, the greater_____ vein should be followed along its entire length.

6. If the saphenous vein is not visualized, _____the pressure on the transducer to make sure that the vein is not being compressed inadvertently.

7. The popliteal vein is evaluated from a _____ approach with the patient's knee rotated externally, with the patient in the decubitus position, or with the patient in the prone position with the foot elevated on a pillow to eliminate extrinsic compression of the vein.

8. The popliteal vein usually lies _____ to the popliteal artery.

Exercise 6

Fill in the blank(s) with the word(s) that best completes the statements or provide a short answer about the peripheral venous examination.

1. The most significant diagnostic criterion during venous imaging is how the vein responds to transducer

_____.

2. If the vein still does not _____, remember that visualization of the thrombus is variable.

3. The purpose of superficial vein mapping is to determine the vein's suitability for use as a bypass

_____ and to identify its anatomic route.

4. The purpose of venous reflux testing is to identify the presence and the location of _____ venous valves.

5. The term _____ femoral vein is often used to describe the deep venous system in the thigh in venous duplex imaging reports. It is advisable to use the term *femoral vein* in venous duplex imaging reports when describing the deep venous system in the thigh.

Exercise 7

Provide a short answer for each question after evaluating the images.

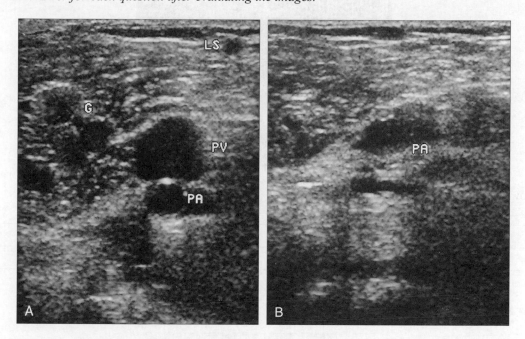

1. Which image (right or left) was made with transducer pressure?

_____

_____

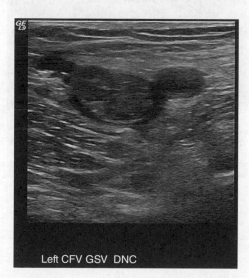

Left CFV GSV DNC

2. This image over the popliteal vein is made with transducer pressure. Describe the sonographic findings. Does this patient have a thrombus?

_____

_____

_____

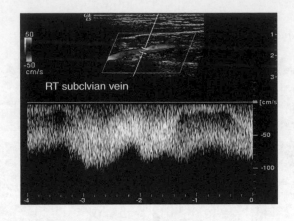

RT subclvian vein

3. Is this flow pattern normal for the subclavian vein?

_____

_____

_____

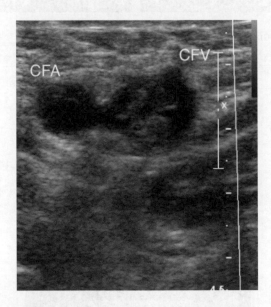

4. This patient presented with tenderness and swelling of the upper thigh. Describe the sonographic findings.

_____

_____

_____

41 Normal Anatomy and Physiology of the Female Pelvis

Exercise 1

Match the following female pelvis anatomy terms with their definitions.

_____ 1. coccygeus muscles

_____ 2. false pelvis

_____ 3. iliacus muscle

_____ 4. iliopectineal line

_____ 5. levator ani

_____ 6. obturator internus muscle

_____ 7. piriformis muscle

_____ 8. psoas major muscle

_____ 9. striations

_____ 10. true pelvis

A. Paired triangular, flat muscles that cover the inner curved surface of the iliac fossae; arise from the iliac fossae, and join the psoas major muscles to form the lateral walls of the pelvis

B. Pelvic cavity found below the brim of the pelvis

C. One of two muscles of the pelvic diaphragm that stretch across the floor of the pelvic cavity like a hammock, supporting the pelvic organs and surrounding the urethra, vagina, and rectum; a broad thin muscle that consists of the pubococcygeus, iliococcygeus, and puborectalis muscles

D. One of two muscles in the pelvic diaphragm; located on the posterior pelvic floor, where it supports the coccyx

E. A flat, pyramidal muscle arising from the anterior sacrum, passing through the greater sciatic notch to insert into the superior aspect of the greater trochanter of the femur; serves to rotate and abduct the thigh

F. Parallel longitudinal lines commonly seen in muscle tissue when imaged sonographically; appear as hyperechoic parallel lines running in the long axis of the hypoechoic muscle tissue

G. A bony ridge on the inner surface of the ilium and pubic bones that divides the true and false pelves

H. Paired muscle that originates at the transverse process of the lumbar vertebrae and extends inferiorly through the false pelvis on the pelvic sidewall, where it unites with the iliacus muscle to form the iliopsoas muscle before inserting into the lesser trochanter of the femur; serves to flex the thigh toward the pelvis

I. Portion of the pelvis found above the brim; that portion of the abdominal cavity cradled by the iliac fossae

J. A triangular sheet of muscle that arises from the anterolateral pelvic wall and surrounds the obturator foramen; passes through the lesser sciatic foramen and inserts into the medial aspect of the greater trochanter of the femur; serves to rotate and abduct the thigh

Exercise 2

Match the following terms related to female pelvic anatomy and uterine positions with their definitions.

_____ 1. anteverted

_____ 2. anteflexed

_____ 3. broad ligament

_____ 4. cardinal ligament

_____ 5. estrogen

_____ 6. mesosalpinx

_____ 7. mesovarium

_____ 8. ovarian ligament

_____ 9. ovum

_____ 10. perimetrium

_____ 11. progesterone

_____ 12. corpus luteum

_____ 13. retroflexed

_____ 14. retroverted

_____ 15. round ligament

_____ 16. space of Retzius

_____ 17. suspensory ligament

_____ 18. uterosacral ligament

A. Position of the uterus when the entire uterus is tipped posteriorly so that the angle formed between the cervix and the vaginal canal is greater than 90 degrees

B. Steroidal hormone secreted by the theca interna and granulosa cells of the ovarian follicle that stimulates the development of female reproductive structures and secondary sexual characteristics; promotes the growth of endometrial tissue during the proliferative phase of the menstrual cycle

C. Female egg; secondary oocyte released from the ovary at ovulation

D. Wide bands of fibromuscular tissue arising from the lateral aspects of the cervix and inserting along the lateral pelvic floor; a continuation of the broad ligament that provides rigid support for the cervix

E. Posterior portion of the broad ligament that is drawn out to enclose and hold the ovary in place

F. Position of the uterus when the uterine fundus bends forward toward the cervix

G. Paired ligaments that extend from the infundibulum of the fallopian tube and the lateral aspect of the ovary to the lateral pelvic wall

H. Anatomic structure on the surface of the ovary, consisting of a spheroid of yellowish tissue that grows within the ruptured ovarian follicle after ovulation; acts as a short-lived endocrine organ that secretes progesterone to maintain the decidual layer of the endometrium should conception occur

I. Broad fold of peritoneum draped over the fallopian tubes, uterus, and ovaries; extends from the sides of the uterus to the side walls of the pelvis, dividing the pelvis from side to side and creating the vesicouterine pouch anterior to the uterus and the rectouterine pouch posteriorly; it is divided into mesometrium, mesosalpinx, and mesovarium

J. Upper portion of the broad ligament that encloses the fallopian tubes

K. Posterior portion of the cardinal ligament that extends from the cervix to the sacrum

L. Serous membrane enveloping the uterus

M. Located between the anterior bladder wall and the pubic symphysis; contains extraperitoneal fat

N. Position of the uterus when the uterus is tipped slightly forward so that the cervix forms a 90-degree angle or less with the vaginal canal; most common uterine position

O. Position of the uterus when the uterine fundus bends posteriorly upon the cervix

P. Paired ligaments that originate at the uterine cornua, anterior to the fallopian tubes, and course anterolaterally within the broad ligament to insert into the fascia of the labia majora; hold the uterus forward in its anteverted position

Q. Steroidal hormone produced by the corpus luteum that helps prepare and maintain the endometrium for arrival and implantation of an embryo

R. Paired ligament that extends from the inferior and/or medial pole of the ovary to the uterine cornua

Exercise 3

Match the following terms related to follicular development, ovulation, and menstruation with their definitions.

_____ 1. amenorrhea

_____ 2. dysmenorrhea

_____ 3. follicle-stimulating hormone

_____ 4. gonadotropin

_____ 5. gonadotropin-releasing hormone

_____ 6. luteinizing hormone

_____ 7. menarche

_____ 8. menopause

_____ 9. menses

_____ 10. menorrhagia

_____ 11. oligomenorrhea

_____ 12. premenarche

A. Hormone secreted by the hypothalamus that stimulates the release of follicle-stimulating hormone and luteinizing hormone by the anterior pituitary gland

B. Hormone secreted by the anterior pituitary gland that stimulates the growth and maturation of graafian follicles in the ovary

C. Abnormally heavy or long menstrual periods

D. Absence of menstruation

E. Refers to cessation of menstruation

F. Abnormally light menstrual periods

G. Pain associated with menstruation

H. Refers to the onset of menstruation and the commencement of cyclic menstrual function; usually occurs between 11 and 13 years of age

I. Hormonal substance that stimulates the function of the testes and the ovaries

J. Periodic flow of blood and cellular debris that occurs during menstruation

K. Time period in young girls before the onset of menstruation

L. Hormone secreted by the anterior pituitary gland that stimulates ovulation and then induces luteinization of the ruptured follicle to form the corpus luteum

ANATOMY AND PHYSIOLOGY

Exercise 4

Label the following illustrations.

A. Pelvic cavity viewed from above.

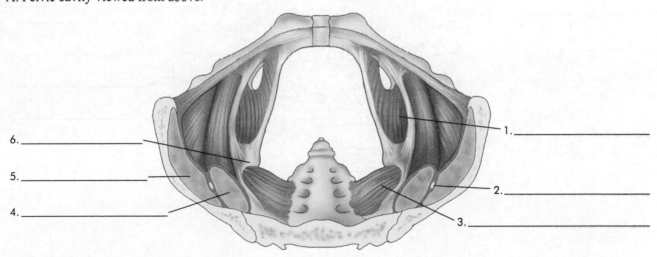

6. _____

5. _____

4. _____

1. _____

2. _____

3. _____

Chapter **41** Normal Anatomy and Physiology of the Female Pelvis

B. The floor of the pelvis.

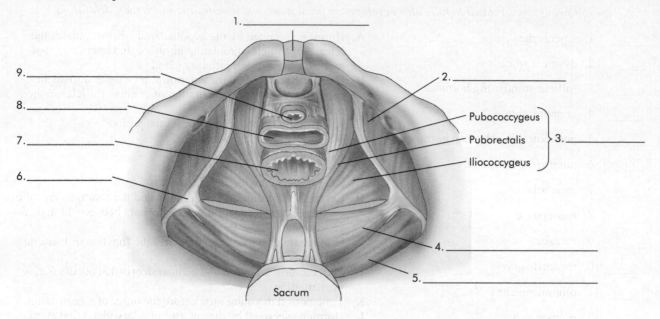

1._____

9._____

8._____

7._____

6._____

2._____

Pubococcygeus

Puborectalis   } 3._____

Iliococcygeus

4._____

5._____

Sacrum

C. Lateral view of the pelvis.

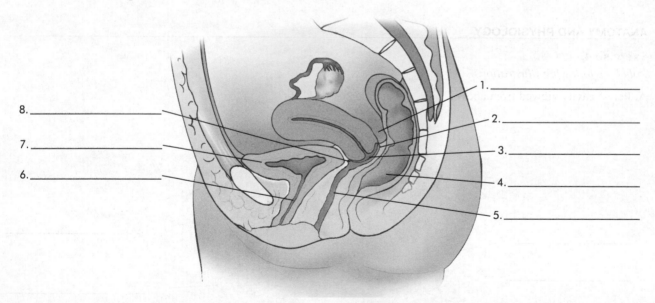

8._____

7._____

6._____

1._____

2._____

3._____

4._____

5._____

D. Coronal view of the vagina, cervix, and uterus.

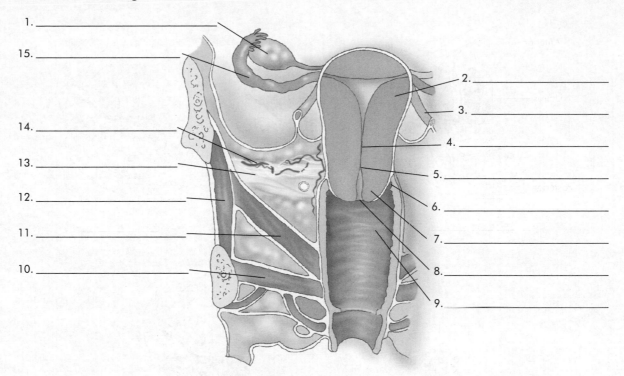

1. _____
15. _____
14. _____
13. _____
12. _____
11. _____
10. _____

2. _____
3. _____
4. _____
5. _____
6. _____
7. _____
8. _____
9. _____

E. Normal female pelvic anatomy.

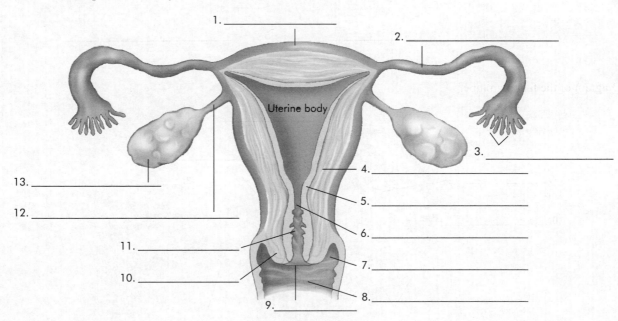

1. _____
2. _____

Uterine body

13. _____
12. _____
11. _____
10. _____
9. _____

3. _____
4. _____
5. _____
6. _____
7. _____
8. _____

F. Identify the uterine positions.

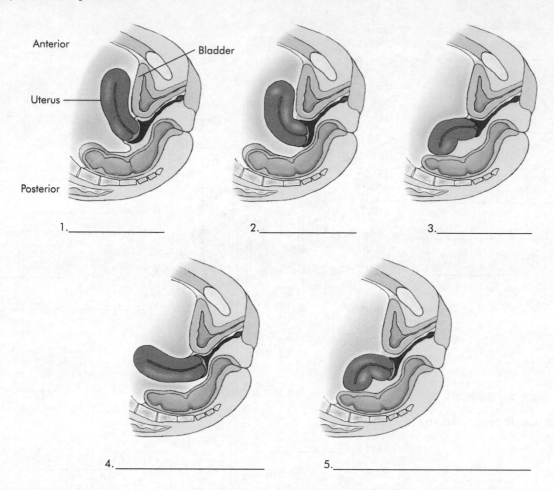

1._____   2._____   3._____

4._____   5._____

G. Diagram of the fallopian tube.

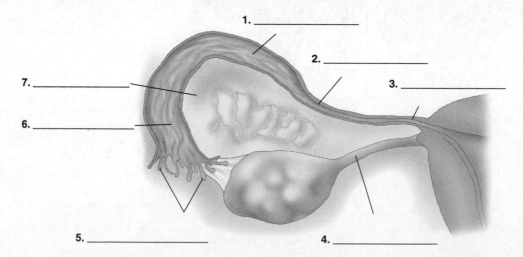

1._____

2._____

3._____

7._____

6._____

5._____   4._____

H. Blood is supplied to the uterus and the vagina by the uterine and vaginal arteries.

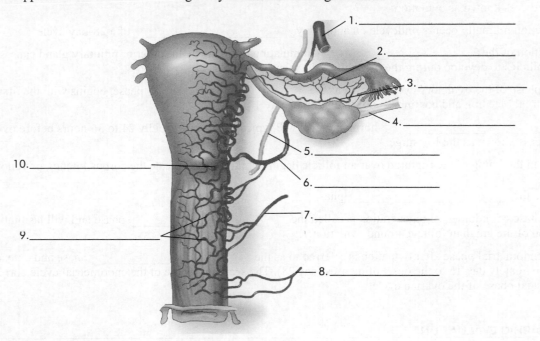

1. _____

2. _____

3. _____

4. _____

5. _____

6. _____

7. _____

8. _____

9. _____

10. _____

Exercise 5

Fill in the blank(s) with the word(s) that best completes the statements about rectouterine spaces.

1. The anterior cul-de-sac, or _____ pouch, is located anterior to the fundus of the uterus between the urinary bladder and the uterus.

2. The posterior cul-de-sac, or _____ pouch, is located posterior to the uterus between the uterus and the rectum.

3. The rectouterine pouch is often referred to as the pouch of _____ and is normally the most inferior and most posterior region of the peritoneal cavity.

4. An additional sonographically significant area is the retropubic space, which is also called the space of

   _____.

5. The retropubic space normally can be identified between the _____ bladder wall and the pubic symphysis.

6. The retropubic space normally contains subcutaneous fat, but a hematoma or abscess in this location may displace

   the urinary bladder _____.

7. The greatest quantity of free fluid in the cul-de-sac normally occurs immediately following

   _____, when the mature follicle ruptures.

Exercise 6

Fill in the blank(s) with the word(s) that best completes the statements about the physiology of the menstrual cycle.

1. The average menstrual cycle is approximately _____ days in length, beginning with the first day of menstrual bleeding.

2. The menstrual cycle is regulated by the _____ and is dependent upon the cyclic release of estrogen and progesterone from the ovaries.

3. During the menarchal years, a(n) _____ is released once a month by one of the two ovaries in a process known as ovulation.

4. Ovulation normally occurs midcycle on about day _____ of a 28-day cycle.

5. Secretion of the _____ stimulating hormone by the anterior pituitary gland causes the ovarian follicles to develop during the first half of the menstrual cycle.

6. This phase of the ovulatory cycle, known as the _____ phase, begins with the first day of menstrual bleeding and continues until ovulation on day 14.

7. The _____ hormone level will typically increase rapidly 24 to 36 hours before ovulation in a process known as the LH surge.

8. Cells in the lining of the ruptured ovarian follicle begin to multiply and create the corpus luteum, or yellow body,

   during the _____ phase.

9. The phase of endometrial regeneration is called the _____ phase and will last until luteinization of the graafian follicle around ovulation.

10. The endometrial phase after ovulation is referred to as the _____ phase and extends from approximately day 15 to the onset of menses (day 28). The secretory phase of the endometrial cycle corresponds to the luteal phase of the ovarian cycle.

SONOGRAPHIC EVALUATION

Exercise 7

Fill in the blank(s) with the word(s) that best completes the statements about the anatomy and sonographic evaluation of the female pelvis.

1. The approach that requires a full urinary bladder for use as an "acoustic window" and typically necessitates the use

   of a 3.5- to 5-MHz transducer for adequate penetration is the _____ approach.

2. A _____ examination is performed with an empty bladder and allows the use of a higher-frequency transducer, typically 7.5 to 10 MHz.

3. The transabdominal scan offers a _____ field of view for a general screening of the pelvic anatomy.

4. The margins of the posterolateral wall of the true pelvis are formed by the _____ and coccygeus muscles.

5. The anterolateral walls of the pelvic cavity are formed by the hip bones and the _____ internus muscles that rim the ischium and pubis.

6. The lower margin of the pelvic cavity, the pelvic floor, is formed by the _____ ani and cocceygeus muscles and is known as the pelvic diaphragm.

7. The area below the pelvic floor is the _____.

8. The muscles of the false pelvis include the _____ major and _____ muscles.

9. The muscles that arise from the lower part of the pubic symphysis and surround the lower part of the rectum,

   forming a sling, are the _____ muscles.

10. A collapsed muscular tube that extends from the external genitalia to the cervix of the uterus is the

   _____.

11. The cervix lies _____ to the urinary bladder and urethra and anterior to the rectum and anus.

12. The largest organ in the normal female pelvis when the urinary bladder is empty is the

_____.

13. At the lateral borders of the uterine fundus are the _____, where the fallopian tubes enter the uterine cavity.

14. The cervix is constricted at its upper end by the _____ os and at its lower end by the external os.

15. The point where the uterus bends anteriorly (anteversion) or posteriorly (retroversion) with an empty bladder is the

_____.

16. The average uterine position is considered to be _____ and anteflexed.

17. The _____ tubes are contained in the upper margin of the broad ligament and extend from the uterine cornua of the uterus laterally where they curve over the ovary.

18. The _____ is often referred to as the fimbriated end of the fallopian tube because it contains fringelike extensions, called fimbriae, which move over the ovary directing the ovum into the fallopian tube after ovulation.

19. The ovaries are usually located _____ to the external iliac vessels and

_____ to the internal iliac vessels and ureter.

20. The cortex of the ovary consists primarily of follicles in varying stages of development and is covered by a layer

of dense connective tissue, the _____.

21. The central _____ is composed of connective tissue containing blood, nerves, lymphatic vessels, and some smooth muscle at the region of the hilum.

22. The _____ arteries extend through the myometrium to the base of the endometrium, where straight and spiral arteries branch off the radial arteries to supply the zona basalis of the endometrium.

42 The Sonographic and Doppler Evaluation of the Female Pelvis

Exercise 1

Match the following patient history and sonographic technique terms with their definitions.

_____ 1. adnexa

_____ 2. anteverted

_____ 3. coronal plane

_____ 4. endometrium

_____ 5. introitus

_____ 6. menarche

_____ 7. menopause

_____ 8. myometrium

_____ 9. parity

_____ 10. premenarche

_____ 11. retroverted

_____ 12. sagittal plane

_____ 13. translabial

_____ 14. transperineal

_____ 15. cornu

A. State after reaching puberty in which menses occurs normally every 21 to 28 days

B. Structure or tissue next to or near another related structure

C. Pregnancy

D. Inner lining of the uterine cavity, which appears echogenic to hypoechoic on ultrasound, depending on the menstrual cycle

E. Across, or through, the labia

F. Refers to a horizontal plane through the longitudinal axis of the body to image structures from anterior to posterior

G. Bending backward

H. Any hornlike projection; refers to the fundus of the uterus, where the fallopian tube arises

I. Across, or through, the perineum

J. Middle layer of the uterine cavity that appears very homogeneous on ultrasound

K. Refers to a vertical plane through the longitudinal axis of the body that divides it into two portions

L. An opening or entrance into a canal or cavity, as the vagina

M. Time before the onset of menses

N. When menses have ceased permanently

O. Tipping forward

Exercise 2

Match the following sonographic evaluation terms with their definitions.

_____ 1. arcuate vessels

_____ 2. internal os

_____ 3. menstruation

_____ 4. Pourcelot resistive index

_____ 5. proliferative phase (early)

_____ 6. proliferative phase (late)

_____ 7. pulsatility index

_____ 8. secretory phase

_____ 9. sonohysterography

_____ 10. S/D ratio

A. Days 1 to 4 of the menstrual cycle; endometrial canal appears as a hypoechoic central line representing blood and tissue

B. Technique that uses a catheter inserted into the endometrial cavity, with instillation of saline solution or contrast medium to fill the endometrial cavity for the purpose of demonstrating abnormalities within the cavity or uterine tubes

C. Days 5 to 9 of the menstrual cycle; endometrium appears as a single thin stripe with a hypoechoic halo encompassing it; creates the "three-line sign"

D. Days 15 to 28 of the menstrual cycle; the endometrium is at its greatest thickness and echogenicity with posterior enhancement

E. Difference between peak systole and end diastole

F. Days 10 to 14 of the menstrual cycle; ovulation occurs; the endometrium increases in thickness and echogenicity

G. Small vessels found along the periphery of the uterus

H. Doppler measurement that takes the highest systolic peak minus the highest diastolic peak divided by the highest systolic peak

I. Doppler measurement that uses peak systole minus peak diastole divided by the mean

J. Inner surface of the cervical os

SAGITTAL AND CORONAL LANDMARKS

Exercise 3

Label the following illustration.

A. Transvaginal sagittal plane. Identify the scanning planes and anatomy.

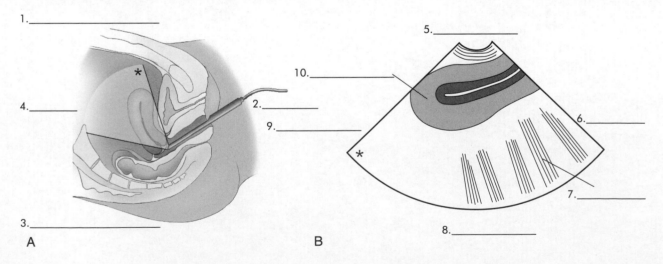

1._____

4._____

3._____

A

5._____

10._____

2._____

9._____

6._____

7._____

8._____

B

B. Transvaginal coronal plane. Identify the scanning planes.

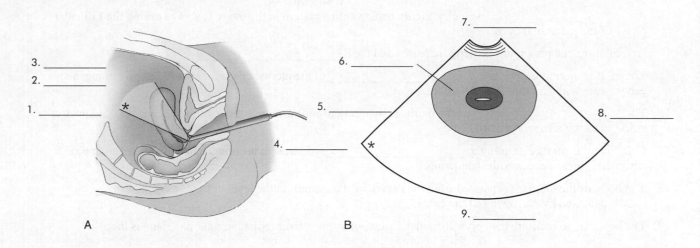

A

B

SONOGRAPHIC EVALUATION

Exercise 4

Fill in the blank(s) with the word(s) that best completes the statements about the sonographic and Doppler evaluation of the female pelvis.

1. The full bladder _____ the bowel and its contained gas from the field of view and

   _____ the anteflexed uterus slightly so that it is more perpendicular to the transducer angle.

2. The bladder shape may be helpful because a well-distended bladder typically has a _____ or elongated shape on midline scans.

3. The _____ vessels can be used as a landmark to identify the lateral adnexal borders.

4. If pathology is present, documentation of the right upper quadrant, (Morison's pouch and subphrenic area), and

   bilateral _____ areas must be obtained.

5. In transvaginal scanning, it is necessary to advance the transducer slightly, angling _____ to

   visualize the fundus, and to withdraw slightly, away from the external os, while angling _____ to see the cervix and the rectouterine recess.

6. These measurements of the uterus and ovaries should be documented: _____,

   _____, and _____.

7. The thickness of the endometrium should be measured in the _____ plane.

8. Pelvic muscles may be mistaken for ovaries, fluid collections, or masses. A _____ bilateral arrangement indicates that they are muscles.

9. Sonographically, sections of the _____ muscle are seen at the posterior lateral corners of the bladder at the level of the vagina and cervix.

10. The muscle that is best visualized sonographically in a transverse plane with caudal angulation at the most inferior

    aspect of the bladder is the _____ muscle.

11. The muscles that are located on either side of the midline posterior to the upper half of the uterine body and fundus

    are the _____ muscles.

Chapter **42** **The Sonographic and Doppler Evaluation of the Female Pelvis**

12. To assess the uterine vessels, the sonographer interrogates just _____ to the cervix and lower uterine segment at the level of the internal os.

13. A _____ velocity, highly resistive flow pattern in the ovary is shown during the follicular phase of the menstrual cycle.

14. At ovulation, the maximum velocity increases and the RI _____.

15. The middle uterine layer is the _____ of the uterus; this layer should have a homogeneous echotexture with smooth-walled borders.

16. The _____ of the uterus is hypoechoic and surrounds the relatively echogenic endometrial stripe, creating a subendometrial halo.

17. Calcifications may be seen in the _____ arteries in postmenopausal women and appear as peripheral linear echoes with shadowing.

18. The body of the uterus is separated from the cervix by the isthmus at the level of the _____ os and is identified by narrowing of the canal.

19. The best way to measure the cervical-fundal dimension of the uterus in the longitudinal plane is the

    _____ technique.

20. During menstruation (days 1 to 4), the _____ canal appears as a hypoechoic central line representing blood and tissue reaching 4 to 8 mm, including the basal layer in this measurement.

21. As menses progress (days 3 to 7), the hypoechoic echo that represented blood disappears, and the endometrial

    stripe is a discrete thin _____ line that is usually only 2 to 3 mm long.

22. In the early proliferative phase (days 5 to 9), the endometrial canal appears as a single _____ stripe.

23. The layer that is seen as a hyperechoic halo encompassing the stripe is the _____ layer.

24. The layer of the endometrium that represents the thin surrounding hyperechoic outermost echo is the _____ layer.

25. During the _____ (luteal) phase (days 15 to 28), the endometrium is at its greatest thickness and echogenicity with posterior enhancement.

26. Sonographically, the postmenopausal endometrial complex is seen as a thin _____ line measuring less than 8 mm, unless a hormone regimen is being followed.

27. If the tubes are distended with or surrounded by a sufficient amount of _____, they can be easily outlined by the contrasting fluid.

28. A useful sonographic marker for the ovary is identification of a _____ cyst, which has the classic appearance of being thin walled and anechoic with through-transmission posteriorly.

29. _____ involves the instillation of sterile saline solution into the endometrial cavity.

Provide a short answer for each question after evaluating the images.

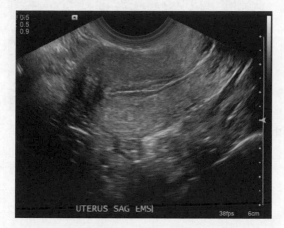

1. Identify the locations of the fundus of the uterus and the cervix in this image.

_____

_____

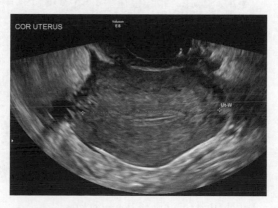

2. Identify the structure in the center of the uterine cavity.

_____

_____

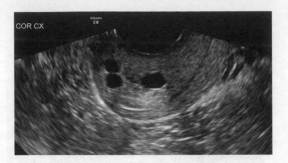

3. Describe the structures seen within the ovary.

_____

_____

_____

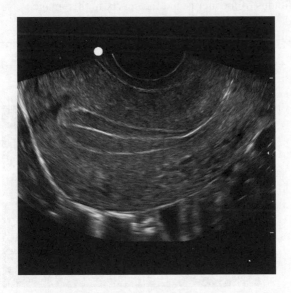

4. Identify the stage of the menstrual cycle that this image demonstrates.

_____

_____

43 Pathology of the Uterus

Exercise 1

Match the following cervical and vaginal pathology terms with their definitions.

_____ 1. cervical polyp

_____ 2. cervical stenosis

_____ 3. dysmenorrhea

_____ 4. ectocervix

_____ 5. ectopic pregnancy

_____ 6. Gartner's duct cyst

_____ 7. leiomyoma

_____ 8. nabothian cyst

_____ 9. squamous cell carcinoma

A. Pain associated with menstruation
B. Small cyst within the vagina
C. Hyperplastic protrusion of the epithelium of the cervix; may be broad-based or pedunculated
D. Portion of the canal of the uterine cervix that is lined with squamous epithelium
E. Benign tiny cyst within the cervix
F. Acquired condition with obstruction of the cervical canal
G. Most common type of cervical cancer
H. Most common benign gynecologic tumor in women during their reproductive years
I. Pregnancy occurring outside the uterine cavity

Exercise 2

Match the following uterine pathology terms with their definitions.

_____ 1. adenomyosis

_____ 2. curettage

_____ 3. intramural leiomyoma

_____ 4. metrorrhea

_____ 5. submucosal leiomyoma

_____ 6. subserosal leiomyoma

A. Type of leiomyoma found to deform the endometrial cavity and cause heavy or irregular menses
B. Benign invasive growth of the endometrium that may cause heavy, painful menstrual bleeding
C. Irregular, acyclic bleeding
D. Scraping with a curette to remove the contents of the uterus, as is done following inevitable or incomplete abortion; to obtain specimens for use in diagnosis; and to remove growths, such as polyps
E. Most common type of leiomyoma; deforms the myometrium
F. Type of leiomyoma that may become pedunculated and appear as an extrauterine mass

297

Exercise 3

Match the following endometrial pathology terms with their definitions.

_____ 1. endometrial carcinoma

_____ 2. endometrial hyperplasia

_____ 3. endometrial polyp

_____ 4. endometritis

_____ 5. hematometra

_____ 6. hydrometra

_____ 7. pyometra

_____ 8. sonohysterography

_____ 9. tamoxifen

A. An antiestrogen drug used in treating some breast carcinomas; reported to cause growth in leiomyomas

B. Pedunculated or sessile well-defined mass attached to the endometrial cavity

C. Obstruction of the uterus and/or the vagina characterized by an accumulation of fluid

D. Malignancy characterized by abnormal thickening of the endometrial cavity; usually associated with irregular bleeding in perimenopausal and in postmenopausal women

E. Obstruction of the uterus and/or the vagina characterized by an accumulation of pus

F. Infection within the endometrium of the uterus

G. Injection of sterile saline into the endometrial cavity under ultrasound guidance

H. Obstruction of the uterus and/or vagina characterized by an accumulation of blood

I. Benign condition that results from estrogen stimulation to the endometrium without the influence of progestin; frequent cause of bleeding

PATHOLOGY

Exercise 4

Fill in the blank(s) with the word(s) that best completes the statements about the pathology of the uterus.

1. The most common finding, seen frequently in middle-aged women, is the presence of _____ cysts.

2. Clinical findings of irregular bleeding may be the result of cervical _____, a condition that arises from the hyperplastic protrusion of the epithelium of the endocervix or ectocervix.

3. An acquired condition with obstruction of the cervical canal at the internal or external os resulting from radiation therapy, previous cone biopsy, postmenopausal cervical atrophy, chronic infection, laser surgery or cryosurgery, or cervical carcinoma is cervical _____.

4. A vaginal _____ is seen in hysterectomy patients after surgery.

5. The most common cystic lesion of the vagina is the _____ duct cyst; it usually is found incidentally during sonographic examination.

6. The most common congenital abnormality of the female genital tract is a(n) _____ hymen, resulting in obstruction.

7. The benign tumor called a _____ is the most common gynecologic tumor, occurring in approximately 20% to 30% of women over the age of 30 with a higher incidence in African American women.

8. Myomas are _____ dependent and may increase in size during pregnancy, although about one half of all myomas show little change during pregnancy.

9. _____ myomas may erode into the endometrial cavity and cause irregular or heavy bleeding, which may lead to anemia.

10. The most common cause of uterine calcification is _____; a less common cause is _____ artery calcification in the periphery of the uterus.

11. The ectopic occurrence of nests of endometrial tissue within the myometrium is _____ and is more extensive in the posterior wall.

12. Uterine _____ malformations (AVMs) consist of a vascular plexus of arteries and veins without an intervening capillary network.

13. The most common cause of abnormal uterine bleeding in both premenopausal and postmenopausal women that develops from unopposed estrogen stimulation is endometrial _____.

14. Ideally a woman using _____ hormones should be studied at the beginning or end of her hormone cycle, when the endometrium is theoretically at its thinnest.

15. Sonographically, _____ appear toward the end of the luteal phase and are represented by a hypoechoic region within the hyperechoic endometrium.

16. _____ most often occurs in association with PID, in the postpartum state, or following instrumentation invasion.

17. Intrauterine _____ (endometrial adhesions, Asherman's syndrome) are found in women with post-traumatic or postsurgical histories, including uterine curettage.

18. The earliest change associated with endometrial _____ is a thickened endometrium; it is also associated with endometrial hypertrophy and polyps.

19. Sonographically, a thickened endometrium (greater than 4 to 5 mm) must be considered _____ until proved otherwise.

20. The _____ _____ device appears as highly echogenic linear structures in the endometrial cavity within the uterine body that are separate from normal, central endometrial echoes.

Exercise 5
Provide a short answer for each question after evaluating the images.

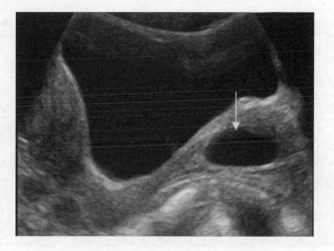

1. Identify the abnormality demonstrated in this transabdominal sagittal image.

_____

_____

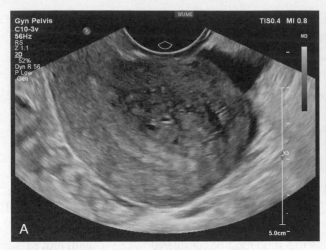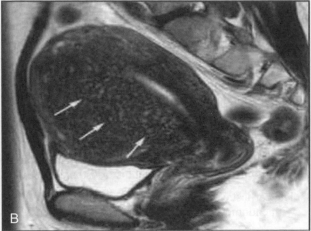

2. What abnormality is shown on this ultrasound and magnetic resonance image?

_____

_____

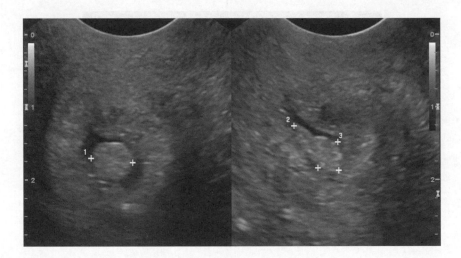

3. What abnormality is seen on these transvaginal images?

_____

_____

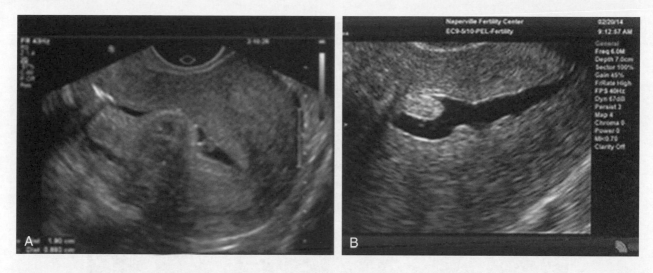

4. Transvaginal images of the uterus demonstrate what abnormality?

_____

_____

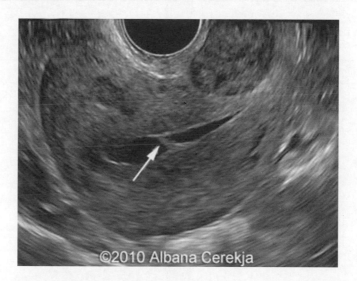

©2010 Albana Cerekja

5. What abnormality is the arrow pointing to in this transvaginal image?

_____

_____

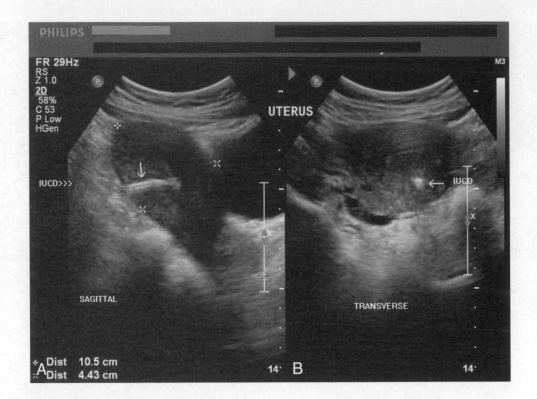

6. A patient presented with pelvic pain. What findings do you see on this ultrasound?

_____

_____

44 Pathology of the Ovaries

KEY TERMS

Exercise 1

Match the following ovarian function and ovarian pathology terms with their definitions.

_____ 1. androgen

_____ 2. cystadenocarcinoma

_____ 3. cystadenoma

_____ 4. estrogen

_____ 5. corpus luteum cyst

_____ 6. dermoid tumor

_____ 7. endometriosis

_____ 8. follicular cyst

_____ 9. functional cyst

_____ 10. Meigs' syndrome

_____ 11. mucinous cystadenocarcinoma

_____ 12. mucinous cystadenoma

_____ 13. ovarian carcinoma

_____ 14. ovarian torsion

_____ 15. paraovarian cyst

_____ 16. polycystic ovarian syndrome

_____ 17. serous cystadenocarcinoma

_____ 18. serous cystadenoma

_____ 19. simple ovarian cyst

_____ 20. surface epithelial-stromal tumors

_____ 21. theca-lutein cysts

A. Second most common benign tumor of the ovary; unilocular or multilocular
B. Cyst that results from the normal function of the ovary
C. Partial or complete rotation of the ovarian pedicle on its axis
D. Multilocular cysts that occur in patients with hyperstimulation
E. Malignant tumor of the ovary with multilocular cysts
F. Smooth, well-defined cystic structure that is filled completely with fluid
G. Condition that occurs when functioning endometrial tissue invades sites outside the uterus
H. Endocrine disorder associated with chronic anovulation
I. Benign tumor of the ovary associated with ascites and pleural effusion
J. Gynecologic tumors that arise from the surface epithelium and cover the ovary and the underlying stroma
K. Malignant tumor of the ovary that may spread beyond the ovary and metastasize to other organs via the peritoneal channels
L. Benign tumor composed of hair, muscle, teeth, and fat
M. Cystic structure that lies adjacent to the ovary
N. Benign tumor of the ovary that contains thin-walled multilocular cysts
O. Most common type of ovarian carcinoma; may be bilateral with multilocular cysts
P. Benign cyst within the ovary that may occur and disappear on a cyclic basis
Q. Benign adenoma containing cysts
R. Small endocrine structure that develops within a ruptured ovarian follicle and secretes progesterone and estrogen
S. Substance that stimulates the development of male characteristics; the ovaries will synthesize some of these substances and convert them to estrogens
T. Female hormone produced by the ovary
U. Malignant tumor that forms cysts

Exercise 2

Label the following illustration.

A. Normal anatomy of the female pelvis.

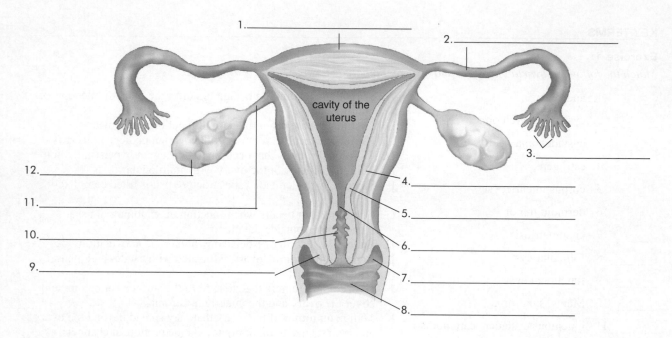

cavity of the uterus

1. _____

2. _____

3. _____

4. _____

5. _____

6. _____

7. _____

8. _____

9. _____

10. _____

11. _____

12. _____

PATHOLOGY

Exercise 3

Fill in the blank(s) with the word(s) that best completes the statements about the pathology and sonographic evaluation of the ovaries.

1. In the anteflexed midline uterus, the ovaries are usually identified _____ to the cornu of the uterus.

2. Following hysterectomy, the ovaries tend to be located more _____ and directly superior to the vaginal cuff.

3. The normal ovary has a(n) _____ echotexture, which may exhibit a central, more echogenic medulla with small anechoic or cystic follicles seen in the cortex.

4. Small anechoic or cystic follicles may be seen _____ in the cortex.

5. During the early _____ phase, many follicles develop and increase in size until about day 8 or 9 of the menstrual cycle.

6. The cumulus _____ may occasionally be detected as an eccentrically located, cystlike, 1-mm internal mural protrusion.

7. If the fluid in the nondominant follicles is not reabsorbed, a(n) _____ cyst develops.

8. The occurrence of fluid in the cul-de-sac is commonly seen after ovulation and peaks in the early _____ phase.

9. Following ovulation in the luteal phase, a mature _____ _____ develops and may be identified sonographically as a small hypoechoic or isoechoic structure peripherally within the ovary.

10. Any simple cyst that hemorrhages may appear as a _____ mass.

11. The more sonographically complex the tumor, the more likely it is to be _____, especially if associated with ascites.

12. Patients with normal menstrual cycles are best scanned in the first _____ days of the cycle; this prevents confusion with normal changes in intraovarian blood flow because high diastolic flow occurs in the luteal phase.

13. A mass showing complete absence of or very little diastolic flow (very elevated RI and PI values) is usually

_____.

14. Duplex Doppler reveals prominent _____ flow in corpus luteum cysts. This low-velocity waveform is present throughout the luteal phase of the cycle.

15. Echogenic, free intraperitoneal fluid in the cul-de-sac can help confirm the diagnosis of a _____ or leaking hemorrhagic cyst.

16. The largest of the functional cysts are _____ cysts and appear as very large, bilateral, multiloculated cystic masses. This mass is associated with high levels of human chorionic gonadotropin (hCG) and is seen most frequently in association with gestational trophoblastic disease.

17. A frequent iatrogenic complication of ovulation induction is ovarian _____ syndrome. The ovaries are enlarged but measure less than 5 cm in diameter.

18. An endocrinologic disorder associated with chronic anovulation with an imbalance of LH and FSH resulting in

abnormal estrogen and androgen production is _____ ovarian syndrome

19. Paraovarian cysts account for approximately 10% of adnexal masses; they arise from the _____ ligament and usually are of mesothelial or paramesonephric origin.

20. Endometriosis is a common condition in which functioning _____ tissue is present outside the uterus.

21. The localized form consists of a discrete mass called an endometrioma, or _____ cyst.

22. Endometriosis may appear as bilateral or unilateral ovarian cysts with patterns ranging from anechoic to solid,

depending on the amount of _____ and its organization.

23. Torsion of the ovary is caused by partial or _____ rotation of the ovarian pedicle on its axis.

24. Ovarian torsion produces an enlarged _____ ovary, usually greater than 4 cm in diameter.

25. Unilocular or thinly septated cysts are more likely _____.

26. Multilocular thickly septated masses and masses with solid nodules are more likely _____.

27. Ovarian cancer can present as a complex, cystic, or solid mass, but it is more likely preponderantly

_____.

28. The incidence of ovarian cancer is greatly _____ in women who have had breast and colon cancer.

29. Malignant tumor growth is dependent on _____ with the development of abnormal tumor vessels. This leads to decreased vascular resistance and higher diastolic flow velocity.

30. The _____ are more involved with metastatic disease than any other pelvic organ.

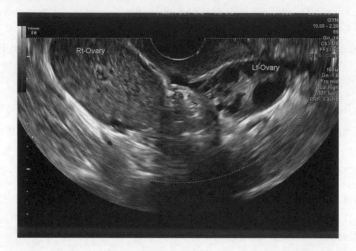

1. Young female presents with severe lower pelvic pain.

_____

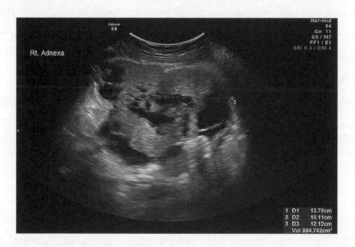

2. A transvaginal ultrasound was performed on a 49-year-old woman whose presenting symptom was a palpable mass. What is your sonographic finding?

_____

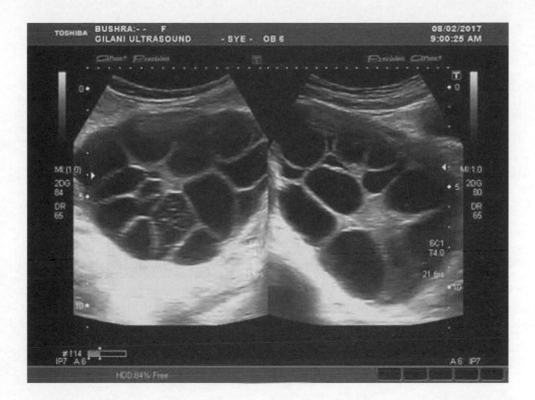

3. Describe your sonographic findings in this transvaginal image of the ovaries in a patient with hydatidiform mole.

_____

_____

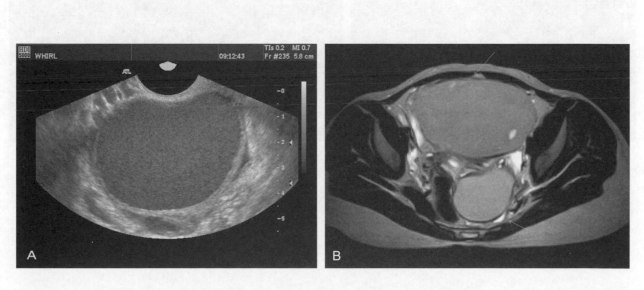

4. A patient with severe pelvic pain. Describe the sonographic findings.

_____

_____

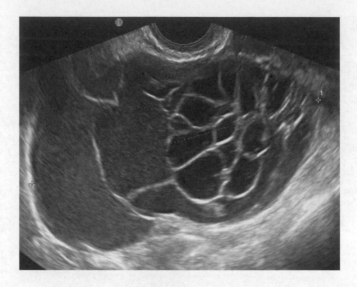

5. A 37-year-old female presented with mild abdominal distention and bloating for 1 month. Describe the sonographic findings.

_____

_____

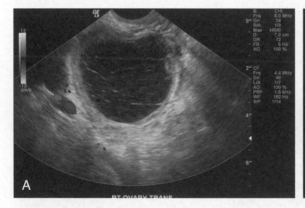
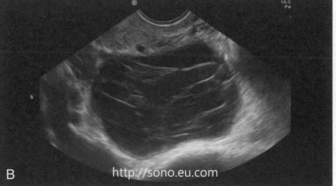

6. What abnormality is most likely represented by these follow-up images of a ovarian cyst?

_____

_____

45 Adenexa

Exercise 1

Match the following adnexa pathology terms with their definitions.

_____ 1. adenomyosis

_____ 2. *Chlamydia trachomatis*

_____ 3. endometrioma

_____ 4. endometriosis

_____ 5. endometritis

_____ 6. hydrosalpinx

_____ 7. myometritis

_____ 8. oophoritis

_____ 9. parametritis

_____ 10. pelvic inflammatory disease

_____ 11. periovarian inflammation

_____ 12. pyosalpinx

_____ 13. salpingitis

_____ 14. tubo-ovarian abscess

_____ 15. tubo-ovarian complex

A. Fluid within the fallopian tube
B. Infection that involves the fallopian tube and the ovary
C. Localized tumor of endometriosis most frequently found in the ovary, cul-de-sac, rectovaginal septum, and peritoneal surface of the posterior wall of the uterus
D. All-inclusive term that refers to all pelvic infections
E. Infection within the endometrium of the uterus
F. Infection within the fallopian tubes
G. Condition that occurs when functioning endometrial tissue invades sites outside the uterus
H. Infection within the ovary
I. Fusion of the inflamed dilated tube and ovary
J. Infection within the uterine serosa and broad ligaments
K. Enlarged ovaries with multiple cysts and indistinct margins
L. Organism that causes a great variety of diseases, including genital infections in men and women
M. Infection within the myometrium of the uterus
N. Benign invasive growth of the endometrium into the muscular layer of the uterus
O. Retained pus within the inflamed fallopian tube

PATHOLOGY

Exercise 2

Fill in the blank(s) with the word(s) that best completes the statements about the pathology of the adnexa.

1. Infrequently, a pelvic infection may ascend the right flank, causing perihepatic inflammation that may mimic liver, gallbladder, or right renal pain. This perihepatic inflammation is called the Fitz- Hugh-_____ syndrome.

2. Sexually transmitted PID is spread via the _____ of the pelvic organs through the cervix into the pelvic cavity.

3. Infection in the uterine endometrium is known as _____; inflammation in the fallopian tubes is called acute

   _____.

4. As the dilated tube becomes obstructed, it becomes filled with pus, a condition known as _____.

5. Clinically, patients with pelvic inflammatory disease may present with intense pelvic _____ and

   tenderness described as dull and aching, with constant _____ discharge.

6. An obstructed tube filled with serous secretions is a _____; this can occur as a result of PID, endometriosis, or postoperative adhesions.

7. Severe and chronic pyosalpinx often contains thick, mucoid pus, which does not transmit sound as well as serous

   fluid or blood. On ultrasound, this would appear _____.

8. When periovarian adhesions that distort anatomy form, the ovary cannot be separated from the inflamed dilated tube and is called the _____ complex.

9. Inflammation of the peritoneum—the serous membrane lining the abdominal cavity and covering the viscera—is called _____.

10. Internal endometriosis is called _____ and occurs within the uterus. External endometriosis is called _____ and occurs outside the uterus (i.e., in the pouch of Douglas, surface of the ovary and fallopian tube and uterus, broad ligaments, and rectovaginal septum).

11. Endometriomas may appear as bilateral or unilateral ovarian cysts with sonographic patterns ranging from _____ to _____, depending on the amount of blood and its organization.

Exercise 3

Provide a short answer for each question after evaluating the images.

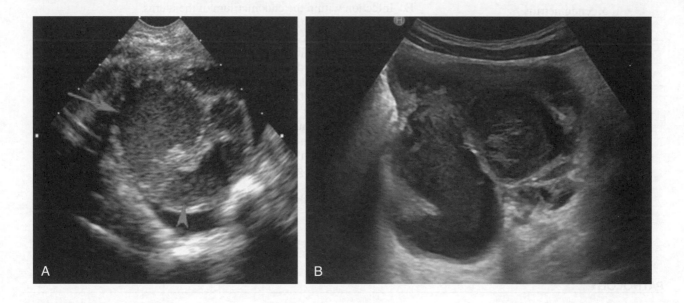

1. This patient presented with pelvic pain for 1 month. Describe your findings.

_____

_____

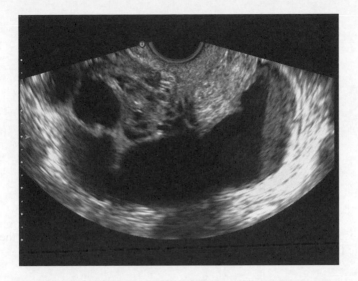

2. A young woman presents with pain, adnexal tenderness, and fever for 2 weeks. What are your sonographic findings of the pelvic ultrasound?

_____

_____

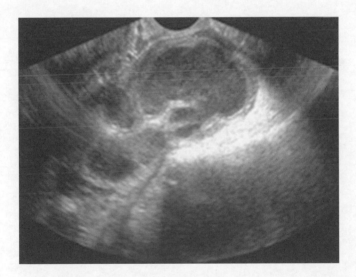

3. Ultrasound of the right lower quadrant was done in a patient with extreme pain and tenderness. What is your finding?

_____

_____

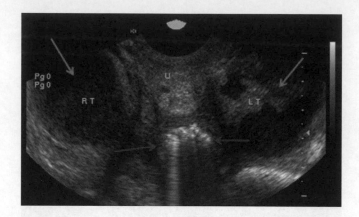

4. A 23-year-old female presented with fever, vaginal discharge, and acute pelvic pain for the past several days. Describe the sonographic findings.

_____

_____

KEY TERMS

Exercise 1

Match the following female infertility terms with their definitions.

_____ 1. assisted reproductive technology

_____ 2. embryo transfer

_____ 3. gonadotropin

_____ 4. human chorionic gonadotropin

_____ 5. intrauterine insemination

_____ 6. in vitro fertilization (IVF)

_____ 7. ovarian hyperstimulation syndrome (OHSS)

_____ 8. ovulation induction therapy

A. Method of fertilizing the human ova outside the body by collecting the mature ova and placing them in a dish with a sample of spermatozoa

B. Technique that follows IVF in which the fertilized ova are injected into the uterus through the cervix

C. Syndrome that presents sonographically as enlarged ovaries with multiple cysts, abdominal ascites, and pleural effusions. Often seen in patients who have undergone ovulation induction, post administration of follicle-stimulating hormone, or with a GnRH analog followed by hCG.

D. Technologies employed using male and female gametes to assist the infertility patient to become pregnant.

E. Hormonal substance that stimulates the function of the testes and ovaries

F. Introduction of semen into the uterus by mechanical or instrumental means rather than by sexual intercourse

G. Controlled ovarian stimulation with clomiphene citrate or parenterally administered gonadotropins

H. Glycoprotein secreted from placental trophoblastic cells; this chemical component is found in maternal urine during pregnancy

FEMALE INFERTILITY

Exercise 2

Fill in the blank(s) with the word(s) that best completes the statements about female infertility.

1. Infertility is the inability to conceive within _____ months with regular coitus.

2. The role of the cervix in fertility is to provide a(n) _____ environment to harbor sperm.

3. When assessing the endometrium, the sonographer wants to evaluate the thickness and echogenicity characteristics and to include evaluation for any _____ lesions.

4. The congenital anomalies most easily assessed with ultrasound require evaluation for _____ uterus and didelphys uterus.

5. _____ uterus is associated with a low incidence of fertility complications.

6. The fallopian tubes can be examined by ultrasound to evaluate for a hydrosalpinx and assess _____ by injecting saline into the tube and looking for spillage of fluid into the cul-de-sac or by using contrast to evaluate for spillage.

7. A follicle is selected to develop into a _____ follicle in response to follicle-stimulating hormone (FSH) and an increase in estradiol.

8. The dominant follicle will grow at a rate of approximately 2 to 3 mm per day until it reaches an average diameter of _____ mm.

9. If serum estradiol is (elevated/decreased) and a large ovarian cyst is present, then oral contraceptives may be indicated to suppress follicular activity before ovarian stimulation therapy is started.

10. A normal endometrial response associated with ovarian stimulation is increasing thickness from 2 to 3 mm to

   _____ mm.

11. Complications associated with assisted reproductive technologies include ovarian _____ syndrome, multiple gestations, and ectopic pregnancy.

12. Ovarian _____ is a syndrome that presents sonographically as enlarged ovaries with multiple cysts, abdominal ascites, and pleural effusions.

13. An ectopic pregnancy coexisting with an intrauterine pregnancy is a(n) _____ pregnancy.

Exercise 3

Provide a short answer for each question after evaluating the images.

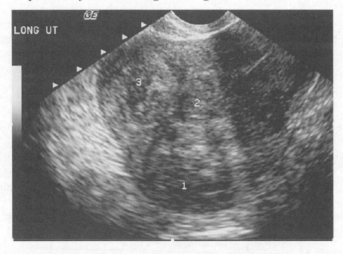

1. Identify the abnormality demonstrated in this infusion sonography image.

_____

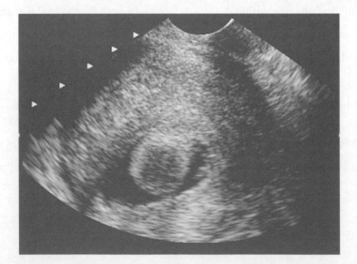

2. Which abnormality, demonstrated in this infusion sonography image, may interfere with implantation?

_____

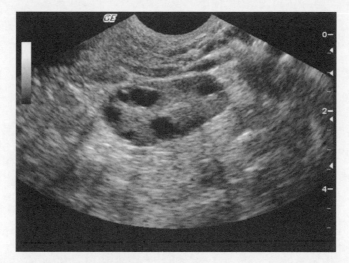

3. Identify the phase of the ovary shown in this image.

_____

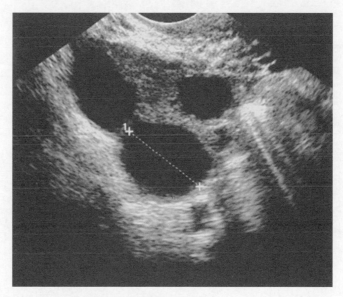

4. This transvaginal image of the ovary is found in what situation?

_____

47 The Role of Sonography in Obstetrics

Exercise 1

Match the following terms related to indications for obstetric sonography with their definitions.

_____ 1. abruptio placentae

_____ 2. amniocentesis

_____ 3. anencephaly

_____ 4. cerclage

_____ 5. embryonic age (or conception age)

_____ 6. gestational age

_____ 7. hydatidiform mole

_____ 8. incompetent cervix

_____ 9. intrauterine growth restriction (IUGR)

_____ 10. macrosomia

_____ 11. maternal serum alpha-fetoprotein (MSAFP)

_____ 12. oligohydramnios

_____ 13. placenta

_____ 14. placenta previa

_____ 15. polyhydramnios

_____ 16. aneuploidy

_____ 17. quad screen

A. Age of embryo stated as time from day of conception

B. Length of pregnancy defined in the as number of weeks from first day of last normal menstrual period (LNMP)

C. Neural tube defect characterized by absence of the brain, including the cerebrum, the cerebellum, and basal ganglia

D. One of several biochemical tests used to assess fetal risk for aneuploidy or fetal defect; a component of the "triple screen," the normal value of MSAFP, varies with gestational age, and assessment of gestational age is essential for accurate interpretation of results

E. Bleeding from a normally situated placenta as a result of its complete or partial detachment after the 20th week of gestation

F. Condition in which the cervix dilates silently during the second trimester; without intervention, the membranes bulge through the cervix and rupture, and the fetus drops out, resulting in a premature preterm delivery

G. Ligatures around the cervix uteri to treat cervical incompetence during pregnancy

H. Reduced growth rate or abnormal growth pattern of the fetus, resulting in a small for gestational age fetus

I. Aspiration of a sample of amniotic fluid through the mother's abdomen for diagnostic analysis of fetal genetics, maturity, and/or disease

J. Exceptionally large infant with excessive fat deposition in the subcutaneous tissue; most frequently seen in fetuses of diabetic mothers

K. Abnormal conception in which there is partial or complete conversion of the chorionic villi into grapelike vesicles

L. Placental implantation encroaches upon the lower uterine segment; if the placenta presents first in late pregnancy, bleeding is inevitable

M. Organ of communication whereby nutrition and products of metabolism are interchanged between the fetal and maternal blood systems; is formed from the chorion frondosum with a maternal decidual contribution

N. Excessive amount of amniotic fluid

O. Reduced amount of amniotic fluid

P. Maternal serum biochemical levels in the second trimester of human chorionic gonadotropin, alpha-fetoprotein, estriol, and inhibin A

Q. Fetal syndrome associated with abnormal number of chromosomes

Exercise 2

Match the following terms related to obstetric sonography during the first, second, and third trimesters with their definitions.

_____ 1. amnion

_____ 2. cervix

_____ 3. chorion

_____ 4. corpus luteum

_____ 5. ductus venosum

_____ 6. embryo

_____ 7. gestational sac

_____ 8. lower uterine segment

_____ 9. trimester

_____ 10. umbilical cord

_____ 11. yolk sac

_____ 12. zygote

A. Cellular, outermost extraembryonic membrane, composed of trophoblast lined with mesoderm
B. Products of conception from fertilization through implantation; the zygotic stage of pregnancy lasts for approximately 12 days after conception
C. Vascular structure within the fetal liver that connects the umbilical vein to the inferior vena cava and allows oxygenated blood to bypass the liver and return directly to the heart
D. Functional structure within the normal ovary that is formed from cells lining the graafian follicle after ovulation; it produces estrogen and progesterone and may become enlarged and appear cystic during early pregnancy
E. Inferior segment of the uterus, which normally is more than 3.5 cm long during pregnancy and decreases in length during labor
F. Connecting lifeline between the fetus and the placenta; it contains two umbilical arteries, which carry deoxygenated fetal blood, and one umbilical vein, which carries oxygenated fetal blood encased in Wharton's jelly
G. Developing individual from implantation to the end of the ninth week of gestation
H. Smooth membrane enclosing the fetus and amniotic fluid; it is loosely fused with the outer chorionic membrane except at the placental insertion of the umbilical cord, where it is contiguous with the membranes surrounding the umbilical cord
I. Thin expanded lower portion of the uterus that forms in the last trimester of pregnancy
J. Circular structure within the gestational sac seen sonographically between 4 and 10 weeks' gestational age; supplies nutrition, facilitates waste removal, and is the site of origin of early hematopoietic stem cells in the embryo
K. A 40-week pregnancy is divided into three 13-week periods from the first day of the last normal menstrual period
L. Structure lined by the chorion that normally implants within the uterine decidua and contains the developing embryo

48 Clinical Ethics for Obstetric Sonography

KEY TERMS

Exercise 1

Match the following clinical ethics terms with their definitions.

_____ 1. autonomy

_____ 2. beneficence

_____ 3. confidentiality

_____ 4. ethics

_____ 5. informed consent

_____ 6. integrity

_____ 7. justice

_____ 8. morality

_____ 9. nonmaleficence

_____ 10. respect for persons

_____ 11. veracity

A. The study of what is good and bad and of moral duty and obligation; systematic reflection on and analysis of morality

B. Bringing about good by maximizing benefits and minimizing possible harm

C. Truthfulness, honesty

D. Refraining from harming oneself or others

E. Incorporates both respect for the autonomy of individuals and the requirement to protect those with diminished autonomy

F. Self-governing or self-directing freedom and especially moral independence; the right of persons to choose and to have their choices respected

G. Adherence to moral and ethical principles

H. The protection of cherished values that relate to how persons interact and live in peace

I. Holding information in confidence; respect for privacy

J. The ethical principle that requires fair distribution of benefits and burdens

K. Providing complete information and ensuring comprehension and voluntary consent by a patient or subject to a required or experimental medical procedure

PRINCIPLES OF MEDICAL ETHICS

Exercise 2

Fill in the blank(s) with the word(s) that best completes the statements about medical ethics.

1. Ethics is defined as systematic reflection on and analysis of _____.

2. Morality concerns _____ and wrong conduct (what we ought to or ought not to do) and _____ and bad character (the kinds of persons we should become and the virtues we should cultivate in doing so).

3. Morality reflects duties and _____.

4. To demonstrate values, a person has to have rights of expression, so freedom and _____ are also integral parts of morality.

5. Discussion, reflection, and discourse on morality are known as _____.

6. Hippocrates cautioned his students to *primum non nocere*, which means, "_____ ___ _____ _____."

7. The principle of _____ directs the sonographer to not cause harm.

8. Application of the principle of nonmaleficence requires the sonographer to obtain appropriate _____ and clinical skills to ensure competence in performing each examination required.

9. Use of obstetric ultrasound must be justified by the goal of seeking the greater balance of clinical "goods" over "harms," not simply preventing harm to the patient at all cost. This ethical principle is called _____ and provides a more comprehensive basis for ethics in sonography than is provided by nonmaleficence.

10. Beneficence encourages sonographers to go beyond the _____ standard protocol and to seek additional images and information if achievable and in the best interests of patients.

11. Beneficence requires sonographers to focus on small comforts for the patient, respecting their _____ and the inclusion of family.

12. Beneficence, similar to nonmaleficence, requires _____, _____, and excellent _____ skills to ensure that the patient and the fetus receive the greatest benefit of the examination.

13. A person's capacity to formulate, express, and carry out value-based preferences is referred to as _____.

14. Informed _____ is an autonomy-based right. Each health professional has autonomy-based obligations regarding this process.

15. If a practitioner asks a sonographer to perform an examination that he or she is not competent to do, it is essential for the sonographer to be truthful about his or her limitations to protect the patient. This is an example of

_____.

16. _____ means simply that sonographers must strive to treat all patients equally.

17. Justice and autonomy are the ethical principles that determine the _____ of routine obstetric sonography examinations.

18. The obligation of confidentiality derives from the principles of _____ (the patient will be more forthcoming) and respect for autonomy (the patient's privacy rights are protected).

49 The Normal First Trimester

Exercise 1

Match the following terms related to a normal first trimester with their definitions.

_____ 1. diamniotic

_____ 2. dichorionic

_____ 3. embryologic age

_____ 4. menstrual age

_____ 5. monoamniotic

_____ 6. monochorionic

_____ 7. primary yolk sac

_____ 8. secondary yolk sac

_____ 9. zygote

A. Multiple pregnancy with two chorionic sacs
B. Multiple pregnancy with one chorionic sac
C. Formed at 23 days when the primary yolk sac is pinched off by the extraembryonic coelom
D. Age calculated from when conception occurs
E. Multiple pregnancy with two amniotic sacs
F. First site of formation of red blood cells that will nourish the embryo
G. Multiple pregnancy with one amniotic sac
H. Conceptus resulting from union of male and female gametes
I. Length of time calculated from the first day of the last normal menstrual period to the point at which the pregnancy is being assessed

Exercise 2

Match the following laboratory values and sonographic evaluation terms with their definitions.

_____ 1. amniotic cavity

_____ 2. chorionic cavity

_____ 3. chorionic villi sampling

_____ 4. crown-rump length

_____ 5. decidua basalis

_____ 6. decidua capsularis

_____ 7. double decidual sac sign

_____ 8. embryonic period

_____ 9. hematopoiesis

_____ 10. human chorionic gonadotropin

_____ 11. IUP

_____ 12. MSD

_____ 13. transvaginal transducer

_____ 14. yolk stalk

A. High-frequency transducer that is inserted into the vaginal canal to obtain better definition of first-trimester pregnancy
B. Uterine decidua on the surface of the implantation site
C. Surrounds the amniotic cavity and contains the yolk sac
D. Hormone secreted by the trophoblastic cells of the blastocyst; laboratory test indicates pregnancy when values are elevated
E. Time between 4 and 10 weeks' gestation
F. The umbilical duct connecting the yolk sac with the embryo
G. Most accurate measurement of the embryo in the first trimester
H. Production and development of blood cells
I. Mean sac diameter
J. Interface between the decidua capsularis and the echogenic, highly vascular endometrium
K. Cavity in which the fetus exists; forms early in gestation; fills with amniotic fluid to protect the fetus
L. Intrauterine pregnancy
M. Uterine decidual surface on the maternal side of the placenta
N. Invasive diagnostic genetic testing that involves sampling zygotic cells from developing placental tissue

Exercise 3

Label the following illustrations.

A. Diagram illustrating stages of normal conception.

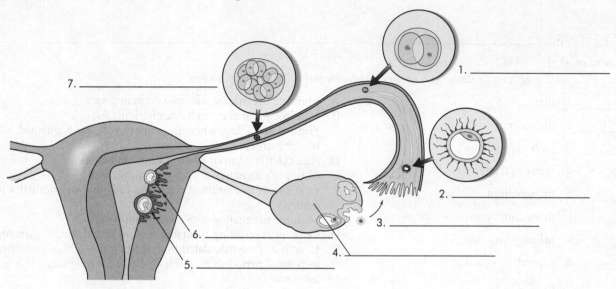

1. _____

2. _____

3. _____

4. _____

5. _____

6. _____

7. _____

B. Schema showing the relation of the fetal membranes and the wall of the uterus.

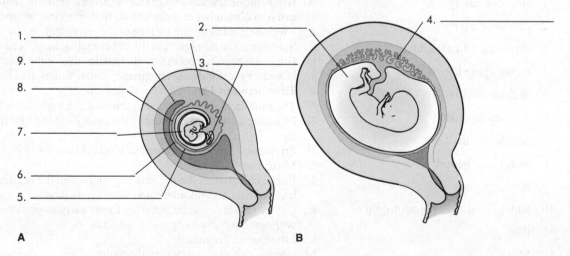

1. _____

2. _____

3. _____

4. _____

5. _____

6. _____

7. _____

8. _____

9. _____

A

B

C. Schematics demonstrating the development of amnion, yolk sac, and embryo.

1. _____
2. _____
3. _____
4. _____
5. _____

6. _____
7. _____
8. _____
9. _____

10. _____
11. _____
12. _____
13. _____

14. _____
15. _____
16. _____
17. _____
18. _____

FIRST TRIMESTER

Exercise 4

Fill in the blank(s) with the word(s) that best completes the statements about early development in the first trimester.

1. Clinicians and sonographers use _____ to date the pregnancy, with the first day of the last menstrual period as the beginning of gestation.

2. In the first 9 menstrual weeks, the conceptus is called a(n) _____.

3. For the time after the first 9 weeks, the embryo is called a(n) _____.

4. The *gestational age* (age known as postmenstrual age) is calculated by adding _____ weeks to conceptional age.

5. The fertilized ovum, which now should be referred to as a _____, undergoes rapid cellular division to form the 16-cell morula.

6. The blastocyst typically enters the uterus 4 to 5 days after fertilization, with implantation occurring _____ days after ovulation.

7. Although the organ function remains as minimal, the _____ system is the first organ to develop rapidly, with the first heartbeats noted between 5.5 and 6 weeks.

8. Gestational sac size and hCG levels increase _____ until 8 menstrual weeks.

9. After 8 weeks, hCG levels _____ and subsequently decline while the gestational sac continues to grow.

10. A normal gestational sac can be consistently demonstrated when the hCG level ranges between _____ mIU/mL.

11. The sonographer must be aware that when the hCG level is elevated and the gestational sac is not seen within the uterus, a(n) _____ pregnancy should be considered.

12. The interface between the decidua capsularis and the echogenic, highly vascularized endometrium forms the _____

    _____ sac sign, which has been reported to be a reliable sign of a viable gestation.

13. The gestational sac size grows at a predictable rate of _____ mm per day in early pregnancy.

14. The first intragestational sac anatomy seen is the sonographic _____ sac, which is routinely visualized between 5 and 5.5 weeks' gestation.

15. The limb buds are embryologically recognizable during the _____ week of gestation.

16. The spine is also developing during the embryonic period, particularly in the _____ week(s) of gestation.

17. The embryonic face undergoes significant evolution starting in the 5th week of gestation, with palate fusion begin-

    ning around the _____ week of gestation.

18. At approximately 10 weeks' gestation, the midgut loop continues to grow and rotate before it descends into the

    fetal abdomen at about the _____ week.

19. The cystic rhomboid fossa can sonographically be imaged routinely from the _____ week of gestation.

20. It is important to note that the _____ ventricles completely fill the cerebral vault in the 8th to 11th week gestation.

Exercise 5

Fill in the blank(s) with the word(s) that best completes the statements about the first trimester of pregnancy.

1. Sonographically, the gestational sac size or mean sac diameter is determined by calculating the average sum of the

    _____, _____, and _____ of the gestational sac.

2. Failure to visualize the yolk sac, with a minimum of _____ mm MSD, using transvaginal sonography, should provoke suspicion of abnormal pregnancy.

3. Transabdominal studies have shown that the yolk sac should be seen within mean sac diameters of _____ mm and should always be visualized with a mean sac diameter of 20 mm.

4. The growth rate of the yolk sac has been reported to be approximately _____ mm per millimeter of growth of the MSD when the MSD is less than 15 mm.

5. The early embryo is not identified with transvaginal sonography until heart motion is detected and the crown-rump

    length measures approximately _____ mm.

6. The embryonic period is the time between _____ and 10 weeks' gestation.

7. The primitive neural tube closes by _____ weeks' gestation.

8. At _____ weeks, three primary vesicles are seen within the fetal brain: the prosencephalon, the mesencephalon, and the rhombencephalon.

9. During development, the midgut loop of the bowel continues to grow and rotate before it descends into the fetal

    abdomen at about the _____ week.

Exercise 6

Fill in the blank(s) with the word(s) that best completes the statements about multiple gestations.

1. Using transvaginal sonography, multiple gestations can readily be diagnosed at very early stages, between _____ weeks.

2. Sonographically, dichorionic and diamniotic twins appear as _____ separate gestational sacs with individual trophoblastic tissue, which allows the appearance of a thick dividing membrane.

3. Monochorionic-diamniotic twins appear to be contained within _____ chorionic sac; _____ amnion(s), yolk sac(s), and _____ embryos are identified.

4. The monozygotic, monoamniotic-monochorionic twin gestation shows _____ gestational sac with _____ amniotic membrane, which may contain one or two yolk sacs and two embryos within the single amniotic membrane.

Exercise 7

Provide a short answer for each question after evaluating the images.

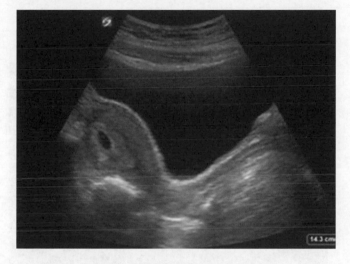

1. Identify the sonographic findings in this early pregnancy.

_____

_____

_____

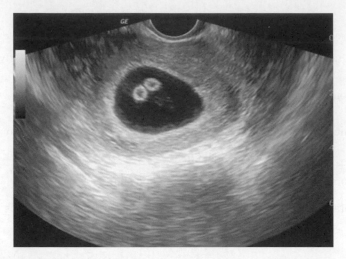

2. What finding is identified in this 6-week gestation?

_____

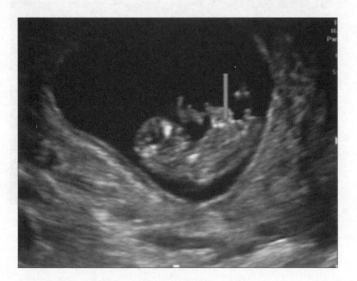

3. Identify the structure (arrow) in this 10-week fetus.

_____

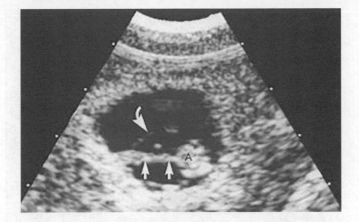

4. In this 8-week gestation, name the structure that the curved arrow is pointing to. Name the structure that the straight arrows are pointing to.

_____

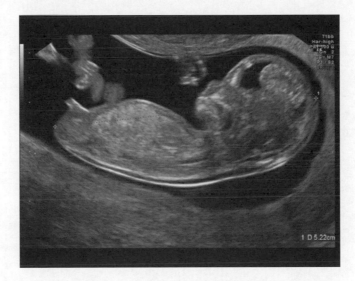

5. What important fetal measurement can be made with this image?

_____

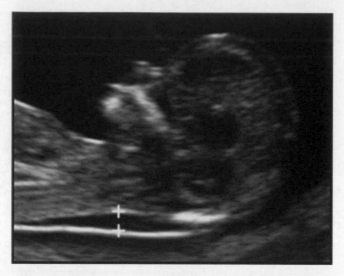

6. This image shows a measurement of what area?

_____

50 First-Trimester Complications

KEY TERMS

Exercise 1

Match the following embryonic abnormality terms with their definitions.

_____ 1. acrania

_____ 2. anencephaly

_____ 3. bowel herniation

_____ 4. cephalocele

_____ 5. cystic hygroma

_____ 6. gastroschisis

_____ 7. holoprosencephaly

_____ 8. iniencephaly

_____ 9. omphalocele

_____ 10. Turner's syndrome

_____ 11. ventriculomegaly

A. Congenital defect of the abdominal wall with protrusion of abdominal contents into the base of the umbilical cord; the cord appears to enter the mass

B. Protrusion of the brain from the cranial cavity

C. Congenital absence of the brain and cranial vault with the cerebral hemispheres missing or reduced to small masses

D. A nonlethal genetic abnormality in which chromosomal makeup is 45 XO instead of the normal 46 XX or XY

E. Congenital defective opening in the wall of the abdomen just to the right of the umbilical cord; bowel and other organs may protrude outside the abdomen from this opening

F. During the first trimester, the bowel normally herniates outside the abdominal cavity between 8 and 12 weeks

G. A rare neural tube defect in which brain tissue protrudes through a fissure in the occiput so that the brain and spinal cord occupy a single cavity

H. Dilation of the cerebral ventricles without enlargement of the cranium

I. Partial or complete absence of the cranium

J. Fluid-filled structure, initially surrounding the neck; may extend upward to the head or laterally to the body

K. Failure of forebrain to divide into cerebral hemispheres, which results in a single large ventricle with varying amounts of cerebral cortex that has been known to occur with trisomies 13 to 15 and trisomy 18

Exercise 2

Match the following first-trimester terms with their definitions.

_____ 1. anembryonic pregnancy

_____ 2. spontaneous pregnancy loss

_____ 3. corpus luteum cyst

_____ 4. ectopic pregnancy

_____ 5. gestational trophoblastic disease

_____ 6. heterotopic pregnancy

_____ 7. incomplete spontaneous abortion

_____ 8. interstitial pregnancy

_____ 9. pseudogestational sac

A. Pregnancy occurring in the fallopian tube near the cornu of the uterus

B. A physiologic cyst that develops within the ovary after ovulation and that secretes progesterone and prevents menses if fertilization occurs; may persist until the 16th to 18th week of pregnancy

C. Simultaneous intrauterine and extrauterine pregnancy

D. Gestational sac without an embryo

E. Pregnancy that implants somewhere other than the center of the uterus

F. Pregnancy loss with products of conception remaining in the uterus

G. Decidual reaction with fluid present within the uterus in a patient with an ectopic pregnancy

H. Additional term for missed abortion or miscarriage

I. Condition in which trophoblastic tissue overtakes the pregnancy and propagates throughout the uterine cavity

Exercise 3

Fill in the blank(s) with the word(s) that best completes the statements or provide a short answer about the abnormal first trimester.

1. The dominant structure seen within the embryonic cranium within the first trimester is that of the

   _____, which fills the lateral ventricles that in turn fill the cranial vault.

2. _____ of the cranial vault is not complete in the first trimester; the resulting false cranial border definition may give rise to a false-negative diagnosis for cranial anomaly.

3. An abnormality that may be seen near the end of the first trimester when there is absence of the cranium superior to the orbits with preservation of the base of the skull and facial features with the brain projected from the open

   cranial vault is _____.

4. In _____, the choroid plexus is shown to be "dangling" in the dilated dependent lateral ventricle.

5. On ultrasound, a large posterior fossa cyst that is continuous with the fourth ventricle, an elevated tentorium, and

   dilatation of the third and lateral ventricles may be seen in a fetus with _____.

6. The fetal urinary bladder becomes sonographically apparent at _____ weeks' gestation.

7. One of the most common abnormalities seen sonographically in the first trimester is _____.

8. Sonographically, placental hematomas may be difficult to distinguish from _____ hemorrhages.

9. By far the most common ovarian mass seen in the first trimester of pregnancy is a(n) _____ cyst.

10. List the associated risk factors for ectopic pregnancy.

    _____

    _____

    _____

11. The most important finding in scanning for ectopic pregnancy is to determine if there is a normal intrauterine gestation (thus ruling out the possibility of an ectopic pregnancy), or if the uterine cavity is _____

    and an adnexal _____ is present.

12. As many as 20% of patients with ectopic pregnancy demonstrate an intrauterine saclike structure known as the

    _____.

13. Cornual pregnancy, or _____, is potentially the most life-threatening of all ectopic gestations.

14. Embryonic cardiac rates lower than _____ beats per minute at any gestational age within the first trimester have been shown to be a poor prognostic finding.

15. The most common occurrence of bleeding in the first trimester results from _____ hemorrhage.

16. Several sonographic findings may be shown with _____ abortion, ranging from an intact gestational sac with a nonliving embryo to a collapsed gestational sac that is grossly misshapen.

17. A proliferative disease of the trophoblast after a pregnancy is _____ disease.

18. In the above condition, serum levels of beta-hCG are dramatically _____, often to greater than 100,000 IU/ml.

19. The characteristic "_____" appearance of hydatidiform mole, which includes a moderately echogenic soft tissue mass filling the uterine cavity and studded with small cystic spaces representing hydropic chorionic villi, may be seen on ultrasound.

20. Bilateral _____ cysts have been reported in as many as half of molar pregnancies.

Provide a short answer for each question after evaluating the images.

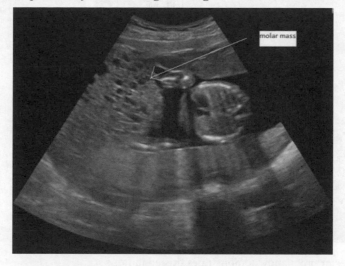

1. The mother presented with an elevated maternal serum alpha-fetoprotein level, larger than appropriate for dates and bleeding. Describe the sonographic findings in this fetus.

   _____

   _____

   _____

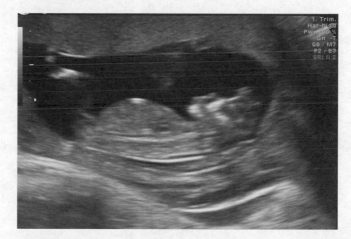

2. A young female in her first trimester presented in the emergency room with elevated human chorionic gonadotropin levels. What is the sonographic finding?

   _____

   _____

   _____

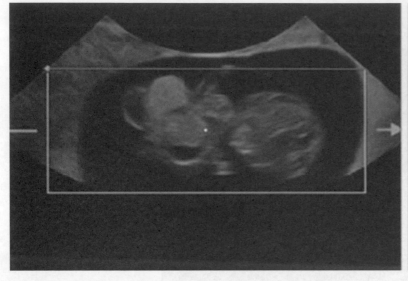
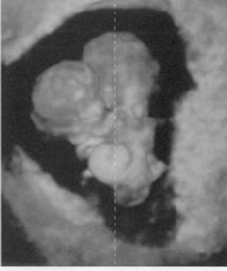

3. Sonogram of a first-trimester pregnancy demonstrates this condition:

_____

_____

_____

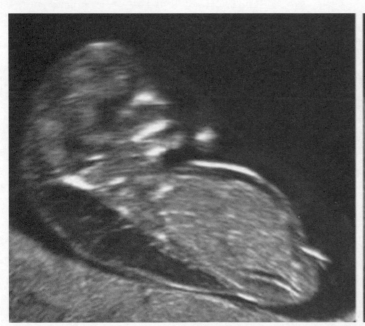
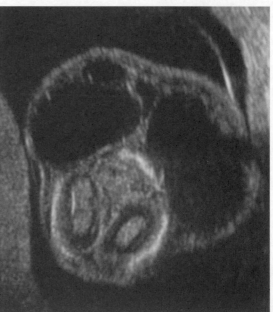

4. Name the abnormal structure in this 13-week embryo.

_____

_____

_____

51 Sonography of the Second and Third Trimesters

KEY TERMS

Exercise 1

Match the following terms related to fetal presentation and fetal anatomy with their definitions.

_____ 1. apex

_____ 2. breech

_____ 3. choroid plexus

_____ 4. ductus arteriosus

_____ 5. ductus venosus

_____ 6. echogenic intracardiac focus

_____ 7. frontal bossing

_____ 8. hyperechoic bowel

_____ 9. micrognathia

_____ 10. midline echo

_____ 11. nomogram

_____ 12. normal situs

_____ 13. nuchal skin fold

_____ 14. transverse fetal lie

_____ 15. vertex

A. Linear echoes located centrally in the fetal head that are produced by the borders of opposing cerebral hemispheres

B. Structure that carries oxygenated blood from the umbilical vein to the inferior vena cava

C. Indicates that fetus is lying transversely in the uterus, horizontal or perpendicular to the maternal sagittal axis

D. Structure that carries oxygenated blood from the pulmonary artery to the descending aorta

E. Typical position of the abdominal organs with the liver and IVC on the right, the stomach on the left, and the apex of the heart directed toward the left

F. Where the ventricles of the heart come to a point; normally directed toward the left hip

G. Abnormally small chin

H. Protrusion or bulging of the forehead

I. Indicates that the fetus is positioned head-down in the uterus

J. Indicates that the fetal head is toward the fundus of the uterus

K. Written representation by graphs, diagrams, or charts of the relationship between numeric variables

L. Increased echogenicity of the bowel associated with aneuploidy risk and fetal pathology

M. Thickness of the fetal skin at the back of the neck; may be visualized to assess aneuploidy risk

N. Echogenic tissue within the lateral ventricles that produces CNS fluid

O. Echo within a fetal heart chamber that is as bright as bone and persists despite changes in the sonographic plane

OBSTETRIC PARAMETERS

Exercise 2

Fill in the blank(s) with the word(s) that best completes the statements about obstetric parameters, gravidity, and parity of the first, second, and third trimesters.

1. Pregnancy can be clinically verified approximately 6 to 8 days after ovulation by the presence of

   _____ within the maternal urine or serum.

2. The number of pregnancies, including the present one, is _____.

3. A numeric system that describes all possible pregnancies is used to report _____.

4. A G4P2103 describes a patient undergoing her fourth pregnancy. She has had _____ full-term

   deliveries, _____ premature births, _____ early pregnancy losses, and

   _____ living children.

Exercise 3

Fill in the blank(s) with the word(s) that best completes the statements about the normal fetoplacental anatomy of the second and third trimesters.

1. The sonographer should initially determine the position of the fetus in relationship to the position of the

    _____.

2. It is important to remember to view _____ activity at the beginning of each study to ensure that the fetus is alive.

3. After fetal position is conceptualized, the sonographer determines the _____ of the fetus.

4. The fetal position changes less frequently after _____ weeks.

5. If the fetus is lying perpendicular to the long axis of the mother, it is described as a _____ fetal lie.

6. If the fetus is lying longitudinal or parallel to the maternal long axis, it is described as a _____ (head-down) presentation or a _____ (head-up) presentation.

7. A _____ breech occurs when the hips are extended and one or both feet are the presenting parts closest to the cervix.

8. If the fetus is in a vertex presentation with the fetal spine toward the maternal right side, the right side of the fetus is _____, and the left side is _____.

Exercise 4

Fill in the blank(s) with the word(s) that best completes the statements about the normal fetoplacental anatomy of the cranium of the fetus.

1. Fetal brain tissue, a solid structure, may appear _____ or cystic because of the low density of the tissue.

2. As the brain develops, structures change their sonographic appearances (e.g., the choroid plexuses seem _____ early in pregnancy), but as the brain grows, these structures appear _____ in relationship to the entire brain.

3. By the 12th week of gestation, the cranial bones _____.

4. Two types of brain tissues are highly echogenic, the _____ and the pia _____, which cover the inner and outer brain surfaces.

5. In a transverse plane, at the most cephalad level within the skull, the contour of the skull should be _____ (depending on exact level) and should have a _____ surface.

6. At the most superior level in the skull, the interhemispheric fissure, or _____ cerebri, is observed as a membrane separating the brain into two equal hemispheres.

7. The fetal ventricles are important to assess because ventriculomegaly, or hydrocephalus (dilated ventricular system), is a sign of central _____ system abnormalities.

8. If the _____ of the choroid plexus appears to float or dangle within the cavity, measurements of ventricular size are recommended to exclude abnormally enlarged or dilated ventricles (ventriculomegaly).

9. Any ventricle measuring greater than _____ mm is considered outside of normal error ranges and therefore is abnormal, warranting further consultation and prenatal testing.

10. The widest transverse diameter of the skull is the _____ echo complex and is therefore the proper level at which to measure the biparietal diameter and to assess the development of midline brain structures.

11. Between the thalamic structures lies the cavity of the _____ ventricle.

12. The circle of _____ may be seen anterior to the midbrain and appears as a triangular region that is highly pulsatile as a result of the midline-positioned anterior cerebral artery and lateral convergence of the middle cerebral arteries.

13. The _____ is located in back of the cerebral peduncles within the posterior fossa.

14. The cisterna _____ (a posterior fossa cistern filled with CSF) lies directly behind the cerebellum.

15. The above structure measures _____ mm, with an average size of 5 to 6 mm.

16. In second-trimester sonographic examinations, the thickness of the nuchal skin fold is measured in a plane containing the cavum septi pellucidi, the _____, and the cisterna magna.

Exercise 5
Fill in the blank(s) with the word(s) that best completes the statements or provide a short answer about the face, spine, and thorax of the fetus.

1. Facial morphology becomes more apparent in the second trimester, but visualization is heavily dependent on fetal positioning, adequate amounts of _____ fluid, and excellent acoustic window.

2. In a normally proportioned face, each of the segments containing the forehead, the eyes and nose, and the mouth and chin forms approximately _____ of the profile.

3. The oral cavity and the tongue are frequently outlined during fetal _____.

4. Fetal hair is often observed along the _____ of the skull and must not be included in the biparietal diameter measurement.

5. Standard antepartum obstetric examination guidelines require the sonographer to image and record the cervical, thoracic, lumbar, and _____ spine.

6. There are _____ ossification points in each vertebra.

7. The double-line appearance of the spine is referred to as the "_____ sign" and is generated by echoes from the posterior and anterior laminae and the spinal cord.

8. In a transverse plane, all three ossification points are visible; the points are spaced _____, and the spinal column appears as a closed circle, indicating closure of the neural tube.

9. Three echoes form a circle that represents the _____ of the vertebral body and the posterior elements (laminae or pedicles).

10. Optimal viewing of the spine occurs when the fetus is lying on its side in a _____ direction with its back a slight distance from the uterine wall.

Exercise 6
Fill in the blank(s) with the word(s) that best completes the statements about the diaphragm, fetal circulation, and the abdomen.

1. The diaphragm is the muscle that separates the thorax and abdomen and is commonly viewed in the _____ plane.

2. The esophagus and oropharynx help determine the location of the carotid arteries and are outlined when amniotic fluid is _____ by the fetus.

Chapter **51 Sonography of the Second and Third Trimesters**

3. The sonographer should recognize the characteristic arterial _____ from the aorta and its branches.

4. The inferior vena cava is identified coursing to the _____ and parallel with the aorta.

5. Fetal _____ occurs in the placenta, where small fetal vessels on the surface of the villi are bathed by maternal blood within the intervillous spaces.

6. Concentrations of waste products, such as urea and creatinine, are (lower/higher) in fetal blood, and these products diffuse into the maternal circulation.

7. Fetal circulation _____ the lungs because fetal lungs do not oxygenate blood.

8. The ductus arteriosus shunts blood _____ from the lungs.

9. Fetal circulation shunts oxygenated blood arriving from the placenta away from the abdomen _____ to the heart and then to the brain.

10. The hepatobiliary system serves the important function of shunting oxygen-rich blood arriving from the placenta directly to the heart through the _____.

11. Oxygenated blood from the placenta flows through the _____ vein, within the umbilical cord, to the fetal cord insertion, where it enters the abdomen.

12. From the umbilicus, the umbilical vein courses cephalad along the _____ ligament to the liver, where it connects with the left portal vein.

13. This blood then filters into the liver sinusoids, returning to the inferior vena cava by drainage into the _____ veins.

14. Inferior vena cava blood flows from the right atrium through the left atrium by way of the _____ ovale.

15. After birth, the foramen ovale, the ductus _____, and the ductus arteriosus close, and fetal circulation converts to the pattern seen throughout the rest of life.

16. The _____ lobe of the liver is larger than the right lobe because of the large quantity of oxygenated blood flowing through it.

17. The fetal _____ appears as a cone-shaped or teardrop-shaped cystic structure located in the right upper abdomen just below the left portal vein.

18. The spleen may be observed by scanning transversely and posteriorly to the left of the _____.

19. The stomach becomes apparent as early as the _____ week of gestation as swallowed amniotic fluid fills the stomach cavity. The full stomach should be seen in all fetuses beyond the _____ week of gestation.

20. The large bowel typically contains _____ particles and may measure up to 20 mm in the preterm fetus and even larger near the time of birth or in the postdate fetus.

21. The kidneys are located on either side of the spine in the posterior abdomen and are apparent as early as the _____ week of pregnancy.

22. The _____ center may be difficult to define in early pregnancy, whereas with continued maturation of the kidneys, the borders become more defined and the renal pelvis becomes more distinct.

23. A renal pelvis that measures greater than _____ mm beyond 20 weeks' gestation is considered abnormal.

24. The center of the adrenal gland appears as a central _____ line surrounded by tissue that is less echogenic.

25. A fetus generally voids at least _____ an hour, so failure to see the bladder should prompt the investigator to recheck for bladder filling.

26. The bladder should be visualized in all _____ fetuses and is an important indicator of renal function.

27. Identification of the male and female genitalia is possible provided the fetal legs are _____ and a sufficient quantity of amniotic fluid is present.

28. The gender of the fetus may be appreciated as early as _____ weeks' gestation, although clear delineation may not be possible until the _____ week(s).

29. The male genitalia may be differentiated as early as the _____ week of pregnancy.

30. The scrotal sac is seen as a mass of _____ between the hips with the scrotal septum.

Exercise 7
Fill in the blank(s) with the word(s) that best completes the statements about the musculoskeletal system of the fetus.

1. The sonographer must attempt not only to measure fetal limb bones but also to survey the anatomic configurations of the individual bones whenever possible for evidence of _____, fractures, or demineralization, as seen in several common forms of skeletal dysplasias.

2. The _____ is found in a sagittal plane by moving the probe laterally away from the ribs and scapula.

3. Epiphyseal ossification centers may be apparent around the _____ week of pregnancy.

4. The laterally positioned _____ projects deeper into the elbow, which is helpful in differentiating this bone from the medially located radius.

5. Coronally, the hands and fingers may be viewed when they are _____.

6. The distal femoral epiphysis is seen within the cartilage at the knee, and this signifies a gestational age beyond _____ weeks' gestation.

Exercise 8
Provide a short answer for each question after evaluating the images.

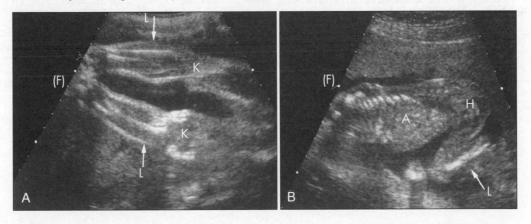

1. What position is the fetus lying in?

_____

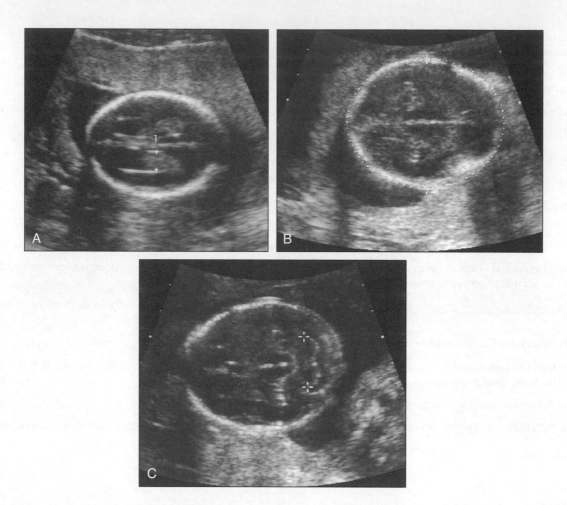

2. What is the echogenic structure within the ventricle in image *A*? What is the hypoechoic structure in the center of the fetal head in image *B*? Name the structure that is being measured in image *C*. Identify the level at which the biparietal diameter should be measured.

A. _____

B. _____

C. _____

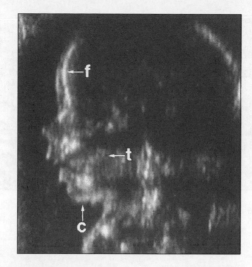

3. Identify the anatomic parts denoted by *f*, *t*, and *c*.

_____

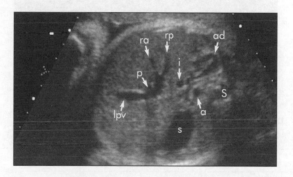

4. Which fetal side is lying closest to the transducer?

_____

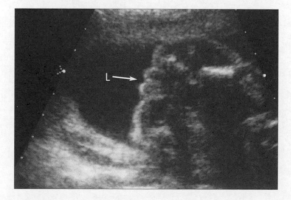

5. Identify what the letter "L" is pointing to in this fetus.

_____

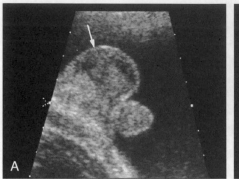 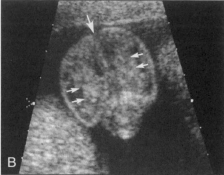

6. Which two anatomic structures are demonstrated here?

_____

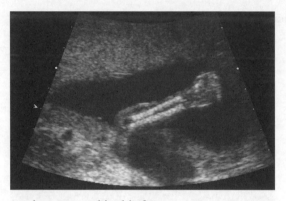

7. Name the two echogenic structures demonstrated in this fetus.

_____

_____

52 Obstetric Measurements and Gestational Age

KEY TERMS

Exercise 1

Match the following terms related to gestational age assessment with their definitions.

_____ 1. abdominal circumference

_____ 2. age range analysis

_____ 3. average age

_____ 4. binocular distance

_____ 5. biparietal diameter

_____ 6. crown-rump length

_____ 7. embryonic heart rate

_____ 8. femoral length

_____ 9. gestational sac diameter

_____ 10. growth-adjusted sonar age

_____ 11. humeral length

_____ 12. last menstrual period

_____ 13. small for gestational age

A. Measurement that includes both fetal orbits at the same time to predict gestational age

B. Used in the first trimester to estimate appropriate gestational age with menstrual dates

C. Method whereby the fetus is categorized into small, average, or large growth percentile

D. Fetal transverse cranial diameter at the level of the thalamus and cavum septum pellucidum

E. Most accurate measurement for determining gestational age; made in the first trimester

F. Used to determine the start date for human pregnancies

G. Measurement at the level of the stomach, left portal vein, and left umbilical sign

H. Heart rate before the 9th week of gestation

I. Measurement from the humeral head to the distal end of the humerus

J. Size and proportionality of the fetal parameter expressed as age

K. Normal fetus that measures smaller than dates

L. Average age of multiple fetal parameter's age

M. Measurement of the femoral diaphysis

Exercise 2

Match the following abnormal finding terms with their definitions.

_____ 1. anophthalmus

_____ 2. banana sign

_____ 3. brachycephaly

_____ 4. dolichocephaly

_____ 5. hypertelorism

_____ 6. intrauterine growth restriction

_____ 7. lemon sign

_____ 8. microphthalmos

_____ 9. oxycephaly

_____ 10. platycephaly

_____ 11. spina bifida

A. Flattening of the vertex of the skull

B. Condition in which the orbits are spaced far apart

C. Refers to the shape of the cerebellum when a spinal defect is present

D. Failure of the vertebrae to close

E. Absence of one or both eyes

F. Fetal head is relatively narrow in the transverse plane and is elongated in the anteroposterior plane

G. Condition of having a relatively high cranial vault with a high or peaked appearance

H. Abnormally small eyes

I. Fetal head is relatively wide in the transverse diameter and shortened in the anteroposterior plane

J. Occurs with spina bifida; frontal lobes collapse inward

K. Condition in which fetus is not growing as fast as normal; usually considered malnourished or abnormal

Exercise 3

Fill in the blank(s) with the word(s) that best completes the statements about gestational age assessment in the first trimester.

1. Sonographically, the earliest sign of intrauterine pregnancy is the _____, which appears as an echogenic, thickening filling of the fundal region of the endometrial cavity occurring at approximately 3 to 4 weeks' gestation.

2. At 5 weeks, the average of the three perpendicular internal diameters of the gestational sac, calculated as the mean of the anteroposterior diameter, the _____ diameter, and the _____ diameter, can provide an adequate estimation of menstrual age.

3. The sac grows rapidly in the first _____ weeks, with an average increase of 1 mm per day.

4. When the gestational sac exceeds _____ mm in mean internal diameter, a yolk sac should be seen.

5. Normal yolk sac size should be less than _____ mm; greater than _____ mm has been associated with poor pregnancy outcome.

6. When the mean gestational sac diameter exceeds _____ mm, an embryo with definite cardiac activity should be well visualized with transvaginal scanning.

7. The embryonic echoes can be identified as early as 38 to 39 days' menstrual age, and the crown-rump length is usually _____ mm at this stage.

8. The most accurate sonographic technique for establishing gestational age in the first trimester is _____ _____ _____.

9. In general, the CRL should increase at a rate of _____ mm per day.

10. Absence of an embryo by 7 to 8 weeks' gestation is consistent with an embryonic demise or an _____ pregnancy.

GESTATIONAL AGE ASSESSMENT: SECOND AND THIRD TRIMESTERS

Exercise 4

Fill in the blank(s) with the word(s) that best completes the statements about gestational age assessment in the second and third trimesters.

1. In the second trimester, the gestational age parameters extend to

   a._____ diameter,

   b._____ circumference,

   c._____ circumference,

   d._____ length.

2. The fetal head should be imaged in a transverse _____ section, ideally with the fetus in a direct occiput transverse position.

3. The BPD should be measured perpendicular to the fetal skull at the level of the _____ and cavum septi _____.

4. The head shape should be _____, not round, because this can lead to overestimation of gestational age, just as a flattened or compressed head can lead to underestimation of gestational age.

5. The calipers should be placed from the _____ edge of the parietal bone to the

   _____ edge of the opposite parietal bone, or "outer edge to inner edge."

6. The _____ head circumference is less affected than BPD by head compression; therefore, the head circumference (HC) is a valuable tool in assessing gestational age.

7. The proper coronal view should be _____ to the standard transverse HC view passing through the thalamus.

8. One can _____ gestational age from a dolichocephalic head or _____ with brachy-cephaly.

9. The AC is very useful in monitoring normal fetal growth and detecting fetal growth disturbances, such as

   intrauterine growth restriction (IUGR), and macrosomia; however, it is more useful as a _____ parameter than in predicting gestational age.

10. The fetal abdomen should be measured in a transverse plane at the level of the _____ where the

    _____ vein branches into the left portal sinus.

11. The abdomen should be more _____ than oval because an oval shape indicates an oblique cut resulting in a false estimation of size.

12. The _____ length is an especially useful parameter that can be used to date a pregnancy when a fetal head cannot be measured because of position, or when there is a fetal head anomaly.

13. Humerus length is sometimes more difficult to measure than femur length because the humerus usually is found

    very close to the fetal _____ but can exhibit a wide range of motion.

14. The ulna can be distinguished from the radius because it penetrates much more deeply into the _____.

OBSTETRIC MEASUREMENTS AND GESTATIONAL AGE

Exercise 5

Provide a short answer for each question after evaluating the images.

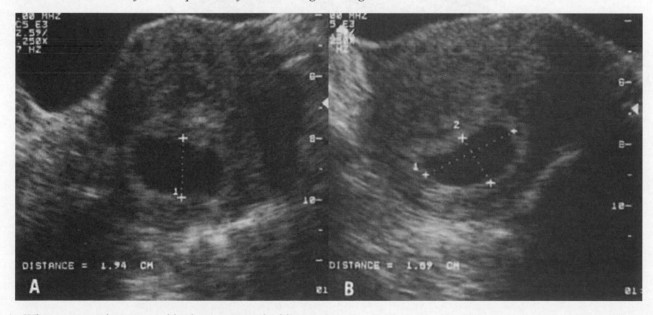

1. What structure is measured in these transvaginal images?

   _____

   _____

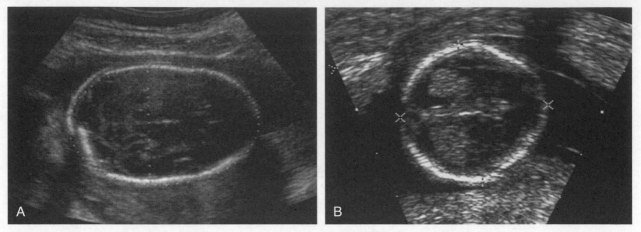

2. Identify which of these images demonstrates a dolichocephalic skull? A or B.

_____

_____

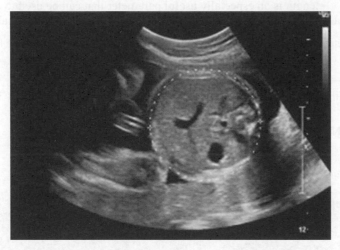

3. Identify three landmarks necessary to measure the abdominal circumference.

   a. _____

   b. _____

   c. _____

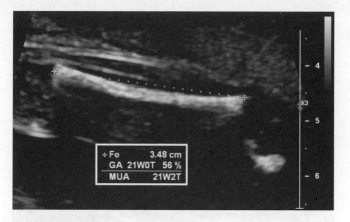

4. This is a measurement of what structure? _____

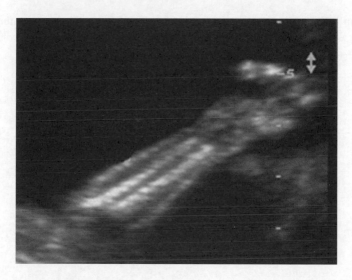

5. What structures are shown in this image?

   a. _____

   b. _____

   c. _____

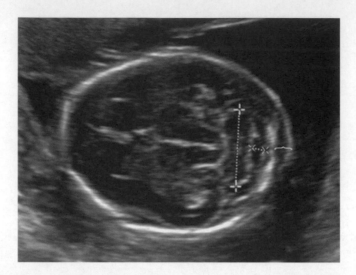

6. The vertical measurement is the _____. The horizontal measurement is the

_____.

53 Fetal Growth Assessment by Sonography

Exercise 1

Match the following fetal growth terms with their definitions.

_____ 1. amniotic fluid index

_____ 2. biophysical profile

_____ 3. estimated fetal weight

_____ 4. intrauterine growth restriction

_____ 5. large for gestational age

_____ 6. macrosomia

_____ 7. nonstress test

_____ 8. placental grade

_____ 9. postterm

_____ 10. preterm

_____ 11. pulsed wave Doppler

_____ 12. small for gestational age

A. Type of Doppler used in most fetal examinations; the transducer can both send and receive signals
B. Technique of grading the placenta for maturity
C. Decreased rate of fetal growth; may be symmetrical or asymmetrical
D. Fetus born earlier than the normal 38- to 42-week gestational period
E. Assessment of fetus to determine fetal well-being; includes evaluation of cardiac nonstress test, fetal breathing movement, gross fetal body movements, fetal tone, and amniotic fluid volume
F. Birth weight greater than 4000 g or above the 90th percentile for the estimated gestational age
G. Fetus born later than the 42-week gestational period
H. Incorporation of all fetal growth parameters
I. Normal fetus measures smaller than dates
J. Uses Doptone to record the fetal heart rate and its reactivity to the stress of uterine contraction
K. Sum of the four quadrants of amniotic fluid
L. Fetus measures larger than dates (diabetic fetus)

FETAL GROWTH ASSESSMENT

Exercise 2

Fill in the blank(s) with the word(s) that best completes the statements or provide a short answer about intrauterine growth restriction.

1. Intrauterine growth restriction is most commonly defined as a fetal weight at or below _____% for a given gestational age.

2. _____ IUGR is usually the result of a first-trimester insult, such as a chromosomal abnormality or infection.

3. _____ IUGR begins late in the second or third trimester and usually results from placental insufficiency.

4. Symmetrical growth restriction is characterized by a fetus that is _____ in all physical parameters (e.g., BPD, HC, AC, FL).

5. Asymmetrical IUGR is characterized by an appropriate BPD and HC and a disproportionately small

    _____.

Exercise 3

Fill in the blank(s) with the word(s) that best completes the statements or provide a short answer about ultrasound diagnostic criteria for fetal growth parameters.

1. Fetal blood is shunted away from other vital organs to nourish the fetal brain, giving the fetus an appropriate BPD

   (±1 standard deviation) for the true gestational age in the _____ theory.

2. A problem with using the biparietal diameter as a predictor of IUGR is the potential alteration in fetal

   _____ shape secondary to oligohydramnios.

3. In IUGR, the fetal _____ is one of the most severely affected body organs, which alters the circumference of the fetal abdomen.

4. The association between IUGR and _____ is well recognized and has been associated with fetal renal anomalies, rupture of the intrauterine membranes, and postdate pregnancy.

Exercise 4

Fill in the blank(s) with the word(s) that best completes the statements or provide a short answer about the biophysical profile and intrauterine growth restriction.

1. Identify and circle the requirements to be obtained in the biophysical profile:

   a. cardiac nonstress test

   b. cardiac stress test

   c. fetal heart rate increase

   d. observation of fetal breathing movements

   e. full bladder

   f. gross fetal body movements

   g. fetal tone

   h. amniotic fluid volume

2. Doppler ultrasound has shown that in fetuses with asymmetrical IUGR, the vascular resistance

   _____ in the aorta and umbilical artery and _____ in the fetal middle cerebral artery.

3. In the umbilical circulation, extreme cases of elevated _____ causing absent or reverse end-diastolic flow velocity waveforms are associated with high rates of morbidity and mortality.

4. Macrosomia has classically been defined as a birth weight of _____ g or greater or above the 90th percentile for estimated gestational age.

5. Macrosomia is also a common result of poorly controlled maternal _____.

Exercise 5

Provide a short answer for each question after evaluating the images.

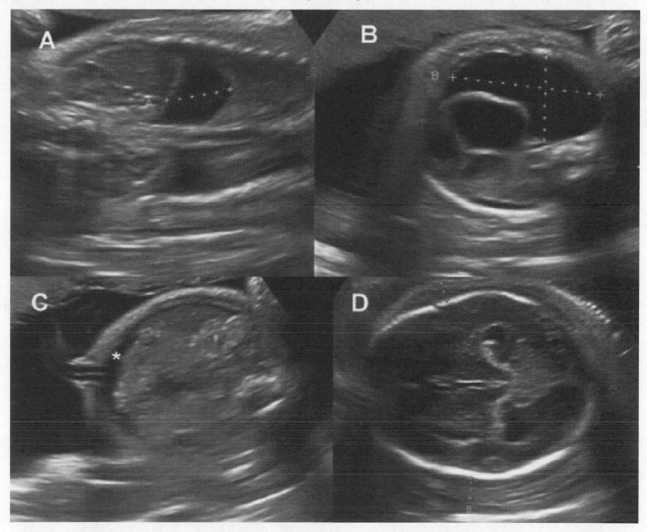

1. This is a 27-week fetus with signs of what condition?

_____

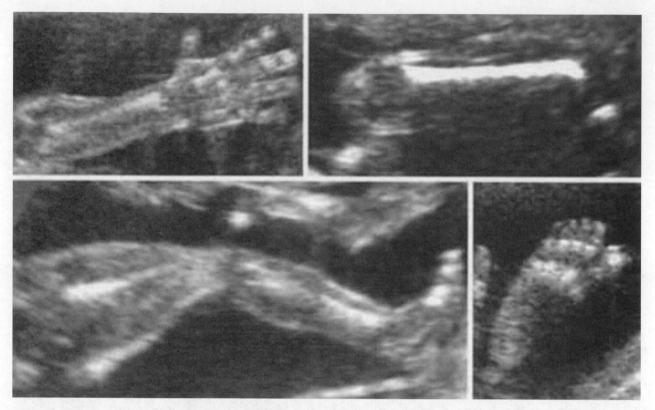

2. Fetal body and trunk gross movements must be observed within what time period as part of the biophysical profile?

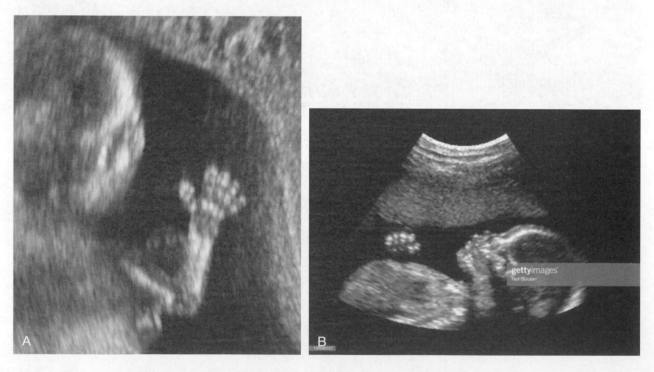

3. One active extension and flexion of an open and closed hand would be a good example of

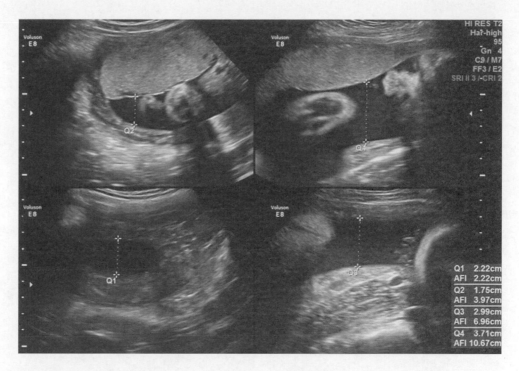

Q1	2.22cm
AFI	2.22cm
Q2	1.75cm
AFI	3.97cm
Q3	2.99cm
AFI	6.96cm
Q4	3.71cm
AFI	10.67cm

4. What is this measurement called?

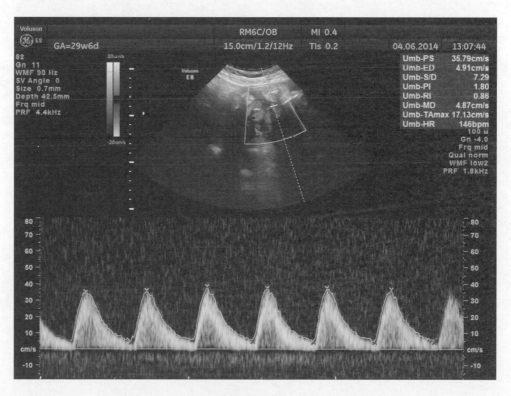

5. Is this measurement of the uterine artery normal or abnormal? _____.

Chapter **53** **Fetal Growth Assessment by Sonography**

54 Sonography and High-Risk Pregnancy

KEY TERMS

Exercise 1

Match the following terms related to high-risk pregnancy with their definitions.

_____ 1. anasarca

_____ 2. caudal regression syndrome

_____ 3. conjoined twins

_____ 4. dizygotic

_____ 5. eclampsia

_____ 6. fetus papyraceus

_____ 7. hydrops fetalis

_____ 8. hyperemesis gravidarum

_____ 9. maternal serum alpha-fetoprotein

_____ 10. maternal serum quad screen

_____ 11. monozygotic

_____ 12. nonimmune hydrops

_____ 13. oligohydramnios

_____ 14. polyhydramnios

_____ 15. preeclampsia

_____ 16. pregnancy-induced hypertension

_____ 17. premature rupture of the membranes

_____ 18. Rh blood group

_____ 19. Spalding's sign

_____ 20. systemic lupus erythematosus

_____ 21. twin–twin transfusion syndrome

A. Too little amniotic fluid; fluid measures less than 5 on the amniotic fluid index

B. Coma and seizures in the second- or third-trimester patient secondary to pregnancy-induced hypertension

C. System of antigens that may be found on the surface of red blood cells

D. Occurs when division of the egg occurs after 13 days

E. Blood test conducted during the second trimester to identify pregnancies at higher risk for chromosomal anomalies and neural tube defects

F. Elevation of maternal blood pressure that may put fetus at risk

G. Inflammatory disease involving multiple organ systems

H. Fluid occurring in at least two areas: pleural effusion, pericardial effusion, ascites, or skin edema

I. Group of conditions in which hydrops is present in the fetus but not as a result of fetomaternal blood group incompatibility

J. Twins that arise from two separately fertilized ova

K. Too much amniotic fluid; fluid measures greater than 22 on the amniotic fluid index

L. Lack of development of the caudal spine and cord that may occur in the fetus of a diabetic mother

M. Overlapping of the skull bones; indicates fetal death

N. Twins that arise from a single fertilized egg, which divides to produce two identical fetuses

O. Excessive vomiting that leads to dehydration and electrolyte imbalance

P. Fetal death that occurs after the fetus has reached a certain growth that is too large to resorb into the uterus

Q. Complication of pregnancy characterized by increasing hypertension, proteinuria, and edema

R. Antigen present in the fetus

S. Leaking or breaking of the amniotic membranes causing loss of amniotic fluid that may lead to premature delivery or infection

T. Severe generalized massive edema often seen with fetal hydrops

U. Monozygotic twin pregnancy with single placenta and arteriovenous shunt within the placenta

Exercise 2

Fill in the blank(s) with the word(s) that best completes the statements or provide a short answer about infertility.

1. A patient who will be 35 or older at the time of delivery is described as _____.

2. In the first trimester, testing is performed by looking for the pattern of biochemical markers associated with plasma protein A (PAPP-A) and free **BhCG3. These laboratory values are used in conjunction with an ultrasound

   (performed between 11 and 14 weeks) to measure the _____ translucency.

3. Second-trimester screening can be performed with the maternal serum _____ screen laboratory value and a targeted ultrasound examination.

4. A detailed evaluation of all fetal anatomy that can be seen at the time between 18 and 20 weeks' gestation is the

   _____ sonogram.

5. A condition in which excessive fluid accumulates within the fetal body cavities is _____ fetalis.

6. Any substance that elicits an immunologic response, such as production of an antibody to that substance, is a(n)

   _____.

7. A procedure in which a needle is placed into the fetal umbilical vein and a blood sample obtained is

   _____.

8. Infants with _____ are at increased risk for intracerebral hemorrhage in utero and spontaneous bleeding.

9. A group of conditions in which hydrops is present in the fetus but is not a result of fetomaternal blood group

   incompatibility is _____ hydrops.

10. Cardiovascular lesions are often the most frequent causes of NIH. Congestive heart failure may result from

    functional cardiac problems, such as dysrhythmias, tachycardias, and myocarditis, and from

    _____ anomalies, such as hypoplastic left heart and other types of congenital heart disease.

11. If glucose levels are very high and uncontrolled, the fetus may also become _____.

12. Caudal regression syndrome (lack of development of the caudal spine and cord) is seen almost exclusively in

    _____ individuals.

13. Hypertensive pregnancies may be associated with _____ placentas because of the effects of hypertension on the blood vessels.

14. The occurrence of seizures or coma in a preeclamptic patient is representative of _____.

15. A chronic autoimmune disorder that can affect almost all organ systems in the body is _____.

16. _____ gravidarum exists when a pregnant woman vomits so much that she develops dehydration and electrolyte imbalance.

PREGNANCY COMPLICATIONS

Exercise 3

Fill in the blank(s) with the word(s) that best completes the statements or provide a short answer about complications of pregnancy.

1. Intrauterine fetal death accounts for roughly _____ of all perinatal mortality.

2. At 20 weeks' gestation, the uterine fundal height should have risen to the umbilicus, and the uterus should measure

   approximately _____ cm above the symphysis pubis.

3. The mother should also perceive fetal movements on a daily basis beginning between _____
   weeks' gestation.

MULTIPLE GESTATION PREGNANCY

Exercise 4

Fill in the blank(s) with the word(s) that best completes the statements about multiple gestation pregnancy.

1. A twin has a _____ times greater chance of perinatal death than a singleton fetus.

2. During the first trimester, multiple pregnancy can be identified by visualizing more than one

   _____ sac within the uterus.

3. _____ twins arise from two separately fertilized ova.

4. In a dizygotic pregnancy each ovum implants separately in the uterus and develops its own placenta and chorion,

   that is called _____. A separate amnion is called _____.

5. Identical or _____ twins arise from a single fertilized egg, which divides, resulting in two genetically identical fetuses.

6. Depending on whether the fertilized egg divides _____ or _____, there may be one or two placentas, chorions, and amniotic sacs.

7. If division occurs _____ 0 to 4 days post conception, two amnions and two chorions (dichorionic, diamniotic) will be present.

8. If division occurs at _____ days, one chorion and two amniotic sacs (monochorionic, diamniotic) will be present.

9. If division occurs after 8 days, two fetuses will be present but only one chorion and one amnion or _____

   chorionic or _____ amniotic.

10. If division occurs after 13 days, the division may be incomplete and _____ twins may result.

11. Stuck twin syndrome, or _____ sequence, is characterized by a diamniotic pregnancy with polyhydramnios in one sac and severe oligohydramnios and a smaller twin in the other sac.

12. Twin–twin transfusion syndrome exists when an _____ shunt is placed within the placenta.

13. By definition, a rare anomaly occurring in monochorionic twins in which one twin develops without a heart and

    often with absence of the upper half of the body is an _____ anomaly.

14. When scanning multiple gestations, the sonographer should always attempt to determine whether one or two

    _____ sacs are present by locating the membrane that separates the sacs.

15. It is important to keep in mind that a fetus from a multiple gestation is usually _____ than a singleton fetus.

16. No flow and _____ flow during diastole are signs of fetal jeopardy that may prompt the obstetrician to do further fetal well-being testing or even to deliver the fetuses.

Exercise 5

Provide a short answer for each question after evaluating the images.

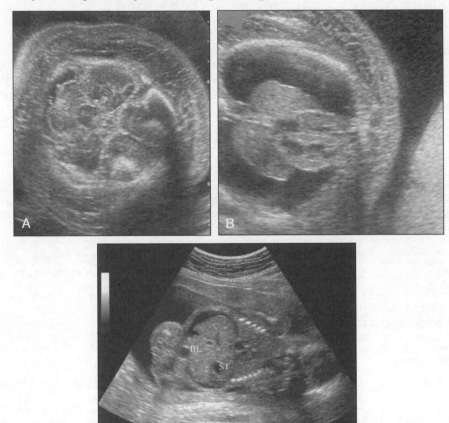

1. Erythroblastosis fetalis is a condition marked by several sonographic findings. Identify which abnormality is shown in each image *(A, B, C).*

    A. _____

    B. _____

    C. _____

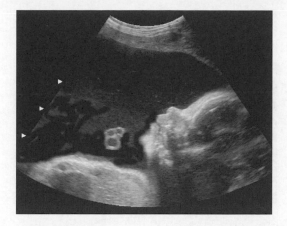

2. Name the abnormality demonstrated in this image.

_____

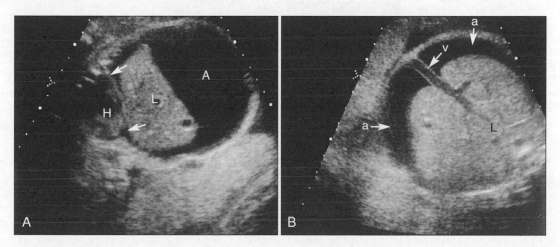

3. Identify the abnormality demonstrated in this fetus with nonimmune hydrops. Identify *v* in image *B*.

_____

_____

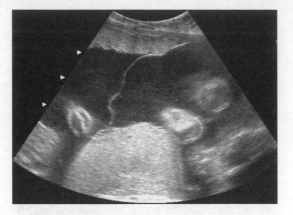

4. This sonogram represents what type of twin gestation?

_____

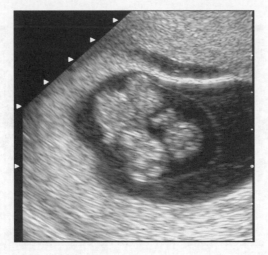

5. This sonogram depicts what type of twinning?

_____

55 Prenatal Diagnosis of Congenital Anomalies

KEY TERMS

Exercise 1

Match the following prenatal diagnosis terms with their definitions.

_____ 1. alpha-fetoprotein

_____ 2. amniocentesis

_____ 3. cystic hygroma

_____ 4. hypertelorism

_____ 5. hypoplasia

_____ 6. hypotelorism

_____ 7. intrauterine growth restriction

_____ 8. micrognathia

_____ 9. omphalocele

_____ 10. polydactyly

_____ 11. TORCH

A. Abnormally small chin; commonly associated with other fetal anomalies

B. Transabdominal removal of amniotic fluid from the amniotic cavity using ultrasound

C. Underdevelopment of a tissue, organ, or body

D. An acronym originally coined from the first letters of toxoplasmosis, rubella, cytomegalovirus, and herpesvirus type 2

E. Dilatation of jugular lymph sacs caused by improper drainage of the lymphatic system into the venous system

F. Anterior abdominal wall defect in which abdominal organs are atypically located within the umbilical cord; highly associated with cardiac, central nervous system, renal, and chromosomal anomalies

G. Abnormally wide-spaced orbits usually found in conjunction with congenital anomalies and mental retardation

H. Abnormally closely spaced orbits; associated with holoprosencephaly, chromosomal and central nervous system disorders, and cleft palate

I. Anomalies of the hands or feet in which there is an addition of a digit; may be found in association with certain skeletal dysplasias

J. Decreased rate of fetal growth, usually fetal weight below the 10th percentile for a given gestational age

K. Protein manufactured by the fetus, which can be studied in amniotic fluid and maternal serum

GENETIC TESTING

Exercise 2

Fill in the blank(s) with the word(s) that best completes the statements about genetic testing.

1. A major congenital anomaly is found in _____ of every 100 births, and an additional 10% to 15% of births are complicated by minor birth defects.

2. An ultrasound-directed biopsy of the placenta or chorionic villi (chorion frondosum) in the first trimester is

   _____.

3. A specialized prenatal test that permits direct viewing of the developing embryo using a transcervical endoscope

   inserted into the extracoelomic cavity during the first trimester of pregnancy is _____.

4. The technique first used to relieve polyhydramnios, to predict Rh isoimmunization, and to document fetal lung

   maturity is _____.

5. The amniocentesis technique for multiple gestations is similar to the singleton method, except that

   _____ fetal sac is entered.

6. Another method in which chromosomes are analyzed is _____.

7. The major protein in fetal serum that is also produced by the yolk sac in early gestation and later by the fetal liver

   is _____.

8. AFP is transported into the _____ fluid by fetal urination and reaches maternal circulation or blood through the fetal membranes.

9. Common reasons for high AFP levels are _____, such as anencephaly and open spina bifida.

10. Two common abdominal wall defects, _____ and _____, produce elevations of AFP.

11. It is expected that the AFP level in a twin pregnancy will be _____ that of a singleton pregnancy.

MEDICAL GENETICS

Exercise 3

Fill in the blank(s) with the word(s) that best completes the statements about medical genetics.

1. A normal karyotype consists of _____ chromosomes, _____ pairs of autosomes, and a pair of sex chromosomes.

2. An abnormality of the number of chromosomes is _____.

3. One of the most common aneuploid conditions is _____ syndrome, in which an individual has an extra chromosome number 21.

4. An inherited dominant disorder carries a _____% chance that each time pregnancy occurs, the fetus will have the condition.

5. A recessive disorder is caused by a pair of defective genes, one inherited from each parent. With each pregnancy,

   the parents have a _____% chance of having a fetus with the disorder.

6. X-linked disorders are inherited by _____ from their mothers.

7. Each of the _____ of female carriers of X-linked disorders has a 50% chance of being affected,

   and each of the _____ has a 50% chance of being a carrier.

8. An abnormal event that arises because of the interaction of one or more genes and environmental factors is a(n)

   _____ condition.

9. The occurrence of a gene mutation or chromosomal abnormality in a portion of an individual's cells is

   _____.

CHROMOSOMAL ABNORMALITIES

Exercise 4

Fill in the blank(s) with the word(s) that best completes the statements or provide a short answer about chromosomal abnormalities.

1. An abnormal fluid collection behind the fetal neck has been strongly associated with _____.

2. A nuchal translucency of _____ mm or greater has been used to define an abnormal thickness.

3. The translucency should be oriented perpendicular to the ultrasound beam, and the measurement should be taken from inside the fetal _____ to inside the _____ membrane.

4. A measurement of _____ mm increases the risk of aneuploidy four times, and nuchal translucencies of _____ mm and greater carry an even greater risk.

5. A genetic abnormality marked by absence of the X or Y chromosome is _____ syndrome (45,X).

6. The most pathognomonic finding for the above disorder is _____.

7. A fetus with Turner's syndrome may have cardiac anomalies, the most common is _____ of the aorta.

CONGENITAL ANOMALIES

Exercise 5

Provide a short answer for each question after evaluating the images.

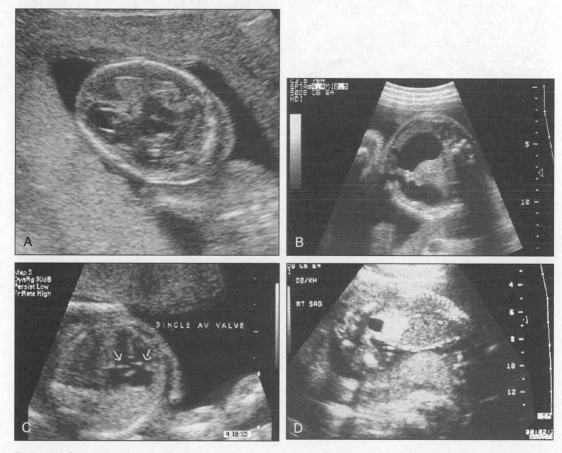

(Image *A* from Henningsen C: *Clinical guide to ultrasonography,* St Louis, 2004, Mosby.) (Image *C* courtesy G. Goreczky, RDMS, Maternal Fetal Center at Florida Hospital, Orlando, Fla.)

1. Describe the sonographic findings in each of these images of different fetuses with trisomy 21.

   A. _____

   B. _____

   C. _____

   D. _____

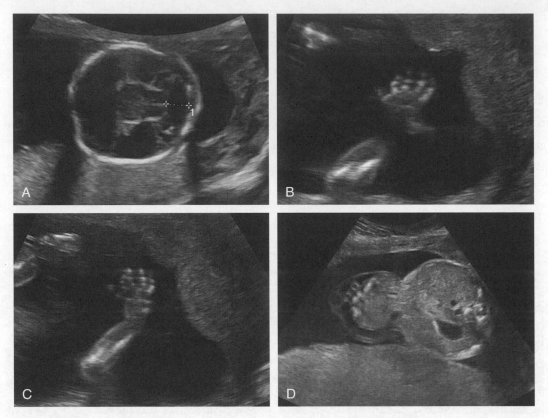

2. A fetus with trisomy 13 presented with alobar holoprosencephaly. Describe the other sonographic findings.

_____

_____

_____

_____

_____

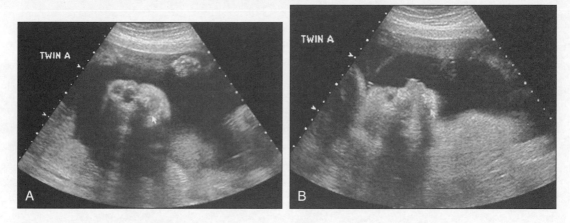

(From Henningsen C: *Clinical guide to ultrasonography,* St. Louis, 2004, Mosby.)

3. A fetus with trisomy 13 is presented for ultrasound examination. Describe the sonographic findings.

_____

_____

_____

_____

_____

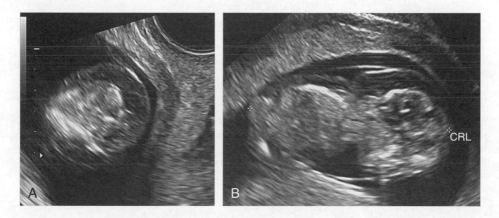

4. A fetus with Turner's syndrome is presented. Describe the sonographic findings.

_____

_____

_____

Chapter **55** **Prenatal Diagnosis of Congenital Anomalies**

56 The Placenta

KEY TERMS

Exercise 1

Match the following terms related to embryogenesis with their definitions.

_____ 1. basal plate
_____ 2. battledore placenta
_____ 3. chorion frondosum
_____ 4. chorionic plate
_____ 5. chorionic villi
_____ 6. decidua basalis
_____ 7. decidua capsularis
_____ 8. placenta previa

A. Portion of the chorion that develops into the fetal portion of the placenta
B. Placenta grows in the lower uterine segment and covers all or part of the cervix
C. Microscopic vascular projections from the chorion that combine with maternal uterine tissue to form the placenta
D. Maternal surface of the placenta that lies contiguous with the decidua basalis
E. Part of the decidua that surrounds the chorionic sac
F. Part of the decidua that unites with the chorion to form the placenta
G. Cord insertion into the margin of the placenta
H. Part of the chorionic membrane that covers the placenta

Exercise 2

Match the following terms associated with sonographic evaluation of the umbilical cord and placenta with their definitions.

_____ 1. abruptio placentae
_____ 2. Braxton Hicks contractions
_____ 3. Circum-marginate placenta
_____ 4. circumvallate placenta
_____ 5. ductus venosus
_____ 6. ligamentum venosum
_____ 7. lower uterine segment (LUS)
_____ 8. molar pregnancy
_____ 9. placenta accreta
_____ 10. placenta increta
_____ 11. placenta percreta
_____ 12. placental migration
_____ 13. succenturiate placenta
_____ 14. vasa previa
_____ 15. Wharton's jelly

A. Also known as gestational trophoblastic disease; abnormal proliferation of trophoblastic cells in the first trimester
B. Fibrous remains of the ductus venosus from fetal circulation
C. Growth of the chorionic villi superficially to the myometrium; does not penetrate through the myometrium
D. Spontaneous painless uterine contractions that occur throughout a pregnancy
E. Occurs when the intramembranous vessels course across the internal cervical os
F. The placenta is attached to the uterine wall; as the uterus enlarges, the placenta "moves" with it. Therefore a low-lying placenta may move out of the uterine segment in the second trimester.
G. Lower part of the uterine cavity, which expands during pregnancy and joins with the cervical canal
H. Mucoid connective tissue that surrounds the vessels within the umbilical cord
I. Growth of the chorionic villi deep into the myometrium
J. Placental condition in which the chorionic plate is smaller than the basal plate; the margin is raised with a rolled edge
K. One or more accessory lobes connected to the body of the placenta by blood vessels
L. Connection that is patent during fetal life from the left portal vein to the systemic veins (inferior vena cava)
M. Premature detachment of the placenta from the maternal wall
N. Growth of the chorionic villi through the myometrium to the uterine serosa
O. Placental condition in which the chorionic plate is smaller than the basal plate, with a flat interface between the fetal membranes and the placenta

Exercise 3

Label the following illustrations.

A. The fetal portion of the placenta.

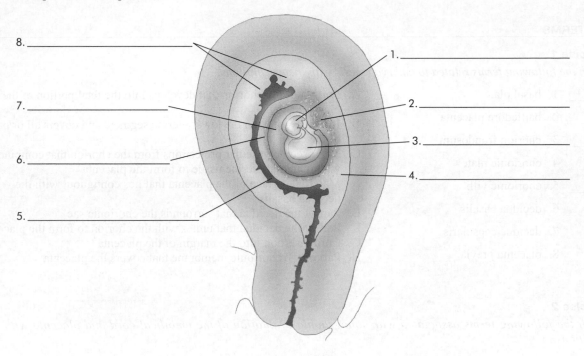

8. _____

7. _____

6. _____

5. _____

1. _____

2. _____

3. _____

4. _____

B. The maternal portion of the placenta.

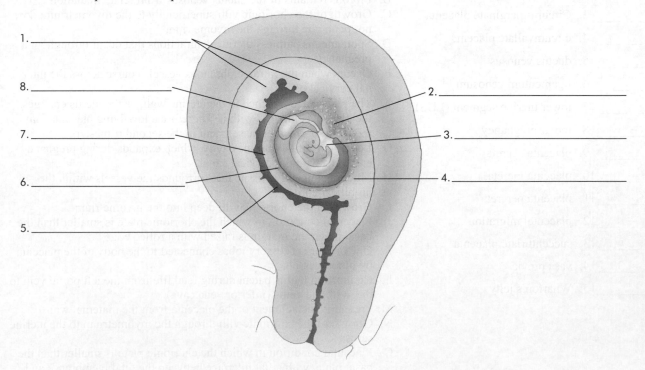

1. _____

8. _____

7. _____

6. _____

5. _____

2. _____

3. _____

4. _____

C. The major functioning unit of the placenta is the chorionic villus.

1._____ 2._____ 3._____

4._____

5._____

6._____

12._____

11._____

10._____

7._____

8._____

9._____

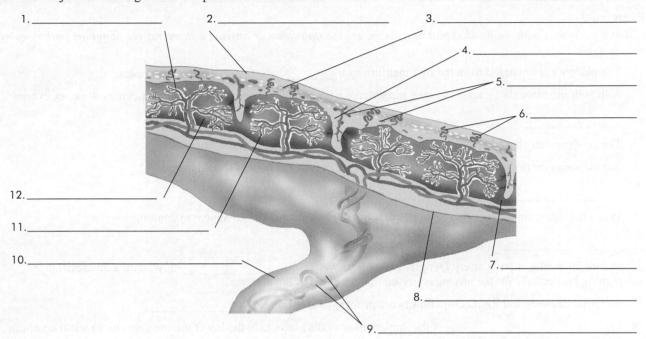

Exercise 4

Fill in the blank(s) with the word(s) that best completes the statements or provide a short answer about the anatomy and physiology of the placenta.

1. The major role of the placenta is to permit the exchange of _____ maternal blood (rich in oxygen and nutrients) with _____ fetal blood.

2. Maternal vessels course posterior to the placenta and circulate blood into the placenta, whereas blood from the fetus reaches this point through the _____ _____.

3. The fetal surface of the placenta, which is contiguous with the surrounding chorion, is termed the _____ _____.

4. The maternal portion of the placenta that lies contiguous with the decidua basalis is termed the _____ plate villus.

5. Oxygenated maternal blood is brought to the placenta through 80 to 100 end branches of the uterine arteries known as the _____ arteries.

6. The maternal placental circulation may be reduced by a variety of conditions that decrease uterine blood flow, such as severe _____, renal disease, or placental infarction.

7. The attachment of the cord is usually near the _____ of the placenta.

8. Most of the amniotic fluid comes from the maternal _____ by diffusion across the amnion from the decidua parietalis and intervillous spaces of the placenta.

9. In the first trimester, the fetus begins to _____ urine into the sac to fill the amniotic cavity; the fetus _____ this fluid, and the cycle continues throughout pregnancy.

Exercise 5

Fill in the blank(s) with the word(s) that best completes the statements or provide a short answer about the pathology of the placenta.

1. The placenta is separated from the myometrium by a _____ venous complex.

2. Although the placenta increases in size and volume with gestational age, the maximum thickness does not exceed

   _____.

3. The sonographer should always describe the _____ of the placenta.

4. For the sonographer to visualize the internal os of the cervix, the patient should have a _____

   _____.

5. When the sonographer sees two separate parts of the placenta that do not appear to communicate, a

   _____ placenta should be considered.

6. Before 20 weeks, uterine artery Doppler typically shows a _____ flow, with a low resistance pattern, particularly for the uterine artery on the same side as the placenta.

7. Maternal diabetes and Rh incompatibility are primary causes for _____.

8. Placenta _____ is the implantation of the placenta in the lower uterine segment in advance of the fetus.

9. With _____ previa, the cervical internal os is completely covered by placental tissue.

10. Other approaches that are useful in evaluating the lower uterine segment with ultrasound when the definition of the

    placenta needs to be clarified include _____ and translabial.

11. A potentially life-threatening fetal complication of the placenta that occurs when large fetal vessels run in the fetal

    membranes across the cervical os is _____ previa, which places them at risk of rupture and hemorrhage.

12. Abnormal adherence of part or all of the placenta with partial or complete absence of the decidua basalis is

    _____ accreta.

13. The risk of placenta accreta increases in patients with placenta previa and uterine scar from previous

    _____.

14. Placenta _____ results from underdeveloped decidualization of the endometrium.

15. The attachment of the placental membranes to the fetal surface of the placenta rather than to the placental margin is

    a(n) _____ placenta.

16. The separation of a normally implanted placenta before term delivery is referred to as placental

    _____.

17. _____ abruption results from the rupture of spiral arteries and is a "high-pressure" bleed.

18. _____ abruption results from tears of the marginal veins and represents a "low-pressure" bleed.

19. A focal discrete lesion caused by ischemic necrosis is placental _____.

20. In gestational _____ disease, the sonogram shows a uterine size larger than dates, no identifiable parts, and an inhomogeneous texture with variously sized cystic structures of the placenta that represent multiple vesicular changes throughout the placenta.

21. The second most common tumor of the placenta is known as _____.

Provide a short answer for each question after evaluating the images.

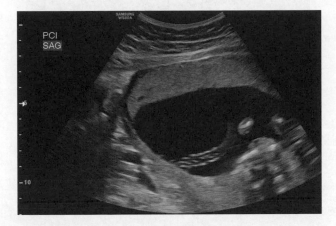

1. Where is the cord insertion in this sonographic image.

_____

_____

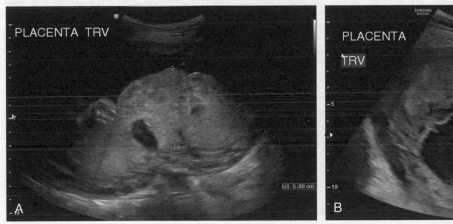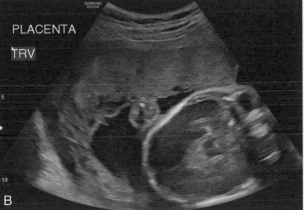

2. Describe the findings in these two images of the placenta.

_____

_____

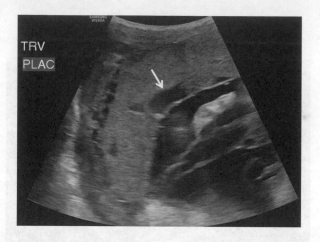

3. What structure is the arrow pointing to?

_____

_____

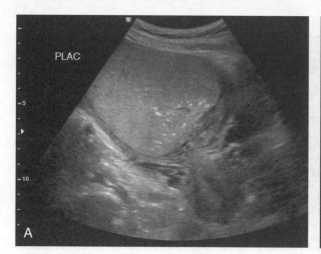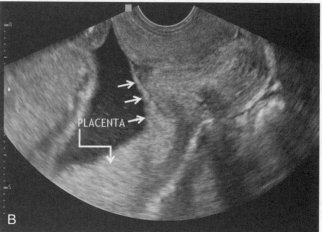

4. This is an image of the lower uterine segment in a patient who has been bleeding for 3 days with bright red blood. Describe the sonographic finding.

_____

_____

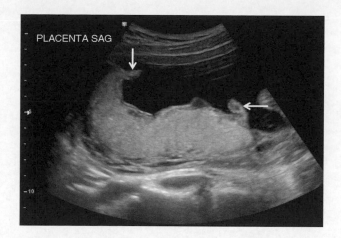

PLACENTA SAG

5. This patient presented with a posterior placenta. What are the arrows pointing to?

_____

_____

KEY TERMS

Exercise 1

Match the following terms related to the umbilical cord with their definitions.

_____ 1. allantoic duct

_____ 2. battledore placenta

_____ 3. ductus venosus

_____ 4. false knots of the umbilical cord

_____ 5. gastroschisis

_____ 6. hemangioma of the cord

_____ 7. membranous (velamentous) insertion of the cord

_____ 8. nuchal cord

_____ 9. omphalocele

_____ 10. omphalomesenteric cyst

_____ 11. single umbilical artery

_____ 12. superior vesical arteries

_____ 13. true knots of the umbilical cord

_____ 14. umbilical herniation

_____ 15. vasa previa

_____ 16. Wharton's jelly

_____ 17. yolk stalk

A. Cord inserts into the membranes before it enters the placenta

B. Failure of the bowel, stomach, and liver to return to the abdominal cavity; completely covered by a peritoneal-amniotic membrane

C. The smaller, shorter, and posterior of the two branches into which the umbilical vein divides after entering the abdomen. It empties into the inferior vena cava

D. Marginal or eccentric insertion of the umbilical cord into the placenta

E. Umbilical duct connecting the yolk sac with the embryo

F. Failure of the anterior abdominal wall to close completely at the level of the umbilicus

G. Myxomatous connective tissue that surrounds the umbilical vessels and varies in size

H. Elongated duct that contributes to development of the umbilical cord and placenta during the first trimester

I. High association of congenital anomalies with this

J. Occurs when blood vessels are longer than the cord; they fold on themselves and produce nodulations on the surface of the cord

K. Cystic lesion of the umbilical cord

L. Occurs when the cord is wrapped around the fetal neck

M. Vascular tumor within the umbilical cord

N. Arise from fetal movements and are more likely to develop during early pregnancy, when relatively more amniotic fluid is present; associated with advanced maternal age, multiparity, and long umbilical cords

O. Occurs when the umbilical cord vessels cross the internal os of the cervix

P. Anomaly in which part of the bowel remains outside the abdominal wall without a membrane

Q. After birth, the umbilical arteries are known as these

Exercise 2

Fill in the blank(s) with the word(s) that best completes the statements about the development and normal anatomy of the umbilical cord.

1. The umbilical cord is the essential link for _____ and important nutrients among the fetus, the placenta, and the mother.

2. The intestines grow at a faster rate than the abdomen and _____ into the proximal umbilical cord at approximately 7 weeks, where they remain until approximately 10 weeks.

3. The umbilical cord includes _____ umbilical arteries and _____ umbilical vein and is surrounded by a homogeneous substance called _____ jelly.

4. The intra-abdominal portions of the umbilical vessels degenerate after birth; the umbilical arteries become the lateral ligaments of the _____, and the umbilical vein becomes the round ligament of the _____.

5. From the left portal vein, the umbilical blood flows through the ductus _____ to the systemic veins, bypassing the liver, or through the right portal sinus to the right portal vein.

6. The ductus venosus forms the conduit between the _____ system and the _____ veins.

7. The ductus venosus is patent during fetal life until shortly after birth, when transformation of the ductus into the ligamentum _____ occurs (beginning in the second week after birth).

8. The umbilical arteries run along the _____ margin of the fetal bladder and are well imaged with color flow Doppler. In the postpartum stage, the umbilical arteries become the superior vesical arteries.

PATHOLOGY

Exercise 3

Fill in the blank(s) with the word(s) that best completes the statements about the pathology of the umbilical cord.

1. _____ knots of the umbilical cord have been associated with long cords, polyhydramnios, intra-uterine growth restriction, and monoamniotic twins.

2. _____ knots of the umbilical cord are seen when the blood vessels are longer than the cord.

3. The most common cord entanglement in the fetus is _____ cord.

4. When the cord implants into the edge of the placenta instead of into the middle, the condition is called _____ placenta.

5. Membranous, or _____, insertion of the cord occurs when the cord inserts into the membranes before it enters the placenta, rather than inserting directly into the placenta.

6. When the cord lies below the presenting part, _____ of the umbilical cord occurs.

7. _____ of the cord reduces or cuts off the blood supply to the fetus and may result in fetal demise.

8. The sonographic detection of a _____ umbilical artery should prompt the investigation of further fetal anomalies.

Provide a short answer for each question after evaluating the images.

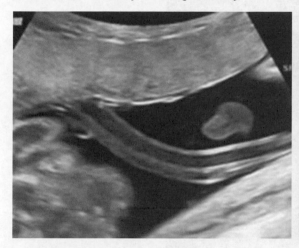 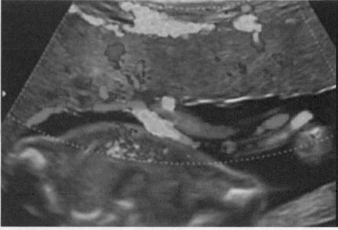

1. Describe the findings in these images in a third-trimester fetus.

   _____

   _____

   _____

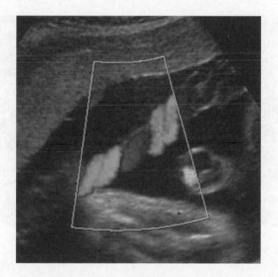

2. Does this image have a right or left twist to the umbilical cord.

   _____

   _____

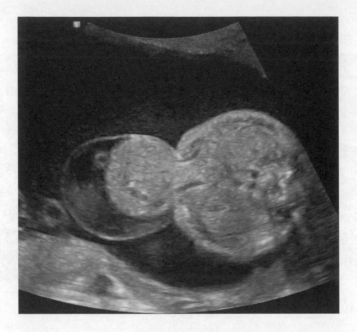

3. This mass was seen to project outside the fetal abdomen. The abnormality you suspect is:

_____

_____

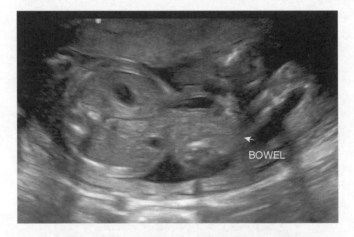

4. Which abnormality is visible on this image of a fetal abdomen?

_____

_____

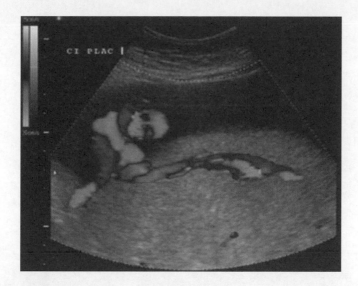

5. How would you describe this cord insertion?

_____

_____

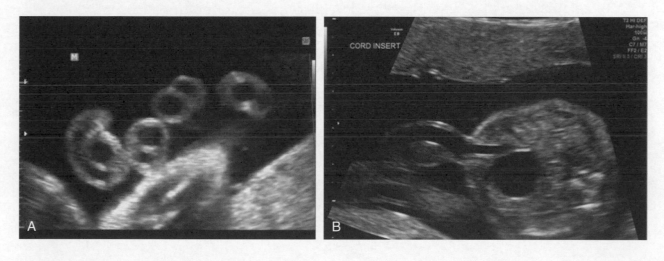

6. Describe these images of the umbilical cord.

_____

_____

58 Amniotic Fluid, Fetal Membranes, and Fetal Hydrops

Exercise 1

Match the following terms related to amniotic fluid assessment and abnormal volumes with their definitions.

_____ 1. amniotic cavity

_____ 2. amniotic fluid

_____ 3. amniotic fluid index

_____ 4. maximum vertical pocket

_____ 5. placental insufficiency

_____ 6. polyhydramnios

_____ 7. oligohydramnios

_____ 8. subjective assessment of fluid

_____ 9. vernix caseosa

A. Sonographer surveys uterine cavity for visual determination of amniotic fluid present

B. Produced by the umbilical cord and membranes, the fetal lung, skin, and kidney

C. Each of the four uterine quadrants is evaluated with the transducer perpendicular to the table in the deepest vertical pocket without fetal parts; the four quadrants are added together to determine this

D. Too little amniotic fluid; associated with intrauterine growth restriction, renal anomalies, premature rupture of membranes, postdate pregnancy, and other factors

E. Fatty material found on fetal skin and in amniotic fluid late in pregnancy

F. Method used to determine the amount of amniotic fluid

G. Structure that forms early in gestation and surrounds the embryo

H. Too much amniotic fluid; associated with central nervous system disorder, gastrointestinal anomalies, fetal hydrops, skeletal anomalies, renal disorders, and other factors

I. Inability of the placenta to provide adequate blood/nutrient supply to the fetus because of underlying maternal disease

Exercise 2

Match the following terms related to fetal membranes with their definitions.

_____ 1. amniotic band syndrome

_____ 2. anasarca

_____ 3. ascites

_____ 4. Asherman's syndrome

_____ 5. chorioamnionitis

_____ 6. corticosteroid therapy

_____ 7. hydrops fetalis

_____ 8. immune hydrops fetalis

_____ 9. nonimmune hydrops fetalis

_____ 10. pericardial effusion

A. Condition in which the amniotic bag breaks, labor has not begun, and the pregnancy is less than 37 weeks' gestation

B. Condition in which the amniotic bag breaks with labor or just after labor begins

C. Scars within the uterus secondary to previous gynecologic surgery

D. Abnormal serous fluid collection found in the abdomen or pelvis

E. Accumulation of abnormal fluid collections caused by rhesus incompatibility

F. Generalized swelling and edema of skin throughout the body

G. Abnormal collection of fluid surrounding the heart measuring greater than 2 mm

379

_____11. pleural effusion

_____12. premature rupture of membranes

_____13. spontaneous premature rupture of membranes

_____14. uterine synechiae

H. Multiple fibrous strands of amnion that develop in utero that may entangle fetal parts to cause amputations or malformations of the fetus

I. Bacterial infection of the fetal membranes usually due to upward ascent of a vaginal infection

J. Accumulation of abnormal fluid collections not caused by rhesus incompatibility

K. Abnormal fluid collection in the thoracic cavity

L. Administered to pregnant women to help accelerate fetal lung maturity

M. Abnormal accumulation of fluid or edema found in at least two fetal areas

N. Acquired uterine condition characterized by the presence of intrauterine scars

AMNIOTIC FLUID

Exercise 3

Fill in the blank(s) with the word(s) that best completes the statements about amniotic fluid.

1. _____ _____ allows the fetus to move freely within the amniotic cavity while also maintaining intrauterine temperature and protecting the developing fetus from injury.

2. The amnion can be visualized with transvaginal sonography in the early first trimester between 4 and 5 weeks' gestation as a thin membrane separating the _____ cavity (which contains the fetus) from the extraembryonic coelom and the secondary _____ sac.

3. Amniotic fluid is produced by the umbilical cord, the membranes, the _____, the skin, and kidneys.

4. As the fetus and placenta mature, amniotic fluid production and consumption change to include movement of fluid across the chorion _____ and fetal skin, fetal urine output and fetal swallowing, and gastrointestinal absorption.

5. Fetal production of urine and the ability to swallow begins between _____ and 11 weeks of gestation and becomes the major pathway for amniotic fluid production and consumption after this time period.

6. The fetus _____ amniotic fluid, which is absorbed by the digestive tract. The fetus also _____ urine, which is passed into the surrounding amniotic fluid.

7. Fetal urination into the amniotic sac accounts for nearly the total volume of amniotic fluid by the second half of pregnancy, so that the quantity of fluid is directly related to _____ function.

8. Normal lung development depends critically on the _____ of amniotic fluid within the lungs.

9. Inadequate lung development may occur when severe _____ is present, placing the fetus at high risk for developing small or hypoplastic lungs.

10. The volume of amniotic fluid increases progressively until about 33 weeks' gestation, with average increment per week of 25 ml from the 11th to the 15th week and _____ ml from the 15th to the 28th week of gestation.

11. At the end of pregnancy, the amniotic fluid is scanty, and _____ fluid pockets may be the only visible areas of fluid.

12. The small-for-age fetus has _____ amniotic fluid; the large-for-age fetus has _____ volume of fluid.

13. Amniotic fluid generally appears _____ sonographically, although fluid particles (particulate matter) may be seen occasionally.

Exercise 4
Fill in the blank(s) with the word(s) that best completes the statements about the sonographic assessment of amniotic fluid.

1. When the sonographer initially scans the entire uterus to get an overall visual assessment of the fluid present, the lie of the fetus, and the position of the placenta, this is called a(n) _____ assessment.

2. With the four _____ method, the uterine cavity is divided into four equal parts by two imaginary lines perpendicular to each other.

3. The largest vertical pocket of amniotic fluid, excluding fetal limbs or umbilical cord loops, is measured in the four quadrants and added together for the _____ pocket assessment.

4. Subjective assessment of normal amniotic fluid correlates with AFI of 10 to 20 cm; borderline values of _____ cm indicate low fluid, and values of _____ cm indicate increased fluid.

5. The sonographer must be careful to hold the transducer _____ to the table (not the curved skin surface) when assessing these pockets of fluid.

6. The _____ vertical pocket (i.e., fluid should measure greater than 1 cm "rule") assessment of amniotic fluid is done by identifying the largest pocket of amniotic fluid.

7. In twin pregnancies, the two-dimensional pocket measurement appears to be a better predictor of _____ than the AFI or the largest vertical pocket.

Exercise 5
Fill in the blank(s) with the word(s) that best completes the statements or provide a short answer about the abnormalities of amniotic fluid.

1. Hydramnios, or _____, is defined as an amniotic fluid volume greater than 2000 ml.

2. Polyhydramnios is often associated with central _____ system disorders and/or gastrointestinal problems.

3. This central nervous system disorder causes _____ swallowing.

4. An overall reduction in the amount of amniotic fluid resulting in fetal crowding and decreased fetal movement is _____.

5. Oligohydramnios may be defined as a single pocket of fluid with a depth less than _____ cm or an AFI less than _____ cm.

6. The association between _____ and decreased amniotic fluid (oligohydramnios) is well recognized.

7. Evaluation of _____ flow in the umbilical cord, the placenta, and the cerebral vascular system with color and Doppler techniques is critical to determine the presence or absence of intrauterine growth restriction.

8. Cord _____ by the fetus is another potential cause for fetal asphyxia leading to oligohydramnios.

Exercise 6

Fill in the blank(s) with the word(s) that best completes the statements about amniotic band syndrome.

1. A common, nonrecurrent cause of various fetal malformations involving the limbs, craniofacial region, and trunk is

   the _____ _____ syndrome.

2. The site where the amniotic band cuts across the fetus is usually evident after _____.

3. Amniotic sheets are believed to be caused by uterine scars, or _____, from previous instrumentation of the uterus (usually curettage), cesarean section, or episodes of endometritis.

Exercise 7

Provide a short answer for each question after evaluating the images.

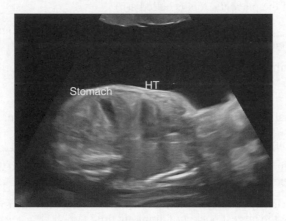

1. Identify the sonographic finding in this 30-week gestation.

   _____

   _____

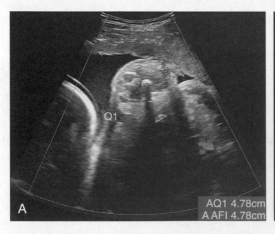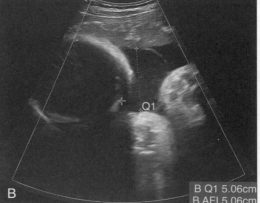

2. Describe the amniotic fluid assessment in twin pregnancies.

   _____

   _____

   _____

Chapter **58 Amniotic Fluid, Fetal Membranes, and Fetal Hydrops**

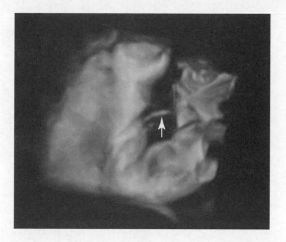

3. Describe the abnormality (arrow) seen in this 3D image.

_____

_____

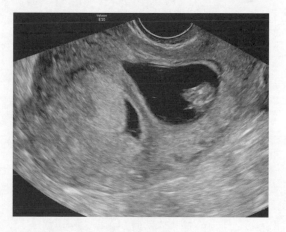

4. Describe the abnormality demonstrated in this fetus.

_____

_____

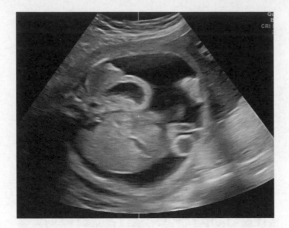

5. Identify the abnormality in this 30-week gestation.

_____

_____

Chapter **58 Amniotic Fluid, Fetal Membranes, and Fetal Hydrops**

59 The Fetal Face and Neck

Exercise 1

Match the following fetal face and neck abnormality terms with their definitions.

_____ 1. anophthalmia

_____ 2. arrhinia

_____ 3. cephalocele

_____ 4. craniosynostoses

_____ 5. dacryocystocele

_____ 6. exophthalmia

_____ 7. fetal cystic hygroma

_____ 8. fetal goiter (thyromegaly)

_____ 9. holoprosencephaly

_____ 10. hypertelorism

_____ 11. microcephaly

_____ 12. micrognathia

_____ 13. nuchal lucency

_____ 14. phenylketonuria (PKU)

_____ 15. Treacher Collins syndrome

A. Malformation of the lymphatic system that leads to single or multiloculated lymph-filled cavities around the neck
B. Premature closure of cranial sutures
C. Underdevelopment of the jaw and cheek bone and abnormal ears
D. Head smaller than the body
E. Cystic dilatation of the lacrimal sac at the nasocanthal angle
F. Absent eyes
G. Small chin
H. Congenital defect caused by an extra chromosome, which causes a deficiency in the forebrain
I. Absence of the nose
J. Increased thickness in the nuchal fold area in the back of the neck associated with trisomy 21
K. Abnormal protrusion of the eyeball
L. Protrusion of the brain from the cranial cavity
M. Enlargement of the thyroid gland
N. Hereditary disease caused by failure to oxidize an amino acid (phenylalanine) to tyrosine because of a defective enzyme; can lead to mental retardation
O. Eyes too far apart

Exercise 2

Match the following fetal face and neck abnormality terms with their definitions.

_____ 1. Beckwith-Wiedemann syndrome

_____ 2. branchial cleft cyst

_____ 3. epignathus

_____ 4. hemifacial microsomia

_____ 5. hypotelorism

_____ 6. macroglossia

_____ 7. microphthalmia

A. Underdevelopment of the eyes, fingers, and mouth
B. A cylindrical protuberance of the face that in cyclopia or ethmocephaly represents the nose
C. Underdevelopment of the jaw that causes the ears to be located close together toward the front of the neck
D. Cystic defect that arises from the primitive branchial apparatus
E. Solid tumor
F. Eyes too close together
G. Small eyes

_____ 8. oculodentodigital dysplasia

_____ 9. otocephaly

_____ 10. Pierre Robin sequence

_____ 11. proboscis

_____ 12. strabismus

_____ 13. teratoma

_____ 14. trigonocephaly

H. Premature closure of the metopic suture
I. Abnormal smallness of one side of the face
J. Group of disorders having in common the coexistence of an omphalocele, macroglossia, and visceromegaly
K. Micrognathia and abnormal smallness of the tongue, usually with a cleft palate
L. Eye disorder in which optic axes cannot be directed to the same object
M. Teratoma located in the oropharynx
N. Hypertrophied tongue

ANATOMY

Exercise 3

Label the following illustrations.

A. Lateral view of the embryo at 28 days.

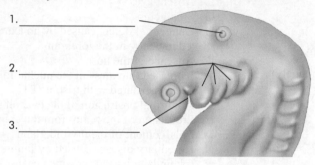

1._____

2._____

3._____

B. Frontal view of the embryo at 24 days.

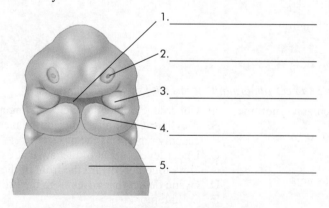

1._____

2._____

3._____

4._____

5._____

C. Frontal view of the embryo at 33 days.

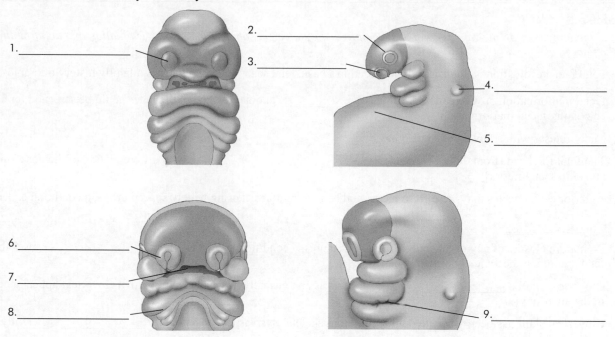

1._____

2._____

3._____

4._____

5._____

6._____

7._____

8._____

9._____

Exercise 4

Fill in the blank(s) with the word(s) that best completes the statements about the embryology of the fetal face and neck.

1. The embryo in the 4th week has characteristic external features of the head and neck area in the form of a series of

   branchial arches, pouches, grooves, and membranes that are referred to as the _____apparatus and bear a resemblance to gills.

2. There are _____ branchial arches.

3. The first branchial arch is also known as the _____ arch; it forms the jaw, zygomatic bone, ear, and temporal bone.

4. The _____ crest cells develop the skeletal parts of the face, and the mesoderm of each arch develops the musculature of the face and neck.

5. The primitive mouth is an indentation on the surface of the _____ (referred to as the *stomodeum*).

6. The maxillary prominences grow _____ between the 5th and 8th weeks. This growth compresses the medial nasal prominences together toward the midline. The two medial nasal prominences and the two maxillary

   prominences lateral to them fuse together to form the _____ lip.

Exercise 5

Fill in the blank(s) with the word(s) that best completes the statements about sonographic evaluation and abnormalities of the fetal face.

1. Fetal facial evaluation is not routinely included in a basic fetal scan, but when there is a family history of cranio-facial malformation or when another _____ anomaly is found, the face should be screened for a coexisting facial malformation.

2. Many fetuses with a facial defect also have _____ abnormalities.

3. The fetal forehead (frontal bone) appears as a _____ surface with differentiation of the nose, lips, and chin seen inferiorly.

4. Anterior cephaloceles may arise from the frontal bone or midface causing widely spaced orbits, a condition called

   _____.

5. Premature closure of any or all six of the cranial sutures, a condition known as _____, causes the fetal cranium to become abnormally shaped.

6. Cloverleaf skull or _____ appears as an unusually misshapen skull with a cloverleaf appearance in the anterior view.

7. Cloverleaf skull has been associated with numerous skeletal dysplasias, most notably _____ dys-plasia and _____.

8. _____ (premature closure of the metopic suture) may cause the forehead to have an elongated (tall) appearance in the sagittal plane and to appear triangular in the axial plane.

9. _____ may be observed in a fetus with a lemon-shaped skull (from spina bifida) or with skeletal dysplasias.

10. Underdevelopment of the middle structures of the face is midface or _____ hypoplasia with depressed or absent nasal bridge.

11. Midface hypoplasia may be seen in fetuses with chromosome anomalies such as trisomy _____, craniosynostosis syndromes such as Apert's syndrome, or limb and skeletal abnormalities such as achondroplasia, chondrodysplasia punctata, asphyxiating thoracic dysplasia, and others.

12. A median-cleft face syndrome consisting of a range of midline facial defects involving the eyes, forehead, and nose is _____ dysplasia.

13. Tongue protrusion may suggest macroglossia (enlarged tongue), a condition found in _____ syn-drome (congenital overgrowth of tissues).

14. The sonographer must document the presence of both eyes and must assess the overall size of the eyes to exclude

   _____ (small eyes) and _____ (absent eyes).

15. A condition characterized by decreased distance between the orbits is _____.

16. _____ is characterized by abnormally widely spaced orbits.

17. The contour of the nose, upper and lower lips, and chin is observed in a(n) _____ plane.

18. _____ lip with or without cleft palate represents the most common congenital anomaly of the face.

19. Isolated cleft lip may occur as a unilateral or bilateral defect, and when unilateral, it commonly originates on the

   _____ side of the face.

ABNORMALITIES

Exercise 6

Fill in the blank(s) with the word(s) that best completes the statements about abnormalities of the neck.

1. Cleft _____ represents the most common congenital anomaly of the face.

2. When a large neck tumor exists, delivery of the infant is complicated because the tumor may cause delivery

   _____, the inability to deliver the trunk once the head has been delivered.

3. When cystic hygroma is found, there is a high risk for _____ syndrome (45,X).

4. Malformation of the lymphatic system that leads to single or multiloculated lymph-filled cavities around the neck

   results in _____.

5. An accumulation of lymph in the fetal tissues may lead to fetal _____hygroma.

6. A fetal _____ usually appears as a symmetrical (bilobed), solid, homogeneous mass arising from the anterior fetal neck in the region of the fetal thyroid gland.

Exercise 7

Provide a short answer for each question after evaluating the images.

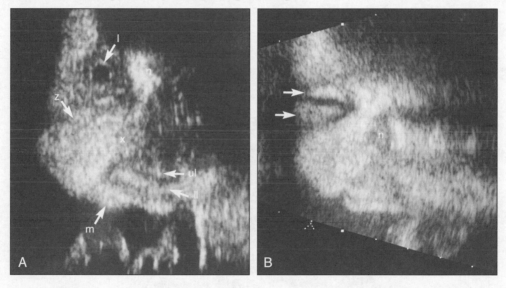

1. What does the letter *l* denote in image *A*? What are the arrows pointing to in image *B*?

   _____

   _____

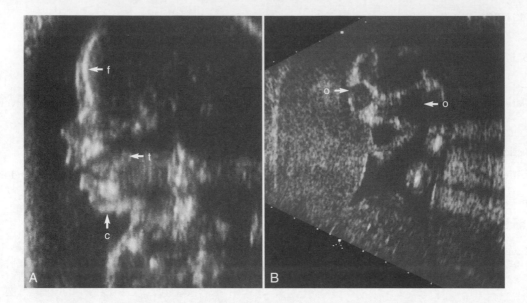

2. What does the *t* stand for in image *A* (a sagittal view of the facial profile)? Identify the view that is demonstrated in image *B*.

A. _____

B. _____

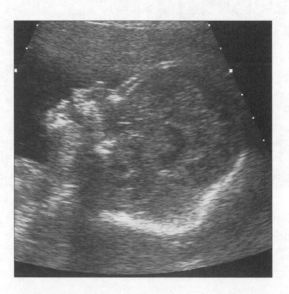

3. Describe this abnormality of the fetal skull.

_____

_____

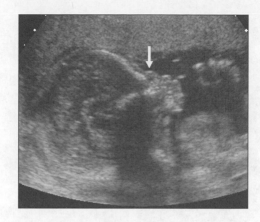

4. Identify what the arrow is pointing to on this fetal face and what it indicates.

_____

_____

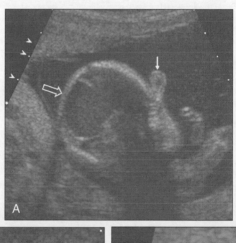

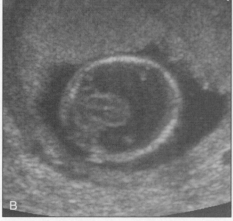

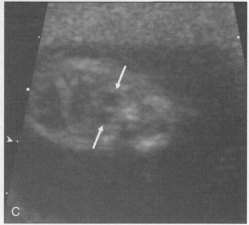

5. Describe the abnormality in this fetal head.

A. _____

B. _____

C. _____

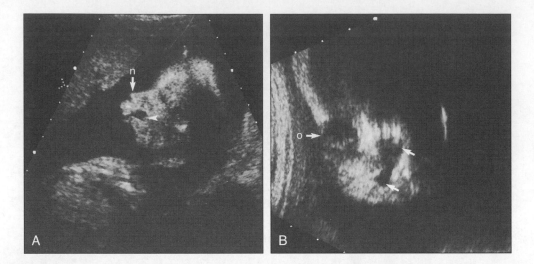

6. Describe the abnormality in this fetal face.

_____

_____

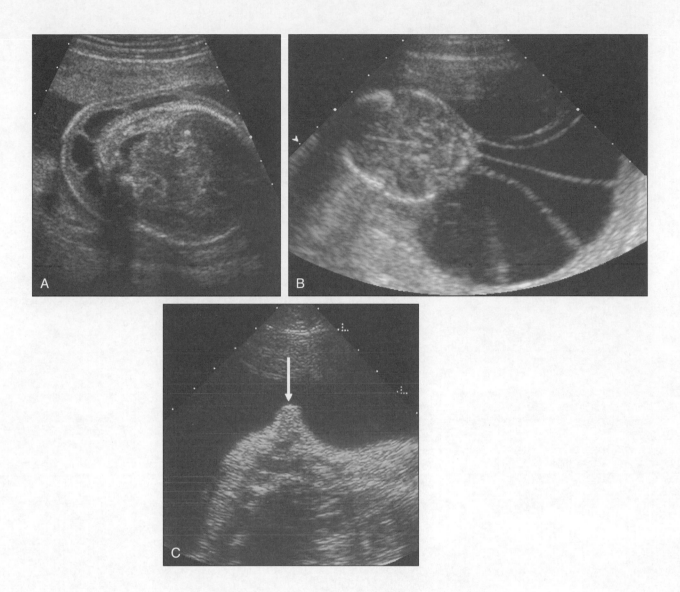

7. Describe the abnormality in each of these fetal images.

_____

_____

KEY TERMS

Exercise 1

Match the following fetal head and spine anomaly terms with their definitions.

_____ 1. acrania

_____ 2. alobar holoprosencephaly

_____ 3. anencephaly

_____ 4. anomaly

_____ 5. cebocephaly

_____ 6. cyclopia

_____ 7. cystic hygroma

_____ 8. holoprosencephaly

_____ 9. hydranencephaly

_____ 10. hydrocephalus

_____ 11. macrocephaly

_____ 12. meningocele

_____ 13. meningomyelocele

_____ 14. spina bifida

_____ 15. spina bifida occulta

_____ 16. ventriculomegaly

A. Enlargement of the fetal cranium as a result of ventriculomegaly

B. Most severe form of holoprosencephaly characterized by a single common ventricle and a malformed brain

C. Increase in size of the jugular lymphatic sacs caused by abnormal development

D. Neural tube defect of the spine in which the dorsal vertebrae fail to fuse together, allowing the protrusion of meninges and/or spinal cord through the defect

E. Abnormal accumulation of cerebrospinal fluid within the cerebral ventricles leading to dilatation of the ventricles; compression of developing brain tissue and brain damage may result; commonly associated with additional fetal anomalies

F. An abnormality or congenital malformation

G. Congenital absence of the cerebral hemispheres caused by occlusion of the carotid arteries; midbrain structures are present, and fluid replaces cerebral tissue

H. Open spinal defect characterized by protrusion of meninges and spinal cord through the defect, usually within a meningeal sac

I. Ventriculomegaly in the neonate; abnormal accumulation of cerebrospinal fluid within the cerebral ventricles resulting in compression and, frequently, destruction of brain tissue

J. Form of holoprosencephaly characterized by a common ventricle, hypotelorism, and a nose with a single nostril

K. Closed defect of the spine without protrusion of meninges or spinal cord

L. Neural tube defect characterized by lack of development of the cerebral and cerebellar hemispheres and cranial vault; this abnormality is incompatible with life

M. Condition associated with anencephaly in which there is complete or partial absence of the cranial bones

N. Severe form of holoprosencephaly characterized by a common ventricle, fusion of the orbits with one or two eyes present, and a proboscis

O. Open spinal defect characterized by protrusion of the spinal meninges

P. Range of abnormalities resulting from abnormal cleavage of the forebrain

Exercise 2

Fill in the blank(s) with the word(s) that best completes the statements or provide a short answer about the fetal neural axis.

1. The cephalic neural plate develops into the _____, and the caudal end forms the _____ cord.

2. The forebrain will continue to develop into the _____.

3. The midbrain will become the _____.

4. The hindbrain will form the _____.

5. Failure of closure of the neural tube at the cranial end is _____.

6. A neural tube defect in which the meninges alone or the meninges and brain herniate through a defect in the calvarium is a(n)_____.

7. The term used to describe herniation of the meninges and brain through the defect is _____.

8. Cranial _____ describes the herniation of only meninges.

9. Fetuses with myelomeningoceles often present with the cranial defects associated with the _____ malformation, which is identified in 90% of patients.

10. _____ holoprosencephaly is characterized by a monoventricle; brain tissue that is small and may have a cup, ball, or pancake configuration; fusion of the thalamus; and absence of the interhemispheric fissure, cavum septi pellucidi, corpus callosum, optic tracts, and olfactory bulbs.

11. _____ holoprosencephaly presents with a single ventricular cavity with partial formation of the occipital horns, partial or complete fusion of the thalamus, a rudimentary flex and interhemispheric fissure, and absent corpus callosum, cavum septi pellucidi, and olfactory bulbs.

12. Almost complete division of the ventricles is seen with a corpus callosum that may be normal, hypoplastic, or absent, although the cavum septi pellucidi will still be absent in _____ holoprosencephaly.

13. A fibrous tract that connects the cerebral hemispheres and aids in learning and memory is the _____ callosum.

14. _____ stenosis results from obstruction, atresia, or stenosis of the aqueduct of Sylvius, causing ventriculomegaly.

15. Porencephaly or _____ cysts are cysts filled with cerebrospinal fluid.

16. A rare disorder characterized by clefts in the cerebral cortex is _____.

17. Enlargement of the ventricles occurs with _____ of cerebrospinal fluid flow.

18. Fetal ventriculomegaly typically progresses from the _____ horns into the temporal and then to the _____ ventricular horns.

19. A ventricle is considered dilated when its diameter exceeds _____ mm.

Provide a short answer for each question after evaluating the images.

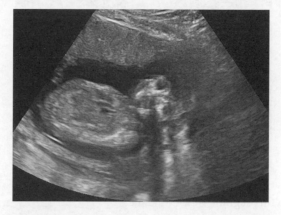

1. Describe your findings in this second-trimester sonogram.

_____

_____

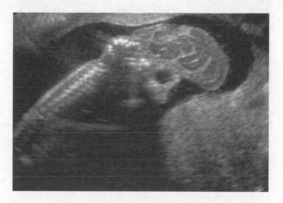

2. Describe the abnormality demonstrated in this sagittal view of the fetal head.

_____

_____

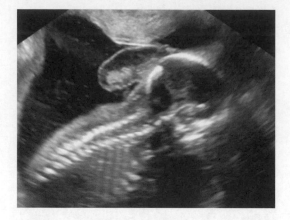

3. Identify the abnormality seen in this sagittal view of the fetus.

_____

_____

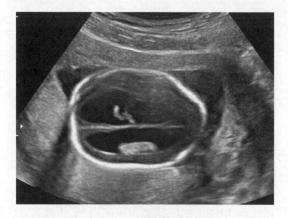

4. Identify this abnormality of the fetal head.

_____

_____

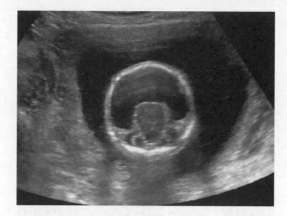

5. Describe this abnormality of the fetal head.

_____

_____

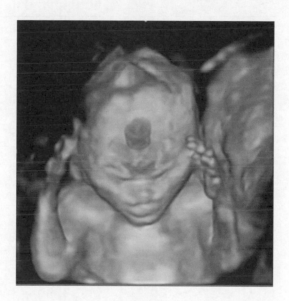

6. Describe this abnormality of the fetal head.

_____

_____

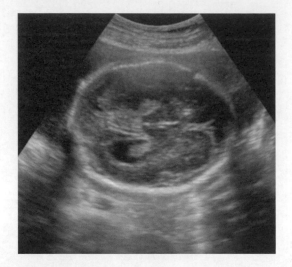

7. Describe the abnormality shown in this fetal head.

_____

_____

KEY TERMS

Exercise 1

Match the following fetal thorax terms with their definitions.

_____ 1. asphyxiating thoracic dystrophy

_____ 2. bronchogenic cyst

_____ 3. congenital bronchial atresia

_____ 4. congenital cystic adenomatoid malformation

_____ 5. congenital diaphragmatic hernia

_____ 6. foramen of Bochdalek

_____ 7. foramen of Morgagni

_____ 8. lymphangiectasia

_____ 9. pleural effusion

_____10. pulmonary hypoplasia

_____11. pulmonary sequestration

A. Dilatation of a lymph node
B. Abnormality in the formation of the bronchial tree with secondary overgrowth of mesenchymal tissue from arrested bronchial development
C. Small, underdeveloped lungs with resultant reduction in lung volume; secondary to prolonged oligohydramnios or as a consequence of a small thoracic cavity
D. Most common lung cyst detected prenatally
E. Type of diaphragmatic defect that occurs posterior and lateral in the diaphragm; usually found in the left side
F. Accumulation of fluid within the thoracic cavity
G. Pulmonary anomaly that results from focal obliteration of a segment of the bronchial lumen
H. Extrapulmonary tissue present within the pleural lung sac or connected to the inferior border of the lung within its own pleural sac
I. Significantly narrow diameter of the chest in the fetus
J. Opening in the pleuroperitoneal membrane that develops in the first trimester
K. Diaphragmatic hernia that occurs anterior and medial in the diaphragm that may communicate with the pericardial sac

EMBRYOLOGY AND SONOGRAPHIC CHARACTERISTICS

Exercise 2

Fill in the blank(s) with the word(s) that best completes the statements about the embryology and sonographic characteristics of the thoracic cavity.

1. The lungs at birth are about half filled with _____ derived from the amniotic cavity, tracheal glands, and lungs.

2. The normal thoracic cavity is symmetrically _____ shaped, with the ribs forming the lateral margins, the _____ forming the upper margins, and the diaphragm forming the lower margins.

3. The thorax is normally slightly _____ than the abdominal cavity.

4. In the presence of oligohydramnios, resultant pulmonary _____ may be seen with a reduction in overall thoracic size.

5. The location of the heart is important to document in a routine sonographic examination because detection of abnormal position may indicate the presence of a chest mass, pleural _____, or cardiac _____.

6. The fetal lungs appear homogeneous on ultrasound with moderate _____.

7. Early in gestation, the lungs are similar to or slightly less echogenic than the _____, and as gestation progresses, there is a trend toward increased pulmonary echogenicity relative to the liver.

8. Fetal breathing becomes most prominent in the _____ and _____ trimesters.

9. Fetal breathing movements are documented as present if characteristic seesaw movements of the fetal chest or abdomen are sustained for at least _____ seconds.

ABNORMALITIES

Exercise 3

Fill in the blank(s) with the word(s) that best completes the statements or provide a short answer about the abnormalities of the thoracic cavity.

1. A decrease in the numbers of lung cells, airways, and alveoli, with a resulting decrease in organ size and weight, causes pulmonary _____.

2. Pulmonary hypoplasia may occur when there is an extreme _____ in amniotic fluid volume.

3. The sonographer may be able to check for pulmonary hypoplasia by measuring the thoracic circumference at the level of the _____ heart view, excluding the skin and subcutaneous tissues.

4. _____ cysts occur as a result of abnormal budding of the foregut and lack of any communication with the trachea or bronchial tree.

5. Accumulation of fluid within the pleural cavity that may appear as isolated lesions or secondary to multiple fetal anomalies is called a _____, or pleural effusion.

6. In pulmonary _____, extrapulmonary tissue is present within the pleural lung sac or is connected to the inferior border of the lung within its own pleural sac.

7. The arterial supply referred to in question 7 is usually derived from the _____ aorta, with venous drainage into the vena cava.

8. A multicystic mass within the lung consisting of primitive lung tissue and abnormal bronchial and bronchiolar-like structures is congenital cystic _____ malformation.

9. Congenital diaphragmatic hernia (CDH) is a herniation of the _____ viscera into the chest, which results from a congenital defect in the fetal diaphragm.

10. The most common type of diaphragmatic defect by far occurs posteriorly and laterally in the diaphragm (herniation through foramen of _____).

11. Diaphragmatic hernias may occur anteriorly and medially in the diaphragm through the foramen of _____ and may communicate with the pericardial sac.

12. Hydrops usually is not present with left-sided congenital diaphragmatic hernias unless associated fetal _____ are present.

13. On sonographic examination, a _____ congenital diaphragmatic hernia usually found when the cardiac silhouette is displaced to the right, and an ectopic stomach is in the chest.

14. The sonographer will see the liver in the chest; collapsed bowel may be present; and the heart may be deviated far to the left in a _____ -sided diaphragmatic hernia.

15. At birth, a majority of infants with congenital diaphragmatic hernia have pulmonary _____ and secondary respiratory insufficiency.

16. Development of the _____ procedure has allowed babies with severe diaphragmatic hernia a chance for survival immediately post delivery.

Exercise 4

Provide a short answer for each question after evaluating the images.

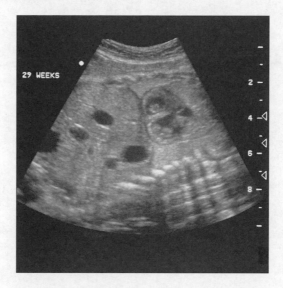

1. State whether the lungs are more or less echogenic than the liver.

_____

_____

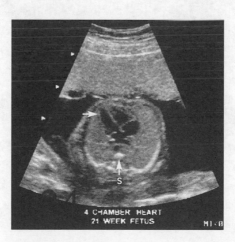

2. Describe where the apex of the fetal heart is in this image. State whether the fetal heart axis is normal in this image.

_____

_____

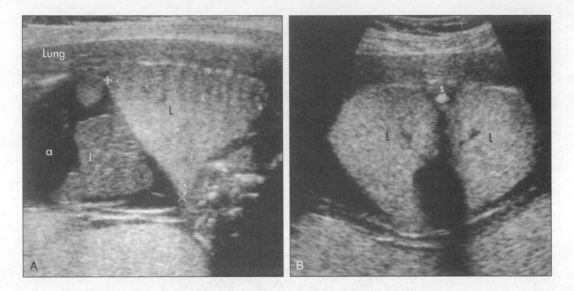

3. Describe the abnormalities seen in these images.

_____

_____

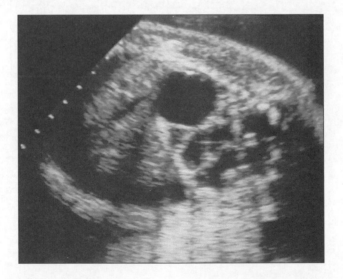

4. Which type of cystic adenomatoid malformation is shown in this fetal lung?

_____

_____

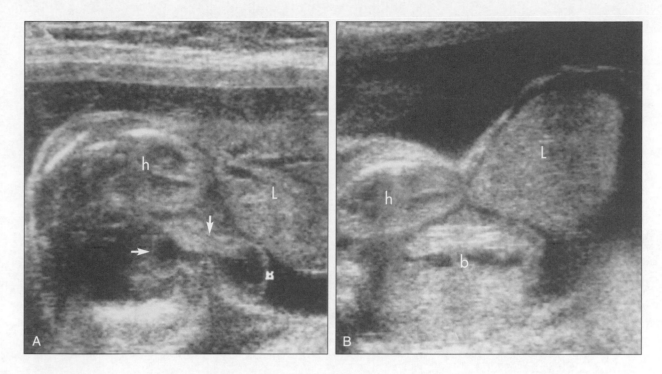

5. Describe the complication in this fetus with a known omphalocele.

_____

_____

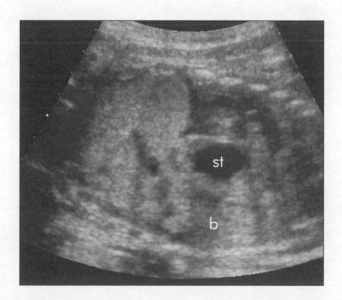

6. Describe the sonographic findings in this 25-week fetus.

_____

_____

62 The Fetal Anterior Abdominal Wall

KEY TERMS

Exercise 1

Match the following terms related to abnormalities of the anterior abdominal wall with their definitions.

_____ 1. amniotic band syndrome

_____ 2. Beckwith-Wiedemann syndrome

_____ 3. cloacal exstrophy

_____ 4. encephalocele

_____ 5. exencephaly

_____ 6. gastroschisis

_____ 7. limb–body wall complex

_____ 8. omphalocele

_____ 9. pentalogy of Cantrell

_____ 10. scoliosis

A. Opening in the layers of the abdominal wall with evisceration of the bowel

B. Rupture of the amnion that leads to entrapment or entanglement of fetal parts by the "sticky" chorion

C. Develops when a midline defect of the abdominal muscles, fascia, and skin results in herniation of intra-abdominal structures into the base of the umbilical cord

D. Defect in the lower abdominal wall and anterior wall of the urinary bladder

E. Anomaly with large cranial defects, facial cleft, large body wall defects, and limb abnormalities

F. Abnormal lateral curvature of the spine

G. Group of disorders having in common the coexistence of an omphalocele, macroglossia, and visceromegaly

H. Abnormal condition in which the brain is located outside the cranium

I. Rare anomaly with five defects: omphalocele, ectopic heart, lower sternum, anterior diaphragm, and diaphragmatic pericardium

J. Protrusion of the brain through a cranial fissure

Exercise 2

Fill in the blank(s) with the word(s) that best completes the statements about the fetal anterior abdominal wall.

1. The embryo is a flat disk consisting of three layers—_____, _____, and _____—that form by the end of the 5th week of development.

2. Umbilical hernia of the _____ occurs during the 8th week of development as the midgut extends to the extraembryonic coelom in the proximal portion of the umbilical cord.

3. The intestines return to the abdominal cavity by the _____ week of gestation.

4. The most common types of abdominal wall defects are _____, _____, and _____.

5. Abdominal wall defects cause _____ of the normal contour of the ventral or anterior surface of the fetal abdomen.

6. When bowel loops fail to return to the abdomen, a bowel-containing _____ occurs.

7. Omphalocele herniation is covered by a(n) _____ that is composed of amnion and peritoneum.

8. Fetuses with an omphalocele that contains only bowel have a higher risk for _____ abnormalities and other anomalies.

9. _____ omphaloceles may contain bowel and may demonstrate a relatively large abdominal wall defect in comparison with the abdominal diameter.

10. Gastroschisis is a periumbilical defect that nearly always is located to the _____ of the umbilicus.

11. _____ bowel is always found in the herniation.

12. _____ levels are significantly higher in gastroschisis compared with omphalocele because of the exposed bowel.

13. In gastroschisis, the edges of the bowel are irregular and free floating _____ a covering membrane, as is seen with omphalocele.

14. Rupture of the amnion, which leads to entrapment or entanglement of fetal parts by the "sticky" chorion, is the _____ _____ syndrome.

15. A rare group of disorders having in common the coexistence of an omphalocele, macroglossia, and visceromegaly is the _____ syndrome.

16. A defect in the lower abdominal wall and the anterior wall of the urinary bladder is a characteristic of bladder _____.

17. The rare condition, _____ _____ _____, is the association of a cleft distal sternum, diaphragmatic defect, midline anterior ventral wall defect, defect of the apical pericardium with communication into the peritoneum, and an internal cardiac defect.

18. The exposed heart presents outside the chest wall through a cleft sternum is called _____ _____.

19. _____ _____ _____ complex anomaly is associated with large cranial defects; facial cleft; body wall complex defects involving the thorax, abdomen, or both; and limb defects.

Provide a short answer for each question after evaluating the images.

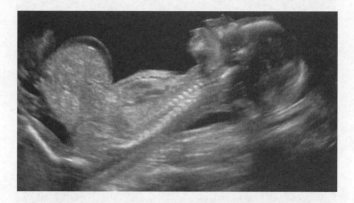

1. Name the abnormality in this fetus.

_____

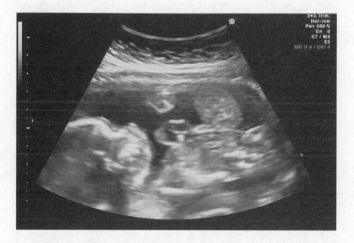

2. This is a fetus with Pentalogy of Cantrell. What abnormalities are seen in these images?

_____

_____

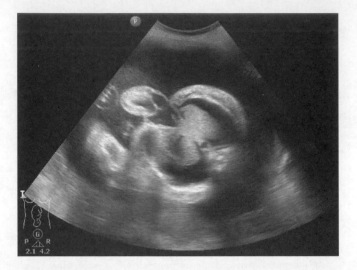

3. Describe the abnormalities seen in this fetus.

_____

_____

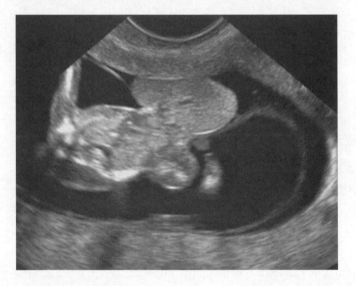

4. Describe the abnormality seen in this fetus.

_____

_____

63 The Fetal Abdomen

KEY TERMS

Exercise 1

Match the following embryology and sonographic evaluation terms with their definitions.

_____ 1. duodenal stenosis

_____ 2. esophageal atresia

_____ 3. esophageal stenosis

_____ 4. gastroschisis

_____ 5. haustral folds

_____ 6. hematopoiesis

_____ 7. Meckel's diverticulum

_____ 8. omphalocele

_____ 9. peristalsis

A. Abnormality of the abdominal wall in which the bowel without a covering membrane protrudes outside of the wall

B. Abnormality of the abdominal wall in which bowel and liver, both covered by a membrane, protrude outside the wall

C. Congenital hypoplasia of the esophagus; usually associated with a tracheoesophageal fistula

D. Narrowing of the esophagus, usually in the distal third segment

E. Remnant of the proximal part of the yolk stalk

F. One of the sacculations of the colon caused by longitudinal bands that are shorter than the gut

G. Narrowing of the pyloric sphincter

H. Formation of blood

I. Movement of the bowel

Exercise 2

Match the following terms related to abnormalities of the hepatobiliary system with their definitions.

_____ 1. anorectal atresia

_____ 2. asplenia

_____ 3. cholcdochal cyst

_____ 4. cholelithiasis

_____ 5. cystic fibrosis

_____ 6. duodenal atresia

_____ 7. Hirschsprung's disease

_____ 8. jejunoileal atresia

_____ 9. meconium ileus

_____ 10. partial situs inversus

_____ 11. polysplenia

_____ 12. pseudoascites

_____ 13. situs inversus

_____ 14. VACTERL

A. Cystic growth of the common bile duct

B. Sonolucent band near the fetal anterior abdominal wall from the abdominal wall muscles in the fetus over 18 weeks

C. A congenital disorder in which there is abnormal innervation of the large intestine

D. Small-bowel disorder marked by the presence of thick echogenic meconium in the distal ileum

E. No development of splenic tissue

F. Complete blockage at the pyloric sphincter

G. Heart and abdominal organs are completely reversed

H. Gallstones

I. More than one spleen; associated with cardiac malformations

J. Vertebral defects, heart defects, renal and limb abnormalities

K. Blockage of the jejunum and ileal bowel segments that appears as multiple cystic structures within the fetal abdomen

L. Congenital condition characterized by mucus buildup within the lungs and other areas of the body

M. Complex disorder of the bowel and genitourinary tract

N. Condition in which only the heart or the abdominal organs are reversed

Exercise 3

Fill in the blank(s) with the word(s) that best completes the statements about the fetal gastrointestinal tract.

1. The derivatives of the _____ are the pharynx, lower respiratory system, esophagus, stomach, part of the duodenum, liver and biliary apparatus, and pancreas.

2. When _____ atresia occurs, amniotic fluid cannot pass to the intestines for absorption, and hydramnios results.

3. The stomach appears as a fusiform dilatation of the caudal part of the _____.

4. The dorsal mesogastrium is carried to the left during rotation of the stomach and formation of a cavity known as the omental bursa or _____ sac of peritoneum.

5. The lesser sac communicates with the main peritoneal cavity or greater peritoneal sac through a small opening, called the _____ foramen.

6. The duodenum develops from the caudal part of the foregut and the cranial part of the _____.

7. The junction of the two embryonic parts of the duodenum in the adult is just _____ to the entrance of the common bile duct.

8. Normally the duodenum is recanalized by the end of the 8th week. Partial or complete failure of this process results in duodenal _____ (narrowing) or duodenal _____ (blockage).

9. The liver grows rapidly and intermingles with the vitelline and _____ veins, divides into _____ parts, and fills most of the abdominal cavity.

10. During the 6th week, _____ (blood formation) begins and accounts for the large size of the liver between the 7th and 9th weeks of development.

11. The derivatives of the _____ are the small intestines (including most of the duodenum), the cecum and vermiform appendix, the ascending colon, and most of the transverse colon. All of these structures are supplied by the superior mesenteric artery.

12. A remnant of the proximal part of the yolk stalk that fails to degenerate and disappear during the early fetal period is a _____ diverticulum.

Exercise 4

Fill in the blank(s) with the word(s) that best completes the statements about the stomach, small bowel, and colon.

1. The stomach should be identified as a(n) _____ structure in the left upper quadrant inferior to the diaphragm.

2. If no fluid is apparent, the stomach should be reevaluated in _____ to _____ minutes to rule out the possibility of a central nervous system problem (swallowing disorders), obstruction, oligohydramnios, or atresia.

3. The abdominal circumference is measured at the level of the _____ sinus and the _____ portion of the left portal vein ("hockey stick" appearance on the sonogram).

4. The insertion of the umbilical cord must be imaged with _____ because it inserts both into the fetal abdomen and into the placenta.

5. The fetus is capable of _____ sufficient amounts of amniotic fluid to permit visualization of the stomach by 11 menstrual weeks.

6. After the 15th to 16th week, _____ begins to accumulate in the distal part of the small intestine as a combination of desquamated cells, bile pigments, and mucoproteins.

7. The region of the small bowel can be seen because it is slightly _____ compared with the liver and may appear "masslike" in the central abdomen and pelvis.

8. After 27 weeks, _____ of normal small bowel is increasingly observed.

9. The _____folds of the colon help to differentiate it from the small bowel.

10. The _____ does not have peristalsis as the small bowel does.

11. The meconium within the lumen of the colon appears _____ relative to the fetal liver and in comparison with the bowel wall.

12. The _____ lobe of the liver is larger than the _____ in utero secondary to the greater supply of oxygenated blood.

13. The normal gallbladder may be seen sonographically after _____ weeks of gestation.

Exercise 5

Fill in the blank(s) with the word(s) that best completes the statements about abnormalities of the fetal abdomen.

1. _____ _____ may present as a total reversal of the thoracic and abdominal organs or as a partial reversal.

2. The stomach may or may not be reversed in _____ _____ _____.

3. True ascites is identified within the peritoneal recesses, whereas _____ is always confined to an anterior or anterolateral aspect of the fetal abdomen.

4. A bowel obstruction results in _____ bowel dilatation that is characteristically recognized as one or more tubular structures within the fetal abdomen.

5. The most reliable criterion for diagnosing dilated bowel is the bowel _____, not the sonographic appearance.

6. A congenital blockage of the esophagus resulting from faulty separation of the foregut into its respiratory and digestive components is _____ atresia.

7. In reference to the diagnosis in question 6, the sonographer may observe the _____ stomach and _____.

8. Blockage of the jejunum and ileal bowel segments (jejunoileal atresia or stenosis) appears as multiple cystic structures _____ to the site of atresia within the fetal abdomen.

9. A small-bowel disorder marked by the presence of thick meconium in the distal ileum is _____ileus.

10. _____ atresia may present as part of the VACTERL association or in caudal regression.

11. Hyperechoic bowel is a(n) _____ impression of unusually echogenic bowel, typically seen during the second trimester.

12. True ascites in the fetal abdomen is always _____; it usually outlines the falciform ligament and umbilical vein.

Exercise 6

Provide a short answer for each question after evaluating the images.

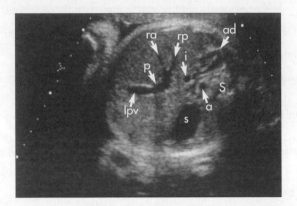

1. This image is representative of the level at which the abdominal circumference should be taken. Identify the following structures: **P, LPV, s, and S.**

_____

_____

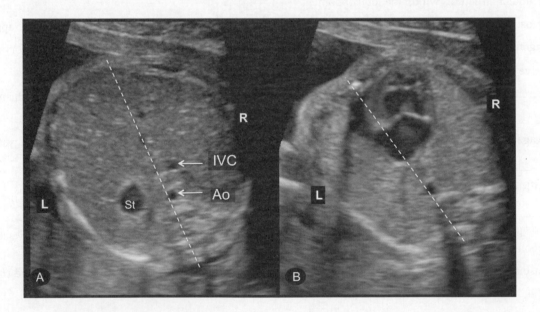

2. What abnormality is demonstrated in this fetus?

_____

_____

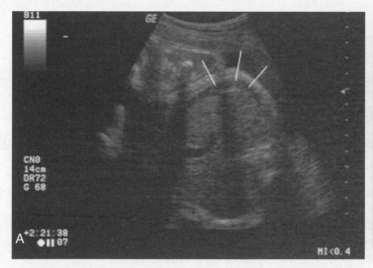 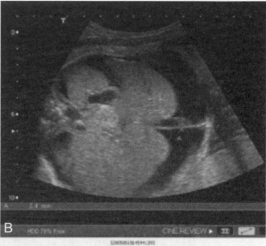

3. Describe the abnormality seen on images A and B.

A. _____

B. _____

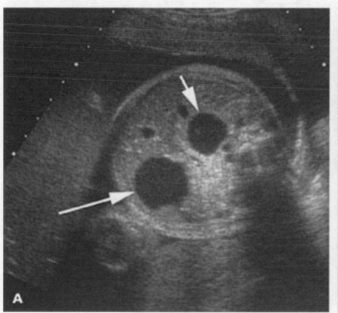 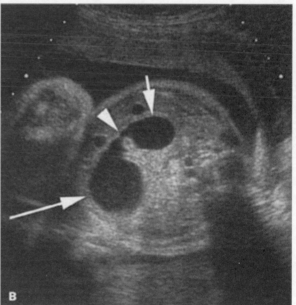

4. Describe the ultrasound findings in this fetal abdomen.

_____

_____

echogenic bowel

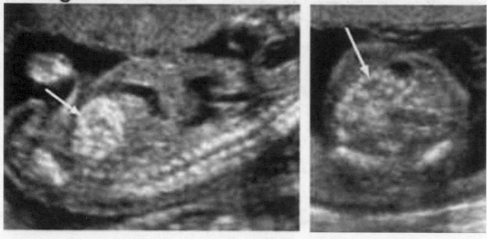

5. Describe the sonographic findings in these images of the fetal abdomen.

_____

_____

64 The Fetal Urogenital System

KEY TERMS

Exercise 1

Match the following terms related to sonographic findings suggesting abnormalities and congenital malformations with their definitions.

_____ 1. cloacal exstrophy

_____ 2. epispadias

_____ 3. horseshoe kidney

_____ 4. hydroureters

_____ 5. hypospadias

_____ 6. pelvic kidney

_____ 7. posterior urethral valve

_____ 8. Potter's syndrome

_____ 9. renal agenesis

_____ 10. urachal cyst

_____ 11. ureterocele

A. Characterized by a group of findings associated with oligohydramnios and renal failure or bilateral renal agenesis

B. Occurs when the kidney does not migrate upward into the retroperitoneal space

C. Small part of the lumen of the allantois that persists while the urachus forms

D. Anatomic structure that occurs only in male fetuses

E. Renal system fails to develop

F. Forms when the inferior poles of the kidney fuse while they are in the pelvis

G. Complex malformation involving lower limb anomalies, spinal defect, anal atresia, and lower abdominal wall defect (exstrophy of the bladder and protrusion of the intestines)

H. Dilated ureters

I. Congenital outpouching of the distal ureter into the bladder

J. Abnormal congenital opening of the male urethra on the undersurface of the penis

K. Abnormal congenital opening of the male urethra on the top side of the penis

Exercise 2

Match the following terms related to obstructive abnormalities, renal cystic disease, and other pelvic masses with their definitions.

_____ 1. cryptorchidism

_____ 2. fetal hydronephrosis

_____ 3. fetal ovarian cyst

_____ 4. hermaphroditism

_____ 5. hydrometrocolpos

_____ 6. infantile polycystic kidney disease

_____ 7. megacystis

_____ 8. megaureter

_____ 9. multicystic dysplastic kidney disease

_____ 10. Potter's sequence

_____ 11. prune belly syndrome

_____ 12. pyelectasis

_____ 13. ureteropelvic junction

_____ 14. ureterovesical junction

_____ 15. urethral atresia

A. Dilated renal pelvis without involvement of the calyces

B. Autosomal recessive disease that affects the fetal kidneys and liver

C. Collection of fluid in the vagina and uterus

D. Junction where the ureter enters the bladder

E. Failure of the testes to descend into the scrotum

F. Dilatation of the fetal abdomen secondary to severe hydronephrosis and fetal ascites

G. Level of the urethra where the urinary tract may become obstructed

H. Junction of the ureter entering the renal pelvis; most common site of obstruction

I. Condition in which both ovarian and testicular tissues are present

J. Condition that causes a massively distended bladder

K. Multiple cysts replace normal renal tissue throughout the kidney

L. Dilated renal pelvis in the fetus

M. Term used to describe renal diseases other than renal agenesis that result in renal failure and facial or structure abnormalities caused by oligohydramnios

N. Dilation of the lower end of the ureter

O. Ovarian mass that results from maternal hormone stimulation

417

Exercise 3

Fill in the blank(s) with the word(s) that best completes the statements about the fetal urinary system.

1. A complete ultrasound examination includes evaluation of both kidneys, documentation of the urinary bladder, and assessment of _____ _____.

2. The urinary system and the genital system develop from the intermediate _____, and the excretory ducts of both systems initially enter a common cavity called the cloaca.

3. The part of the urogenital ridge that gives rise to the urinary system is known as the nephrogenic cord or _____ ridge.

4. The part that gives rise to the genital system is known as the gonadal ridge or _____ ridge.

5. The permanent kidneys or _____ begins to develop early in the 5th week while the mesonephric ducts are still developing.

6. Urine formation begins toward the end of the first trimester, around the _____ or _____ week, and continues actively throughout fetal life.

7. Urine is excreted into the amniotic cavity and forms a major part of the _____.

8. The kidneys do not need to function in utero because the _____ eliminates waste from the fetal blood.

9. The kidneys initially lie very close together in the _____; gradually, they migrate into the abdomen and become separated from one another.

10. In adolescent and adult patients, persistence of the fetal lobulation and groove may be seen on ultrasound as an _____ triangular notch along the anterior wall of the _____ kidney.

Exercise 4

Fill in the blank(s) with the word(s) that best completes the statements about the development of the fetal urinary system.

1. Complete absence of the kidneys is known as renal _____.

2. Division of the ureteric bud at an early stage results in a double or _____ kidney.

3. When the inferior poles of the kidney fuse while they are in the pelvis, a _____ kidney is formed.

4. The fetal urinary bladder is derived from the hindgut derivative known as the _____ sinus.

5. _____ of the bladder occurs primarily in males and is characterized by protrusion of the posterior wall of the urinary bladder, which contains the trigone of the bladder and the ureteric orifices.

6. Early in development, the urinary bladder is continuous with the _____.

7. The allantois regresses to become a fibrous cord known as the _____.

8. If the lumen of the allantois persists while the urachus forms, a urachal _____ develops, which causes urine to drain from the bladder to the umbilicus.

9. If only a small part of the lumen of the allantois persists, it is called a _____ cyst.

Exercise 5

Fill in the blank(s) with the word(s) that best completes the statements about sonographic evaluation of the urinary system.

1. The fetal kidneys and bladder may be well seen on ultrasound by _____ weeks' gestation.

2. At this time period, the kidneys appear as bilateral _____ structures in the paravertebral regions.

3. By _____ weeks, it is possible to distinguish the renal cortex from the medulla, to outline the renal capsule clearly, and to see a central echogenic area in the renal sinus region.

4. The upper limit of normal for the renal pelves is _____ mm up to 33 weeks' gestation and _____ mm from 33 weeks' gestation until term.

5. If the bladder appears too large, it should be evaluated again at the end of the study (assuming the examination takes at least _____ minutes) to see if normal emptying has occurred.

6. When obstruction occurs at the level of the urethra, the bladder wall becomes _____.

7. Dilatation of the posterior _____ is highly suggestive of an obstructive process, such as posterior urethral valve syndrome, known as the "keyhole" sign on sonography because the dilated bladder has the shape of a keyhole superior to the obstructed urethra.

8. It is possible to have unilateral renal agenesis, but the contralateral kidney is usually quite _____ to compensate for this abnormality.

9. The _____ kidney shows a large central cyst with multiple small peripheral cysts that appear as a pelviureteric junction obstruction; however, these cysts do not communicate with one another, as is seen with hydronephrosis.

10. When the kidneys appear enlarged and echogenic, the sonographer should think of infantile _____ renal disease (with oligohydramnios).

11. Dilatation of the renal collecting system suggests either _____ or reflux.

12. Pelviureteric junction obstruction shows dilatation of the renal _____, whereas ureteric dilatation suggests either a _____ junction obstruction or reflux.

13. When the hydronephrosis is _____, the possibility of bladder outlet obstruction should be considered.

Exercise 6

Fill in the blank(s) with the word(s) that best completes the statements about the pathophysiology of the fetal urinary system.

1. A critical marker in the assessment of renal function is _____.

2. It usually takes at least _____ minutes to fill and empty the fetal bladder.

3. Renal agenesis and infantile polycystic kidney disease are fetal conditions _____ with life.

4. In renal agenesis, the _____ glands may be large and may mimic the kidneys.

5. _____ kidneys should be considered when the kidneys are not in their normal retroperitoneal location.

6. _____ syndrome is characterized by renal agenesis, oligohydramnios, pulmonary hypoplasia, abnormal facies, and malformed hands and feet.

7. In the most severe cases of IPKD, renal failure occurs with _____ and an absent urinary bladder.

8. Multicystic dysplastic kidney disease is the most common form of renal _____ disease in childhood and represents one of the most common abdominal masses in the neonate.

9. Multicystic dysplastic kidney disease is composed of multiple, smooth-walled, nonfunctioning, _____ cysts of variable size and number.

10. In autosomal dominant (adult) polycystic kidney disease, the fetal kidneys appear _____ and _____, and, rarely, cysts may be observed prenatally.

11. The urinary tract may be obstructed at the junction of the ureter entering the renal pelvis (_____ junction) or at the junction of the ureter where it enters the bladder _____(junction) or at the level of the urethra (_____).

12. Late obstruction causes _____.

Exercise 7

Fill in the blank(s) with the word(s) that best completes the statements about the dilatation of the fetal urinary system.

1. The dilated anechoic renal pelvis is centrally located and distended with urine. If only the pelvis is seen, the term _____ is used. Hydronephrosis will be identified with dilatation of the renal pelvis and the _____.

2. Unilateral renal hydronephrosis commonly results from an obstruction at the junction of the renal pelvis and the ureter; this is called a(n) _____ junction obstruction.

3. _____junction obstruction commonly presents with dilatation of the lower end of the ureter (megaureter).

4. A dilatation of the intravesical (bladder) segment of the distal ureter is a _____.

5. _____ outlet obstruction is produced by a membrane within the posterior urethra; the bladder wall is severely thickened with a dilated posterior urethra, the "_____ sign."

6. Sonographic findings in prune belly syndrome include _____, mild to severe bilateral hydronephrosis, fetal _____, and hypoplastic lungs.

Exercise 8

Fill in the blank(s) with the word(s) that best completes the statements about fetal genital development.

1. The phallus elongates to form the penis; this sonographic finding is known as the "_____ sign."

2. Both the urethra and the vagina open into the urogenital sinus, the vestibule of the vagina. The urogenital folds become the labia minora, the labioscrotal swellings become the labia majora, and the phallus becomes the clitoris; this sonographic finding is known as the "_____ sign."

3. The female fetus with _____ has a 46,XX karyotype. The most common cause is congenital virilizing adrenal hyperplasia that causes masculinization of the external genitalia.

4. _____ represent the most common cystic mass in female fetuses.

5. _____ occurs in the male fetus and is seen as an accumulation of serous fluid surrounding the testicle resulting from a communication with the peritoneal cavity.

6. Failure of the testes to completely descend into the scrotal sac results in a condition called _____.

7. _____ genitalia is the sonographic finding that describes the inability to delineate fetal gender. There are several congenital malformations that attribute to this finding; the malformations typically result from chromosomal defects or abnormal hormone levels.

8. A collection of fluid in the vagina and uterus is _____.

Provide a short answer for each question after evaluating the images.

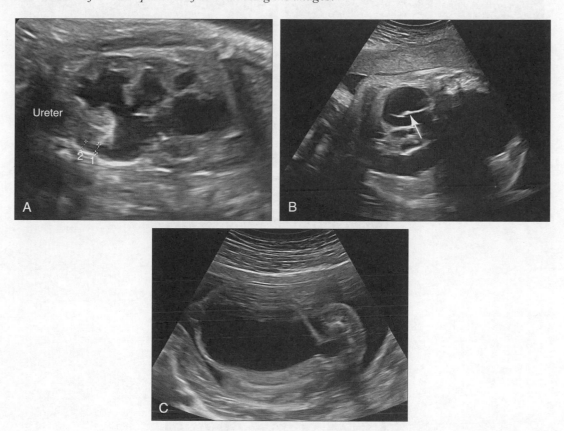

1. From these images of the fetal urinary system, describe the abnormalities.

_____

_____

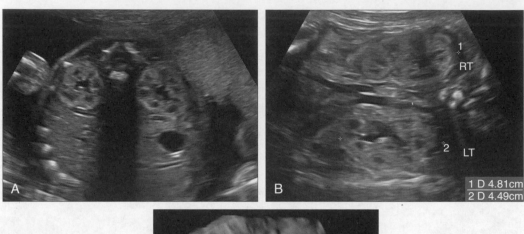

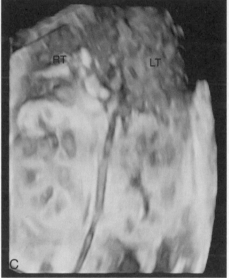

2. Describe the sonographic findings on this image.

_____

_____

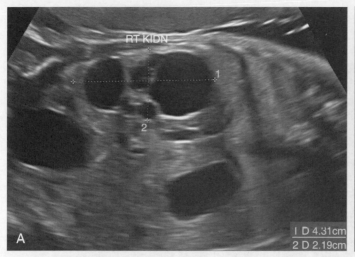
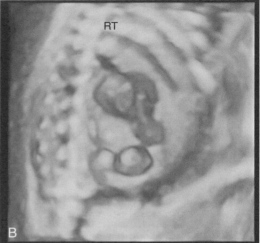

3. Describe the sonographic findings in this 28-week gestation.

_____

_____

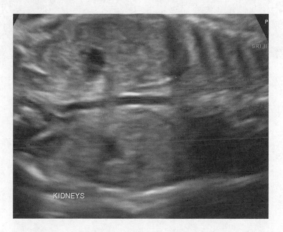

4. This fetus was known to have Beckwith-Wiedemann syndrome. Describe the sonographic findings in this image.

_____

_____

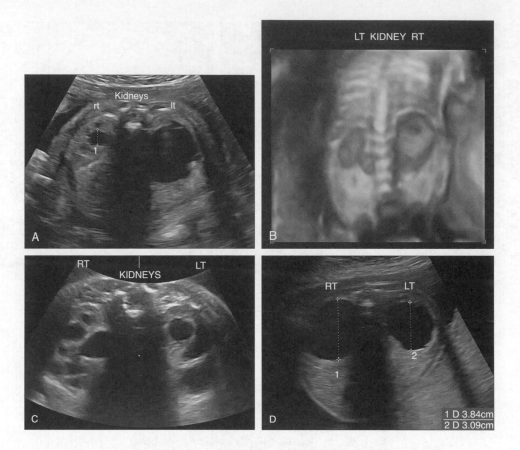

5. Describe the sonographic findings of these fetal kidneys.

_____

_____

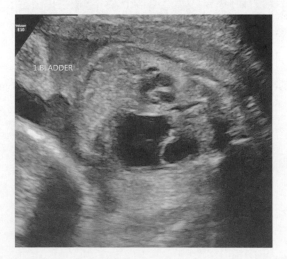

6. Discuss the sonographic findings in this fetal abdomen.

_____

_____

65 The Fetal Skeleton

KEY TERMS

Exercise 1

Match the following fetal skeletal terms with their definitions.

_____ 1. achondrogenesis

_____ 2. achondroplasia

_____ 3. craniosynostosis

_____ 4. hetcrozygous achondroplasia

_____ 5. homozygous achondroplasia

_____ 6. hypophosphatasia

_____ 7. osteogenesis imperfecta

_____ 8. polydactyly

_____ 9. thanatophoric dysplasia

A. Early ossification of the calvarium with destruction of the sutures; hypertelorism frequently found in association; sonographically the fetal cranium may appear brachycephalic

B. Congenital condition characterized by decreased mineralization of the bones resulting in "ribbon-like" and bowed limbs, underossified cranium, and compression of the chest; early death often occurs

C. A defect in the development of the cartilage at the epiphyseal centers of the long bones producing short, square bones

D. Anomalies of the hands or feet in which there is an addition of a digit; may be found in association with certain skeletal dysplasias

E. Lethal autosomal recessive short-limb dwarfism marked by long-bone and trunk shortening, decreased echogenicity of the bones and spine, and "flipper-like" appendages

F. Short-limb dwarfism affecting fetuses of achondroplastic parents

G. Lethal short-limb dwarfism characterized by a notable reduction in the length of the long bones, pear-shaped chest, soft tissue redundancy, and frequently cloverleaf skull deformity and ventriculomegaly

H. Short-limb dysplasia that manifests in the second trimester of pregnancy; conversion abnormality of cartilage to bone affecting the epiphyseal growth centers; extremities are notably shortened at birth, with a normal trunk and frequent enlargement of the head

I. Metabolic disorder affecting the fetal collagen system that leads to varying forms of bone disease: intrauterine bone fractures, shortened long bones, poorly mineralized calvaria, and compression of the chest found in type II forms

FETAL MUSCULOSKELETAL SYSTEM

Exercise 2

Fill in the blank(s) with the word(s) that best completes the statements or provide a short answer about the fetal musculoskeletal system.

1. The majority of the musculoskeletal system is formed from the primitive _____ arising from mesenchymal cells that are the embryonic connective tissues.

2. The vertebral column and ribs arise from the _____, and the limbs arise from the lateral plate _____.

3. Initially the limbs have a paddle shape with a ridge of thickened _____, known as the apical ectodermal ridge, at the apex of each bud.

4. The fingers are distinctly evident by day 49, although they are still webbed, and by the _____ week of development, the fingers are longer.

5. Development of the feet and toes is essentially complete by the _____ week, although the soles of the feet are still turned inward at this time.

6. The term used to describe abnormal growth and density of cartilage and bone is skeletal _____.

425

Exercise 3

Fill in the blank(s) with the word(s) that best completes the statements or provide a short answer about the fetal skeleton.

1. Type I _____ dysplasia is characterized by short, curved femurs and flat vertebral bodies.

2. Type II is characterized by straight, _____ femurs, flat vertebral bodies, and a _____ skull.

3. The most common nonlethal skeletal dysplasia is _____.

4. Achondrogenesis is caused by cartilage abnormalities that result in abnormal _____ formation and

   _____.

5. Osteogenesis imperfecta is a rare disorder of collagen production leading to _____ bones; manifestations in the teeth, skin, and ligaments; and blue _____.

6. Type II osteogenesis is considered the most severe form of osteogenesis _____, having a lethal outcome.

7. A condition that presents with diffuse hypomineralization of the bone caused by an alkaline phosphatase deficiency

   is congenital _____.

8. Camptomelic (bent bone) dysplasia is a group of lethal skeletal dysplasias that are characterized by _____ of the long bones.

9. Short-rib polydactyly syndrome is a lethal skeletal dysplasia characterized by short ribs, short _____, and polydactyly.

10. Ellis–van Creveld syndrome may present with a _____ thorax, causing pulmonary hypoplasia, and heart

    defects, the most common of which is the _____.

11. An anomaly in which there is fusion of the lower extremities is _____.

12. For the VACTERL association to be considered, three features must be identified; a _____ umbilical artery may also be identified.

13. Amputation defects may be identified as total or partial absence and may be associated with _____ syndrome.

14. Clubfoot, also known as _____, describes deformities of the foot and ankle.

15. _____ foot is characterized by a prominent heel and a convex sole.

Exercise 4

Provide a short answer for each question after evaluating the images.

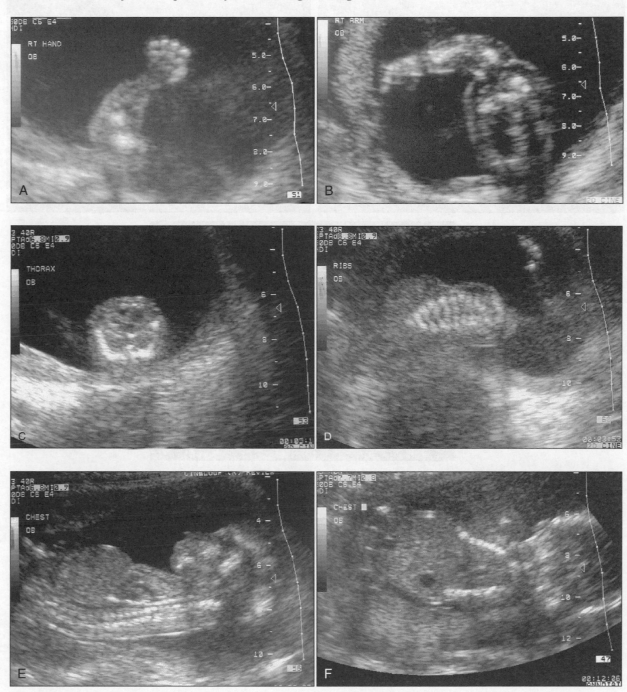

1. Discuss the sonographic findings in this fetus with a lethal skeletal dysplasia.

_____

_____

_____

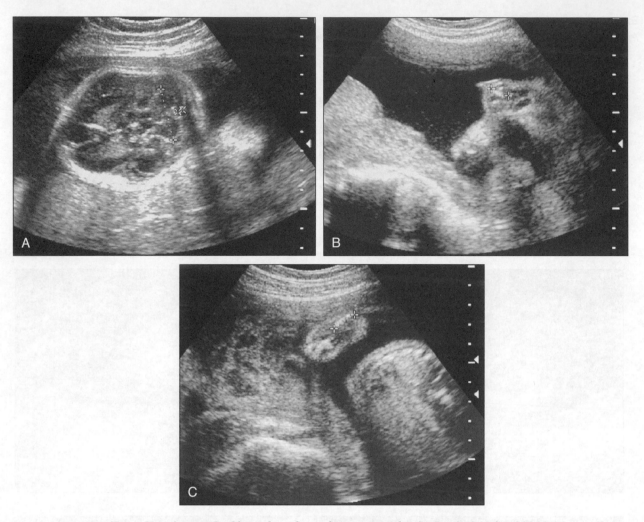

(From Henningsen C: *Clinical guide to ultrasonography*, St. Louis, Mosby, 2004.)

2. Discuss the sonographic findings in this fetus with achondrogenesis.

_____

_____

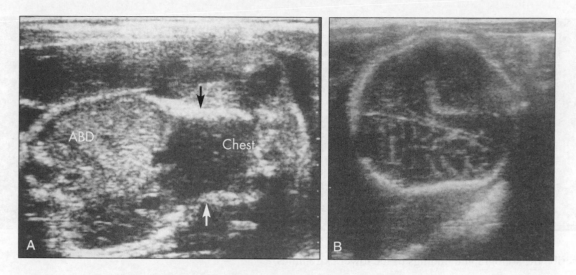

3. This fetus had osteogenesis imperfecta, type II. Describe the sonographic findings.

_____

_____

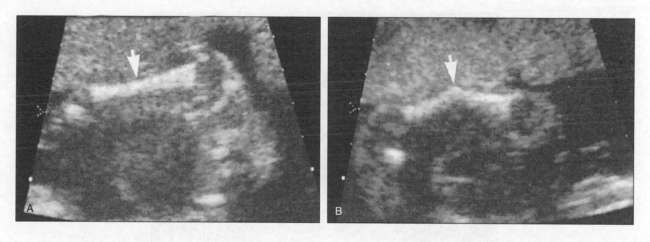

4. Images of both femurs in a 22-week fetus. Describe the sonographic findings.

_____

_____

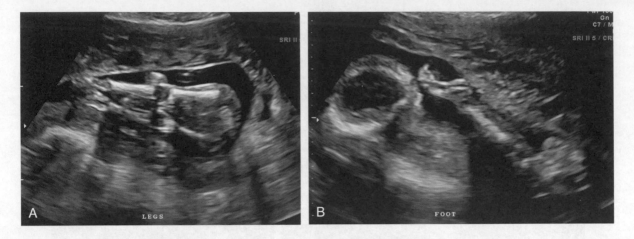

5. Describe the sonographic findings of the lower extremities.

_____

_____

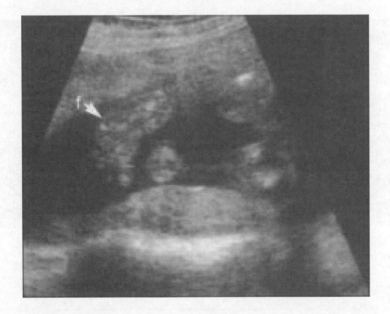

6. Describe the sonographic findings in these images of the fetal feet.

_____

_____

Cardiovascular Anatomy Review

Select the answer that best completes the following questions or statements.

1. The tricuspid valve opens when
   a. the right ventricular pressure drops below the right atrial pressure
   b. the papillary muscle contracts
   c. the velocity of blood flow in the right ventricle exceeds the velocity of flow in the right atrium
   d. the pulmonic valve opens

2. Blood normally flows from the right ventricle to the
   a. pulmonary artery
   b. aorta
   c. right atrium
   d. pulmonary vein

3. Which of the following statements about cardiac anatomy is false?
   a. The heart tends to assume a more vertical position in tall, thin people and a more horizontal position in short, heavy people.
   b. The ligamentum arteriosum runs from the left pulmonary artery to the descending aorta.
   c. The coronary arteries arise from the sinuses within the cusps of the aortic valve.
   d. The left ventricle constitutes most of the ventral surface of the heart.

4. The most posterior chamber to the left of the sternum is the
   a. right atrium
   b. left atrium
   c. right ventricle
   d. left ventricle

5. The medial wall of the right atrium contains the
   a. interventricular septum
   b. interatrial septum
   c. right upper pulmonary vein
   d. right lower pulmonary vein

6. The inferior vena cava is guarded by a fold of tissue called the _____ valve, whereas the coronary sinus is guarded by the _____ valve.
   a. eustachian, coronary
   b. thebesian, eustachian
   c. eustachian, thebesian
   d. eustachian, atrial

7. The interventricular septum is divided primarily into two major sections: membranous and muscular. Which of the terms below would be identified with the muscular septum?

a. inflow

b. outflow

c. infundibular

d. trabecular

8. The wall of the aorta bulges slightly at each semilunar cusp to form

a. coronary arteries

b. sinus of Valsalva

c. chordae tendineae

d. Arantius nodule

9. The _____ valve lies behind the right half of the sternum opposite the 4th ICS.

a. mitral

b. aortic

c. tricuspid

d. pulmonic

10. The pulmonary artery may be distinguished from the aorta by all of the following except that

a. it runs upward and to the left, anterior to the aorta

b. the cusps are thinner than the aorta

c. it bifurcates into right and left branches

d. it runs upward and to the right, posterior to the aorta

11. The point at which the ductus joins the aorta is near the

a. left common carotid artery

b. left subclavian artery

c. brachiocephalic artery

d. crux of the heart

12. Most coronary venous drainage is into the

a. coronary veins

b. coronary sinus

c. thebesian veins

d. atrial sinus

13. Atrial contraction follows the _____ on the ECG.

a. T wave

b. P wave

c. QRS

d. ST segment

14. The brightest returning echo signal on the echocardiogram is from the

a. anterior wall of the heart

b. anterior leaflet of the mitral valve

c. aortic semilunar cusps

d. pericardium

15. To image the aortic root with semilunar cusps, the sonographer should angle the transducer
    a. toward the right shoulder
    b. toward the left shoulder
    c. inferior toward the left hip
    d. toward the 4th left ICS

16. The coronary sinus is often identified as a(n)
    a. vertical tubular structure posterior to the heart
    b. oblique tubular structure posterior and lateral to the heart
    c. vertical tubular structure lateral to the heart
    d. horizontal tubular structure posterior to the atria of the heart

17. The Doppler shift would best be explained in the following way:
    a. If the source is moving toward the listener, it is "catching up" with the wave it just generated; the wavelength becomes shorter, and the listener hears a higher frequency.
    b. If the source is moving away, the wavelength becomes longer, and the listener hears a higher frequency.
    c. If the source is moving toward the listener, the wavelength becomes longer, and the listener hears a higher frequency.
    d. The difference between the frequency generated by the source and that observed by the listener is the Doppler shift.

18. The inflammatory process of the cardiac muscle is known as
    a. endocarditis
    b. pericarditis
    c. epicarditis
    d. myocarditis

19. The term *dyspnea* refers to the condition of
    a. difficulty in digesting food
    b. difficulty in breathing
    c. rapid breathing
    d. deep breathing

20. The amplitude of aortic root motion has been used to assess
    a. the vigor of left ventricular contraction
    b. the degree of aortic stenosis
    c. the degree of aortic insufficiency
    d. the size of the left atrium

21. The best window to image the area of the fossa ovalis is the
    a. apical
    b. subcostal four chamber
    c. parasternal long axis
    d. subcostal short axis

22. Atrial septal defects are classified on the basis of their position in the septum and their embryologic origin. The most common defect is the
    a. ostium primum defect
    b. ostium secundum defect
    c. sinus venosus defect
    d. primum secundum defect

23. The structure that plays a significant role in the development of the septum primum, atrioventricular valves, and membranous septum is the
    a. endocardial cushion
    b. ventral septal endocardium
    c. atrial septal endocardium
    d. endocardial fibroelastocushion

24. The heart is lined by a serous membrane called the
    a. pericardium
    b. endocardium
    c. myocardium
    d. epicardium

25. The middle muscular layer of the heart is the
    a. pericardium
    b. endocardium
    c. myocardium
    d. epicardium

26. The _____ is located between the pericardium and the myocardium and is most prominent around the inflow and outflow arteries of the heart.
    a. epicardium
    b. visceral pericardium
    c. pericardial fat
    d. endocardium

27. Risk factors identified for stroke include all of the following except
    a. age
    b. sex
    c. hypertension
    d. pregnancy

28. The warning signs of stroke include all of the following except
    a. symptoms of weakness or numbness
    b. sudden confusion, trouble speaking or understanding
    c. hypotension
    d. difficulty seeing or walking

29. An ischemic neurologic deficit that lasts less than 24 hours is known as
    a. CVA
    b. TIA
    c. RIND
    d. BEND

30. Blood supply to the brain is provided by the _____ arteries.
    a. internal and external
    b. carotid and vertebral
    c. ophthalmic and posterior communicating
    d. middle cerebral and anterior cerebral

31. Symptoms of lower extremity occlusive arterial disease include
    a. claudication and rest pain
    b. shoulder pain
    c. thoracic pain
    d. lower abdominal pain

32. Characteristics of a normal Doppler arterial waveform include all of the following except
    a. triphasic
    b. high-velocity forward flow during systole
    c. low-velocity forward flow during systole
    d. short flow reversal in early diastole

33. A potentially lethal complication of acute DVT is
    a. pulmonary embolism
    b. claudication
    c. abscess
    d. fistula

34. Dilated, elongated, tortuous superficial veins are
    a. perforating veins
    b. varicose veins
    c. abscessed veins
    d. tortellini veins

35. In the neonatal stage, communication is open between the right and left sides of the fetal heart through the
    _____ _____ and between the aorta and the pulmonary artery via the

    _____ _____.
    a. right atrium, left atrium
    b. ductus venosus, fossa suprema
    c. fossa ovale, ductus arteriosus
    d. pulmonary veins, ductus venosus

36. The normal fetal heart rate is between:
    a. 120 to 160 beats per minute
    b. 90 to 120 beats per minute
    c. 130 to 190 beats per minute
    d. 100 to 140 beats per minute

37. At 20 weeks gestation, the normal fetal ventricles should measure:
    a. 4 mm
    b. 5 mm
    c. 6 mm
    d. 7 mm

38. The fetal survey should demonstrate the following structures before focusing on the fetal heart; select which is incorrect.
    a. The position of the fetus and thorax
    b. The position of the fetal stomach
    c. The location of the great vessels (aorta on right, inferior vena cava on left)
    d. The location of the apex of the heart

39. The pulmonary veins are best imaged in which view:
    a. parasternal short axis
    b. apical four chamber
    c. suprasternal
    d. parasternal long axis with medial angulation

40. In order to consider pericardial effusion, the separation should be greater than:
    a. 2 mm
    b. 4 mm
    c. 6 cmm
    d. 8 mm

41. The best view to image the presence of an atrial septal defect is:
    a. parasternal long axis
    b. apical four chamber
    c. subcostal four chamber
    d. high arch view

42. An abnormal displacement of the tricuspid valve with regurgitation is known as:
    a. Transposition of the Great Arteries
    b. Ebstein's Anomaly
    c. Atrioventricular septal defect
    d. Truncus Arteriosus

43. Which of the following conditions is not seen in a fetus with Tetrology of Fallot:
    a. High,membranous septal defect
    b. Large, anteriorly displaced aort which overrides the septal defect
    c. Pulmonary stenosis
    d. Right ventricular hypertrophy

44. What is the abnormality called when the aorta is connected to the right ventricle and the pulmonary artery is connected to the left ventricle:
    a. Truncus arteriosus
    b. Transposition of the Great Arteries
    c. Single Ventricle
    d. Hypoplastic left heart

General Sonography Review

Select the answer that best completes the following questions or statements.

1. Useful clinical history and clinical symptoms the sonographer should be aware of in a patient who presents with acute abdominal pain include all of the following except
   a. past history
   b. previous diagnostic examinations and pertinent laboratory findings
   c. age and present condition
   d. weight

2. Which of the following would be most useful to the sonographer trying to define the nature of a patient's pain?
   a. Has the pain shifted?
   b. Locate the pain with your hand.
   c. Is there any radiation of the pain?
   d. Is the pain related to food ingestion?

3. All of the following questions relate to vomiting except
   a. Is it related to pain?
   b. How often does it occur?
   c. Is it related to inspiration?
   d. Is it associated with nausea?

4. When a pelvic examination is performed, all of the following questions regarding menstruation should be asked except
   a. What was the date of the LMP?
   b. Was the LMP normal?
   c. How long have you been pregnant?
   d. Do you have pain associated with your period?

5. All of the following terms relate to the past history of a patient except
   a. apnea
   b. jaundice
   c. weight loss
   d. fatigue

6. Central upper abdominal pain most likely would be associated with which of the following diseases?
   a. Crohn's disease
   b. diverticulitis
   c. acute pancreatitis
   d. PID

7. Central pain with shock may be seen in all of the following conditions except
   a. cholelithiasis
   b. ectopic pregnancy
   c. internal hemorrhage
   d. dissecting aneurysm

437

8. An acute abdomen in a pregnant patient may represent any of the following conditions except
   a. degeneration of a fibroid
   b. hydatid disease
   c. ovarian torsion
   d. pelvic peritonitis

9. Patients who present with RUQ pain may have any of the following conditions except
   a. gallbladder disease
   b. hepatitis
   c. Baker's cyst
   d. renal stones

10. An abdominal trauma case may present with any of the following conditions except
    a. rupture of the cerebellum
    b. rupture of the liver, spleen, or kidney
    c. rupture of the bladder
    d. rupture of the intestine

11. Common clinical findings in patients with renal disease include any of the following except
    a. urinary pain, frequency, retention
    b. hematuria
    c. flank pain
    d. pectoralis pain

12. The most specific laboratory value in detecting acute pancreatitis is
    a. serum amylase
    b. serum lipase
    c. BUN
    d. bilirubin

13. Clinical signs of urinary tract infection may include any or all of the following except
    a. fever
    b. tremors
    c. nausea
    d. flank pain

14. Alkaline phosphatase is markedly increased in patients with
    a. hepatocellular disease
    b. early obstruction
    c. hydatid disease
    d. polycystic disease

15. If there is an interruption of the IVC, which vascular structure will take over its "job"?
    a. SVC
    b. azygos
    c. lumbar
    d. iliac

16. Distribution of blood to the liver, spleen, and stomach occurs via the
    a. portal vein
    b. celiac trunk vessels
    c. gastroduodenal artery
    d. superior mesenteric vein

17. Distribution of the proximal half of the colon and small intestine occurs via the
    a. splenic artery
    b. IMA
    c. SMA
    d. hepatic vein

18. A patient who presents with a clot in the main portal vein and hepatopetal flow in the collaterals most likely has
    a. hepatic vein thrombosis
    b. transformation of the portal vein
    c. renal vein thrombosis
    d. Budd-Chiari syndrome

19. When venous obstruction occurs within the liver or in extrahepatic portal veins, which condition exists?
    a. pulmonary hypertension
    b. portal hypertension
    c. superior mesenteric artery obstruction
    d. renal vein thrombosis

20. The most common collaterals in portal hypertension are
    a. left gastric and paraumbilical veins
    b. retroperitoneal and short gastric veins
    c. splenorenal and omental veins
    d. splenoperitoneal and retroperitoneal veins

21. The shunt that is performed via a transjugular approach is called
    a. PITS
    b. SIPS
    c. JITS
    d. TIPS

22. As portal venous flow to the liver decreases, hepatic arterial flow
    a. decreases
    b. increases
    c. stabilizes
    d. remains the same

23. Clinical signs of hepatic vein obstruction are characterized by all of the following except
    a. hepatomegaly
    b. shrunken liver
    c. ascites
    d. pain

24. Ultrasound excels over CT in its ability to image
    a. fascial planes and fat-containing structures
    b. ascites and intraperitoneal abscesses
    c. mesenteric infiltration
    d. omental seeding

25. Intraperitoneal fluid first accumulates in
    a. cul-de-sac or retrovesical fossa
    b. mesentery
    c. omental bursa
    d. pericolic ligaments

26. The location and distribution of intraperitoneal fluid are influenced by all of the following except
    a. patient position
    b. viscosity of the fluid
    c. respiration
    d. peritoneal adhesions

27. When ascites is found unexpectedly, the abdomen must be surveyed to detect all of the following except
    a. malignancy
    b. renal hypertension
    c. portal hypertension
    d. hepatic or portal vein thrombosis

28. Serous fluid is
    a. echogenic
    b. inhomogeneous
    c. anechoic
    d. complex

29. Peritoneal fluid that contains septations, low-level echoes, or debris suggests all of the following except
    a. portal vein thrombosis
    b. infection
    c. hemorrhage
    d. carcinomatosis

30. Which statement is false?
    a. Long-standing ascites may contain internal septations and may be loculated.
    b. Uninfected ascites usually has no mass effect and passively conforms to intraperitoneal compartments.
    c. Abscesses never displace adjacent bowel or organs.
    d. Abscesses usually have significant mass effect.

31. Acute intraperitoneal hemorrhage most often is caused by all of the following except
    a. lymphadenopathy
    b. blunt trauma
    c. ruptured ectopic pregnancy
    d. interventional procedures

32. This layer is a constant anatomic feature of the GI tract and serves as a useful landmark to identify a loop of bowel:
    a. muscularis propria
    b. submucosal layer
    c. muscularis mucosa
    d. adventitial surface

33. Neoplastic invasion of the bowel may cause a target or _____ appearance.
    a. sandwich sign
    b. comet tail
    c. pseudokidney
    d. mirror image

34. Landmarks the sonographer should use to image the appendix include all of the following except
    a. right colon
    b. cecum
    c. left colon
    d. psoas muscle

35. Complications of appendicitis may include all of the following except
    a. gangrenous infection
    b. periappendiceal abscess
    c. appendicolith
    d. cholecystitis

36. A mucocele is the result of
    a. acute appendicitis
    b. phlegmon
    c. chronic obstruction of the appendix
    d. intramural hemorrhage

37. Optimal color flow and spectral Doppler sonography of the liver requires
    a. high-frequency scanning
    b. low-frequency scanning
    c. high PRF
    d. increased scan angle

38. Flash artifact is associated with
    a. wraparound
    b. diaphragm interface
    c. color related to tissue motion
    d. decreased respiration

39. Thicker septations seen within a cyst are usually
    a. complicated cyst or neoplasm
    b. adenoma
    c. polycystic disease
    d. focal nodular hyperplasia

40. The most common benign hepatic neoplasm is
    a. adenoma
    b. hepatoma
    c. cavernous hemangioma
    d. angiomyolipoma

41. The most common liver metastases originate from all of the following except
    a. lung
    b. colon
    c. pancreas
    d. brain

42. The most common primary liver cancer in the United States is
    a. hemangioma
    b. hepatoblastoma
    c. liposarcoma
    d. hepatocellular carcinoma

43. The type of tumor that arises from the bile ducts to account for 10% of all primary liver cancers is
    a. cholangioma
    b. cholangiocarcinoma
    c. cholangiosarcoma
    d. cholangiolipoma

44. This type of abscess should be suspected when a patient presents from a high-risk population (e.g., recent immigrant from an endemic area, patients living in poor sanitary conditions, HIV-positive patients):
    a. pyogenic
    b. echinococcal
    c. fungal microabscess
    d. amebic

45. The most common symptomatic liver tumor in children younger than 5 years is
    a. Wilms' tumor
    b. hepatoblastoma
    c. neuroblastoma
    d. nephroblastoma

46. In chronic viral hepatitis, hepatomegaly and inhomogeneous patchy or diffuse increased echogenicity are common and are related to the
    a. amount of fatty infiltration and fibrosis present
    b. amount of fibrosis present
    c. amount of portal hypertension present
    d. amount of vascular compression present

47. Fatty liver is a nonspecific response to liver injury and may occur in dysnutritional states including any of the following except
    a. obesity
    b. hyperlipidemia
    c. dehydration
    d. diabetes mellitus

48. Fatty infiltration is often patchy or focal. A less affected region of the liver is called
    a. spared
    b. infiltrated
    c. hyperfused
    d. revascularized

49. In sonographic evaluation of patients with cirrhosis of the liver, all of the following should be considered except
    a. ratio of LLL to RLL
    b. nodularity of the liver surface
    c. attenuation of the ultrasound transmission
    d. increased size of the caudate lobe

50. The thyroid gland can be located at the level of the
    a. thyroid cartilage
    b. manubrium
    c. hyoid bone
    d. cricoid cartilage

51. Which of the following is typically the largest vascular structure located in the neck?
    a. common carotid artery
    b. internal jugular vein
    c. internal carotid artery
    d. external jugular vein

52. Which muscle divides the neck into anterior and posterior triangles?
    a. trapezius
    b. platysma
    c. longissimus dorsi
    d. sternocleidomastoid

53. The superior vena cava is formed by the junction of the
    a. internal jugular veins
    b. external jugular veins
    c. subclavian veins
    d. brachiocephalic veins

54. Which of the following makes up the apex of the heart?
    a. right atrium
    b. left atrium
    c. right ventricle
    d. left ventricle

55. Collateral circulation between the IVC and the SVC is supplied by the
    a. thoracic veins
    b. subclavian veins
    c. azygos veins
    d. intercostal veins

56. Which of the following is not considered a mediastinal structure?
    a. heart
    b. lungs
    c. trachea
    d. thymus gland

57. What vein passes anterior to the third part of the duodenum and posterior to the neck of the pancreas?
    a. portal
    b. splenic
    c. superior mesenteric
    d. inferior mesenteric

58. The gastroepiploic artery is a branch of the
    a. left gastric artery
    b. hepatic artery
    c. splenic artery
    d. pancreatic artery

59. The gastroduodenal artery arises from:
    a. right hepatic artery
    b. common hepatic artery
    c. splenic artery
    d. superior mesenteric artery

60. The superior mesenteric artery is the posterior border of:
    a. tail of the pancreas
    b. common bile duct
    c. body of the pancreas
    d. hepatic vein

61. The most common cause for abdominal aneurysm is
    a. cystic medial necrosis
    b. syphilis
    c. atheroma
    d. arteriosclerosis

62. An aneurysm that is connected to the vascular lumen by a neck that varies in size is
    a. fusiform
    b. saccular
    c. berry
    d. cylindroid

63. The triphasic waveform seen in the hepatic veins reflects the contractility of the
    a. right atrium
    b. left atrium
    c. right ventricle
    d. left ventricle

64. Which structure is retroperitoneal?
    a. gallbladder
    b. spleen
    c. pancreas
    d. stomach

65. Which of the following arteries is NOT one of the branches of the celiac axis?
    a. hepatic artery
    b. splenic artery
    c. gastric artery
    d. cystic artery

66. Which part of the pancreas is located in the curve of the duodenum?
    a. head
    b. neck
    c. body
    d. tail

67. What is the smallest lobe of the liver?
    a. right
    b. left
    c. caudate
    d. Riedel's

68. Which thin, tendinous structure connects the two rectus abdominis muscles at the midline?
    a. linea alba
    b. transversus abdominis
    c. internal oblique
    d. ligamentum teres

69. Morison's pouch is located in the
    a. subhepatic space
    b. subphrenic space
    c. paracolic gutter
    d. retroperitoneal space

70. Which of the following does not unite to form the portal vein?
    a. superior mesenteric vein
    b. inferior mesenteric vein
    c. hepatic vein
    d. splenic vein

71. The peritoneum is divided into the _____ layer, which lines the abdominal walls, and the
    _____ layer, which covers the organs.
    a. parietal, visceral
    b. visceral, parietal
    c. serous, mucous
    d. outer, inner

72. The major renal calyces empty urine into the
    a. pyramids
    b. arteries
    c. papilla
    d. pelvis

73. What anatomic area would you examine to rule out a rectus sheath hematoma?
    a. posterior abdominal wall
    b. anterior chest wall
    c. lateral wall
    d. anterior abdominal wall

74. The interlobar arteries of the kidneys can be found
    a. at the base of the medullary pyramids
    b. branching at right angles from the arcuate arteries
    c. coursing toward the cortex along the lateral borders of the pyramids
    d. along the capsule of the kidney

75. The glomerulus is
    a. contained in the loop of Henle
    b. a network of capillaries encased in Bowman's capsule
    c. located in the renal papilla
    d. found in the renal pelvis

76. The apices of the renal pyramids project into the minor calyces as the
    a. convoluted tubules
    b. renal columns of Bertin
    c. renal papillae
    d. glomerulus

77. Which of the following statements is(are) true regarding the sonographic appearance of the neonatal kidney?
    a. The medullary pyramids are larger in relation to the cortex than in adult life.
    b. The kidneys are generally much more echogenic than the liver in the newborn and become increasingly less echogenic with age.
    c. In the normal newborn, the kidneys are often echogenic compared with the liver and spleen.
    d. The kidneys are generally smaller in relation to the other organs than they will appear in adult life.

78. The right adrenal gland is located
    a. anterior to the IVC, superior and medial to the upper pole of the right kidney, and posterior to the crus of the diaphragm
    b. posterior to the IVC, superior and lateral to the upper pole of the right kidney, and anterior to the crus of the diaphragm
    c. medial to the IVC, superior and medial to the upper pole of the right kidney, and posterior to the crus of the diaphragm
    d. posterior to the IVC, superior and medial to the upper pole of the right kidney, and anterior to the crus of the diaphragm

79. Arcuate arteries in the kidney are branches of the
    a. segmental arteries
    b. interlobar arteries
    c. renal arteries
    d. papillary arteries

80. The left renal vein courses
    a. posterior to the IVC
    b. anterior to the IVC
    c. anterior to the AO
    d. anterior to the SMA

81. The common bile duct can be seen at the _____ aspect of the pancreatic head.
    a. anterolateral
    b. superior
    c. anteromedial
    d. posteromedial

82. A choledochal cyst is an abnormality of the
    a. sphincter of Oddi
    b. gallbladder
    c. common bile duct
    d. pancreatic duct

83. The major renal calyces empty urine into the
    a. minor calyces and/or pyramids
    b. arteries
    c. papilla
    d. pelvis

84. Which of the following statements is TRUE regarding the common bile duct?
    a. It crosses the duodenum anteriorly before reaching the pancreas.
    b. It extends from the neck of the gallbladder to the duodenum.
    c. It is formed by the confluence of the cystic and common hepatic ducts.
    d. It courses posterior to the portal vein.

85. A thickened gallbladder wall may be encountered in any of the following states except
    a. ascites
    b. acute cholecystitis
    c. hydrops
    d. cholangiocarcinoma

86. In a 50-year-old female, the intraluminal diameter of the normal distal common bile duct should not exceed
    a. 4 mm
    b. 5 mm
    c. 6 mm
    d. 7 mm

87. Which of the following statements is NOT true regarding the spleen?
    a. The stomach lies on the posterior border of the spleen.
    b. The spleen is positioned posteriorly in the left upper quadrant.
    c. The spleen is bordered posteriorly by the ribs and the left kidney.
    d. The splenic artery is a branch of the portal trunk.

88. Which of the following is NOT true regarding multicystic dysplastic kidney?
    a. The reniform contour of the kidney is maintained.
    b. The cysts are of variable size and have a random distribution.
    c. Contralateral disease occurs in approximately one third of patients.
    d. The normal central echo pattern of the renal pelvis is generally absent.

89. An 8-year-old boy presents with a recent sore throat, hematuria and proteinuria, urinary red cell casts, and a slightly elevated BUN. His history is very suggestive of acute poststreptococcal glomerulonephritis. Which of the following is false?
    a. The renal sonogram may demonstrate a diffuse increase in cortical echogenicity similar to that of the renal sinus.
    b. Acute glomerulonephritis is usually an incidental finding.
    c. The kidneys may be enlarged in acute glomerulonephritis.
    d. The disease may reverse or progress to end-stage renal disease.

90. Which of the following is NOT a true statement about renal allograft rejection?
    a. The allograft increases in size at a greater rate than that associated with compensatory hypertrophy.
    b. Shrinking and increased echogenicity of the renal medullary pyramids occur.
    c. The size and echogenicity of the central renal sinus fat are diminished.
    d. The allograft may lose its elliptical configuration and become more globular in shape.

91. Which of the following is NOT a sign of renal transplant rejection?
    a. enlargement and decreased echogenicity of the pyramids
    b. hyperechoic cortex
    c. localized area of renal parenchyma presenting with an anechoic appearance
    d. hydronephrosis

92. Sonographic findings of acute cholecystitis include all of the following except
    a. positive Murphy's sign
    b. thickened gallbladder wall
    c. hydrops
    d. contracted gallbladder filled with stones

93. A tumor of the adrenal medulla that produces intermittent hypertension is
    a. neuroblastoma
    b. adenoma
    c. pheochromocytoma
    d. hyperplasia

94. A fluid collection that tends to occur 2 to 6 weeks post transplantation and is associated with a chronic diminution in renal function rather than an acute decrease in urine output is the
    a. seroma
    b. abscess
    c. urinoma
    d. lymphocele

95. Which of the following describes the Doppler criteria used to diagnose acute vascular rejection of a renal allograft?

   a. In acute vascular rejection, diastolic flow in the renal, arcuate, and interlobar arteries rises significantly in relation to the systolic value.

   b. In acute vascular rejection, the diastolic value in the renal artery decreases in relation to the systolic value in the interlobar and arcuate arteries.

   c. In acute vascular rejection, the systolic-to-diastolic ratio decreases in the arcuate, interlobar, and renal arteries.

   d. In acute vascular rejection, the diastolic flow decreases, reverses, or becomes absent in the renal, arcuate, and interlobar arteries, increasing the systolic-to-diastolic ratio.

96. Which of the following would most likely cause anterior displacement of the superior mesenteric artery and vein?

   a. pancreatic neoplasm

   b. para-aortic lymphadenopathy

   c. cholelithiasis

   d. small-bowel obstruction

97. Courvoisier's gallbladder is associated with

   a. cholesterolosis

   b. multiple cholesterol polyps

   c. pancreatic head mass

   d. chronic cholecystitis

98. A form of infection seen in patients with obstruction secondary to long-standing calculi and chronic renal infection is

   a. acute lobar nephronia

   b. acute bacterial nephritis

   c. xanthogranulomatous pyelonephritis

   d. chronic atrophic pyelonephritis

99. A localized process in the kidney that forms a wedge-shaped phlegmonous lesion in which no true abscess exists is a

   a. renal carbuncle

   b. acute lobar nephronia

   c. xanthogranulomatous pyelonephritis

   d. chronic atrophic pyelonephritis

100. Empyema of the gallbladder refers to

   a. gas in the gallbladder wall

   b. pus-filled gallbladder

   c. distention of the gallbladder with mucus and stones

   d. calcified gallbladder

101. Which of the following is NOT a true statement regarding adult polycystic disease?

   a. It is a form of primary renal disease transmitted as an autosomal dominant trait.

   b. Patients typically present with a large kidney, which contains multiple cysts of varying sizes, loss of the reniform contour, and no definable central echo complex.

   c. Associated cysts may be found in the liver and pancreas.

   d. Clinically, patients present with deteriorating renal function.

102. The blood supply to the gallbladder is accomplished by the
    a. gastroduodenal artery
    b. right gastric artery
    c. portal vein
    d. cystic artery

103. Cholangitis refers to
    a. inflammation of a bile duct
    b. inflammation of the gallbladder
    c. inflammation of a choledochal cyst
    d. inflammation of the bladder

104. A high level of serum amylase may be a result of
    a. liver disease
    b. dilated intrahepatic ducts
    c. pancreatitis
    d. insulinoma

105. Which of the following is NOT a retroperitoneal structure?
    a. pancreas
    b. kidney
    c. adrenal
    d. liver

106. The PRIMARY hormones produced in the pancreas are
    a. glucagon and insulin
    b. collagen and fibrin
    c. lipase and cholase
    d. pancreatin and secretin

107. The membrane that lines the abdominal cavity is the
    a. retroperitoneum
    b. omentum
    c. mesentery
    d. peritoneum

108. Chronic pancreatitis is usually associated with all of the following sonographic patterns except
    a. hyperechoic, more echogenic than liver
    b. generalized decrease in size
    c. bright, discrete echoes from calcification, dilated pancreatic duct
    d. hypoechoic with diffuse swelling

109. The target-like structure anterior to the aorta and posterior to the left lobe of the liver represents the normal
    a. appendix
    b. pylorus
    c. antrum
    d. esophagogastric junction

110. Which of the following statements about the right crus of the diaphragm is true?
    a. It is larger and longer than the left.
    b. It attaches the psoas muscle to the diaphragm.
    c. It is the frequent site of metastasis in lymphoma.
    d. It is shorter than the left.

111. Which of the following does not describe the pancreas?
    a. It lies within the peritoneal space.
    b. It is a retroperitoneal structure.
    c. It is nonencapsulated.
    d. It is a multilobulated gland.

112. Which of the following is the correct order of abdominal wall structures from the skin inward?
    a. linea alba, rectus muscle, subcutaneous fat
    b. subcutaneous fat, rectus sheath, rectus muscle, peritoneum
    c. peritoneum, linea alba, rectus sheath
    d. rectus muscle, peritoneum, linea alba

113. With aging, the pancreas becomes
    a. smaller and more echogenic
    b. larger and more echogenic
    c. smaller and less echogenic
    d. the same size but less echogenic

114. The most common posthepatic transplant vascular complication is
    a. portal vein thrombosis
    b. hepatic artery thrombosis
    c. portal hypertension
    d. hepatic vein thrombosis

115. The abdominal organ transplant most commonly performed is
    a. pancreas
    b. liver
    c. kidney
    d. heart

116. The aorta is named the "abdominal aorta" when it passes through the
    a. diaphragm
    b. Glisson's capsule
    c. spleen hiatus
    d. aortic arch

117. Atherosclerosis involves accumulation of lipids in the
    a. intima only
    b. media only
    c. intima and media
    d. adventitia only

118. The most common type of aneurysm is
    a. saccular
    b. mycotic
    c. fusiform
    d. pseudoaneurysm

119. A complication of pancreatitis is
    a. formation of islet cell tumor
    b. formation of pseudocyst
    c. formation of cystadenoma
    d. pancreatic carcinoma

120. The most common cause of aortic aneurysm is
    a. infection
    b. atherosclerosis
    c. trauma
    d. congenital

121. The spleen is a peritoneal structure lying between
    a. the right hemidiaphragm and the stomach
    b. the left hemidiaphragm and the stomach
    c. the hepatic flexure of the colon and the left kidney
    d. spleen is not peritoneal

122. The most echogenic organ or structure listed below is the
    a. liver
    b. spleen
    c. renal sinus
    d. pancreas

123. The remnant of the fetal umbilical vein is the
    a. main lobar fissure
    b. ligamentum venosum
    c. falciform ligament
    d. ligamentum teres

124. Focal calcifications seen in the spleen as small, bright, echogenic foci with or without shadow are often the result of
    a. metastasis
    b. primary neoplasm
    c. previous granulomatous infection
    d. hydatid disease

125. Splenomegaly may be associated with diffuse splenic disease that includes all of the following except
    a. sickle cell
    b. hereditary spherocytosis
    c. polycythemia vera
    d. abscess

126. The pancreas is both an exocrine and an endocrine gland. The endocrine function is to produce
    a. insulin
    b. lipase
    c. amylase
    d. trypsin

127. Mild to moderate splenomegaly most often is caused by all of the following except
    a. infection, portal hypertension, or AIDS
    b. metastatic disease
    c. trauma
    d. leukemia

128. A phlegmon of the pancreas represents
    a. an inflammatory process
    b. a malignant neoplasm
    c. a benign adenoma
    d. a functioning islet cell tumor

129. If a mass is found in the head of the pancreas, special attention should be directed to which of the following areas?
    a. the portal vein for portal hypertension
    b. the liver for fatty changes
    c. the spleen for splenomegaly
    d. the bile ducts for dilatation

130. When the gallbladder fundus is folded over on itself, it is called
    a. junctional fold
    b. Hartmann's pouch
    c. phrygian cap
    d. Morison's pouch

131. One sonographic method used to distinguish dilated bile ducts involves demonstrating the
    a. double-barrel shotgun sign
    b. Mirizzi syndrome
    c. Courvoisier's sign
    d. stop sign

132. A congenital insertion of the CBD into the pancreatic duct causing a focal and abnormal dilatation of the CBD is called
    a. sclerosing cholangitis
    b. Courvoisier's gallbladder
    c. choledochal cyst
    d. biliary atresia

133. Adenomyomatosis of the gallbladder is
    a. proliferation and thickening of the epithelial layer with glandlike outpouchings in the wall
    b. an inflammation of the gallbladder wall
    c. strongly associated with a positive Murphy's sign
    d. always accompanied by dilated ducts

134. A 42-year-old female presents with right upper quadrant pain and nausea that comes and goes. Her sonogram reveals a normal-sized gallbladder with a slightly thick wall and contains a small, echogenic focus that casts an acoustic shadow. This most likely represents
    a. choledochal cyst
    b. cholangitis
    c. cholelithiasis with chronic cholecystitis
    d. choledocholithiasis with intermittent jaundice

135. Nonshadowing, nonmobile, echogenic foci attached to the gallbladder wall most likely represent
    a. calculi
    b. gravel
    c. sludge
    d. polyps

136. Thick, viscid bile ("sludge") within the gallbladder indicates
    a. obstruction of the intrahepatic ducts
    b. an incidental finding sometimes linked to gallbladder pathology
    c. the definite presence of calculi
    d. carcinoma of the gallbladder

137. All of the following describe the appearance of a gallbladder filled with stones except
    a. WES triad
    b. double-arc sign
    c. two parallel echogenic lines separated by a thin anechoic space with distal acoustic shadowing
    d. single echogenic line from the falciform ligament with posterior shadowing

138. The usual sonographic appearance of acute pancreatitis is
    a. hyperechoic with generalized decrease in size
    b. hypoechoic with generalized enlargement
    c. isoechoic with generalized enlargement
    d. isoechoic with increase in size

139. Focal gallbladder tenderness is referred to as
    a. Mirizzi syndrome
    b. Courvoisier's sign
    c. Klatskin's sign
    d. positive Murphy's sign

140. Perforation of the gallbladder is strongly associated with
    a. gangrenous cholecystitis
    b. acute cholecystitis
    c. chronic cholecystitis
    d. biliary atresia

141. With regard to bile duct dimensions after a cholecystectomy, the size of the CHD or CBD may be
    a. somewhat larger
    b. somewhat smaller
    c. slow to return to normal size for several months
    d. shortened

142. Jaundice is due to a buildup of _____ in the body.
    a. glycogen
    b. urea
    c. heparin
    d. bilirubin

143. One way to distinguish hepatic veins from portal veins is by
    a. size; the hepatic veins are much smaller than the portal veins
    b. tracing them to their points of origin
    c. noting the decrease in caliber as they approach the IVC
    d. visualizing the wall thickness of the vessels, knowing that hepatic veins have thicker walls

144. A patent umbilical vein may be found in the
    a. ligamentum venosum
    b. main labor fissure
    c. ligamentum teres
    d. intersegmental fissure

145. The portal veins can be distinguished from the hepatic veins by their
    a. thicker wall and echogenic rim surrounding them
    b. thin wall and echo-poor rim surrounding them
    c. close proximity to the periphery
    d. cluster-like appearance close to the hepatic periphery

146. The portal triad consists of
    a. portal vein, hepatic artery, bile duct
    b. left hepatic vein, middle hepatic vein, right hepatic vein
    c. common duct, cystic duct, pancreatic duct
    d. caudate lobe of liver, right lobe of liver, left lobe of liver

147. A high level of serum lipase would be most associated with
    a. liver disease
    b. dilated intrahepatic ducts
    c. pancreatitis
    d. insulinoma

148. Which of the following is the most common site for pseudocyst formation?
    a. iliac fossa
    b. lesser sac
    c. Morison's pouch
    d. pouch of Douglas

149. The celiac axis gives rise to all of the following vessels except
    a. splenic artery
    b. hepatic artery
    c. superior mesenteric artery
    d. left gastric artery

150. A linear echodensity that connects the gallbladder to the main portal vein is the
    a. ligamentum teres
    b. main lobar fissure
    c. ligamentum venosum
    d. coronary ligament

151. Chronic pancreatitis most often is caused by
    a. cholelithiasis
    b. ETOH abuse
    c. trauma
    d. choledocholithiasis

152. The vessel that can be seen posterior to the IVC is the
    a. right renal artery
    b. splenic artery
    c. pancreaticoduodenal artery
    d. left renal vein

153. Which of the following vessels courses between the SMA and the aorta?
    a. right renal vein
    b. right renal artery
    c. gastroduodenal artery
    d. left renal vein

154. Which of the following structures is seen in close relation to the anterolateral aspect of the head of the pancreas?
    a. common bile duct
    b. pancreaticoduodenal artery
    c. right gastric vein
    d. gastroduodenal artery

155. In the liver, the right and left hepatic ducts will join to form the
    a. cystic duct
    b. common bile duct
    c. valves of Heister
    d. common hepatic duct

156. Calcifications, pancreatic duct dilatation, and pseudocyst formation are most consistent with
    a. islet cell tumor
    b. acute and chronic pancreatitis
    c. cholelithiasis
    d. adenocarcinoma

157. Budd-Chiari syndrome may present sonographically as
    a. relative enlargement of the caudate lobe caused by hepatic vein thrombosis of the liver
    b. relative shrinkage of the caudate lobe caused by splenic vein thrombosis
    c. relative enlargement of the quadrate lobe caused by splenic vein thrombosis
    d. relative shrinkage of all lobes of the liver caused by IVC thrombosis

158. The liver is supplied with blood via the
    a. inferior vena cava and hepatic veins
    b. splenic artery and splenic vein
    c. abdominal aorta and iliac artery
    d. hepatic artery and portal vein

159. The normal echographic pattern of the liver is
    a. diffusely inhomogeneous throughout
    b. patchy areas of increased echogenicity
    c. decreased areas of echogenicity diffusely situated
    d. homogeneous throughout without interruption of the echo pattern

160. Lymphocele is a fluid collection caused by
    a. lymph duct obstruction secondary to inflammation
    b. agenesis of a lymphatic chain
    c. lymph-filled spaces secondary to surgery
    d. enlarged lymph nodes secondary to neoplasm

161. The segments of the right lobe of the liver are
    a. medial and lateral
    b. anterior and posterior
    c. cephalad and caudad
    d. caudad and quadrate

162. Loculations within ascites are most commonly the result of
    a. malignancy or inflammation
    b. benign conditions
    c. pedal edema
    d. pleural effusions

163. Riedel's lobe is a normal liver variant defined as a(n)
    a. elongated left lobe of the liver
    b. tonguelike extension of the caudate lobe of the liver
    c. tonguelike extension of the right lobe of the liver
    d. tonguelike extension of the quadrate lobe of the liver

164. Ascites is defined as accumulation of fluid in the
    a. abdominal wall
    b. peritoneal cavity
    c. retroperitoneal cavity
    d. any abdominal cavity

165. The visceral peritoneum refers to the surface that is in contact with the
    a. abdominal wall
    b. organs
    c. skin
    d. retroperitoneum

166. Ultrasound is capable of demonstrating the ligaments and fissures of the liver because
    a. they are hyperechoic
    b. collagen and fat are present within and around these structures
    c. they contain heparin, an echogenic substance
    d. they are perpendicular to the beam

167. Crohn's disease is an inflammatory bowel disease usually affecting the
    a. terminal ileum
    b. stomach
    c. pylorus
    d. esophagus

168. Compared with the adult adrenal gland, the neonatal adrenal gland
    a. appears larger and increased in medullary echogenicity
    b. appears smaller and hypoechoic
    c. appears no different
    d. cannot be seen

169. An echogenic linear echo located immediately anterior to the caudate lobe represents the
    a. main lobar fissure
    b. ligamentum venosum
    c. falciform ligament
    d. ligamentum teres

170. The segments of the left lobe of the liver are
    a. medial and lateral
    b. anterior and posterior
    c. cephalad and caudad
    d. caudate and quadrate

171. When longitudinal scans of the liver are performed with a subcostal approach, the patient is asked to take in a deep breath. This technique displaces the liver
    a. anteriorly
    b. posteriorly
    c. superiorly
    d. inferiorly

172. Sonographic visualization of the anterior wall of the appendix greater than _____ in an adult with RLQ pain is highly suggestive of acute appendicitis.
    a. 1.6 cm
    b. 16 mm
    c. 6 cm
    d. 6 mm

173. Portal vein obstruction may develop as an extension of
    a. hepatocellular carcinoma
    b. Budd-Chiari syndrome
    c. marked dilatation of the interhepatic veins
    d. fatty liver infiltration

174. Portal vein gas is an important diagnosis in the infant associated with
    a. right renal cell carcinoma
    b. ascites
    c. abdominal tumor
    d. necrotizing enterocolitis

175. The reflection of the liver above the diaphragm is due to
    a. reverberation
    b. mirror-image artifact
    c. reflection
    d. ring-down artifact

176. Metastatic lesions in the liver may appear sonographically as any of the following except
    a. anechoic with decreased transmission
    b. hyperechoic with decreased transmission
    c. hypoechoic
    d. anechoic with good transmission

177. Glycogen storage disease is associated with
    a. adenomas
    b. angiomyolipomas
    c. lipomas
    d. pancreatitis

178. An amebic abscess of the liver most frequently is located
    a. superior to the liver
    b. in the right lobe of the liver
    c. in the caudate lobe of the liver
    d. inferior to the liver, posterior to the right kidney

179. Which of the following disorders may not produce a complex sonographic pattern?
    a. infected cyst
    b. hemorrhagic cyst
    c. hematoma
    d. congenital cyst

180. All of the following structures form neighboring structures for the thyroid gland except
    a. superficial and deep fascia
    b. parotid muscle
    c. strap muscles
    d. sternocleidomastoid muscle

181. All of the following statements about thyroid cysts are true except
    a. Cysts account for 20% of all cold thyroid nodules.
    b. Lesions are usually multiple.
    c. The vast majority result from hemorrhage or degenerative changes in an adenoma.
    d. Incidence of carcinoma in cystic lesions less than 4 cm is less than 2%.

182. The most common sonographic finding of a thyroid goiter is
    a. lymph node enlargement
    b. rapidly enlarging mass
    c. fainting
    d. thyroid enlargement

183. All of the following details about thyroid carcinoma are true except
    a. has central sonolucent halo
    b. most common endocrine malignancy
    c. usually found in women older than 40 years of age
    d. rapid growth

184. The most descriptive sonographic finding in thyroid carcinoma is
    a. well-defined borders
    b. lesion is more hyperechoic than normal thyroid tissue
    c. solid complex mass with heterogeneous echo pattern and irregular margins
    d. lymph nodes of normal size

185. The most common feature of a thyroid adenoma is
    a. diffuse echogenicity
    b. hemorrhage
    c. peripheral sonolucent halo
    d. inhomogeneity

186. The most common cause of hyperparathyroidism is
    a. thyroid adenoma
    b. parathyroid adenoma
    c. parathyroid cyst
    d. parathyroid hemorrhagic cyst

187. Fat, Cooper's ligaments, connective tissue, blood vessels, nerves, and lymphatics are found
    a. in the retromammary region
    b. in the parenchyma
    c. in the subcutaneous layer
    d. in the subareolar area

188. The most important signs to look for in identifying a cystic lesion of the breast include all of the following except
    a. well-defined borders
    b. good through-transmission
    c. anechoic
    d. disruption of architecture

189. The most common solid benign tumor of the breast is
    a. cystosarcoma phyllodes
    b. fibroadenoma
    c. papilloma
    d. lipoma

190. A cystic enlargement of a distal duct filled with milk is called a
    a. lactoadenoma
    b. lactoma
    c. galactocele
    d. lactiferoma

191. The most common malignant neoplasm of the breast in women is
    a. lymphoma
    b. adenocarcinoma
    c. mucinous carcinoma
    d. cystosarcoma phyllodes

192. A breast lesion that presents with well-defined borders, low-level internal echoes, and moderate through-transmission most likely represents
    a. infected cyst
    b. simple cyst
    c. fibroadenoma
    d. cystosarcoma phyllodes

193. A linear stripe of variable thickness and echogenicity running through the testis in a craniocaudal direction represents the
    a. Cowper's fascia
    b. mediastinum testis
    c. epithelial fascia
    d. dartos muscle

194. The epididymis is located
    a. anterior and inferior to the testis
    b. anterior and superior to the testis
    c. posterior and inferior to the testis
    d. posterior and lateral to the testis

195. Which fact about undescended testes is false?
    a. The testis originates in the retroperitoneum at the level of the fetal kidney.
    b. All undescended testes are found in the inguinal canal.
    c. There is a 40% to 50% association with testicular malignancy.
    d. The incidence of infertility is increased.

196. Common causes of a secondary hydrocele include all of the following except
    a. trauma
    b. undescended testes
    c. infection
    d. neoplasm

197. Which of the following statements is false regarding varicocele?
    a. Varicoceles refer to dilated, serpiginous, and elongated veins of the pampiniform plexus.
    b. They are more common on the right side.
    c. Primary varicoceles result from incompetent valves in the spermatic vein.
    d. Secondary varicoceles develop from compression of the spermatic vein.

198. A common problem that is viral in origin and affects some adolescent and middle-aged men is
    a. epididymal cyst
    b. epididymitis
    c. spermatocele
    d. testiculitis

199. An infection that has spread to the testicle is
    a. epididymitis
    b. hydrocele
    c. orchitis
    d. spermatocele

200. Sonographic patterns of testicular neoplasms include all of the following except
    a. focal and well-defined homogeneous hypoechoic region
    b. diffuse and ill-defined region of decreased echogenicity
    c. complex mass with internal anechoic and echogenic areas
    d. anechoic pattern with increased transmission

Obstetrics and Gynecology Review

Select the answer that best completes the following questions or statements.

1. The physiologic status of prepuberty is
   a. menarche
   b. menopause
   c. premenarche
   d. postmenarche

2. The bladder is considered adequately filled when
   a. it extends past the endometrial canal
   b. it extends past the uterine fundus
   c. it fills the true pelvic cavity
   d. it covers the fimbria

3. A routine transabdominal image protocol of the pelvis consists of longitudinal and transverse scans of
   a. uterus, cervix, adnexa
   b. cervix, right adnexa, left adnexa, uterus, rectouterine recess
   c. endometrial canal, cervix, adnexa
   d. cervix, uterus, fallopian tubes

4. If pelvic pathology is present, what other areas should be examined?
   a. renal
   b. subphrenic
   c. Morison's pouch, subphrenic, renal
   d. Morison's pouch, renal, pouch of Douglas

5. To image the cervix on the TV examination, the transducer should be
   a. inserted deep and angled anteriorly
   b. withdrawn and angled posteriorly
   c. withdrawn and angled anteriorly
   d. inserted deep and angled posteriorly

6. To image the fundus of the anteverted uterus on the TV examination, the transducer should be
   a. inserted deep and angled anteriorly
   b. withdrawn and angled posteriorly
   c. withdrawn slightly and angled anteriorly
   d. inserted deep and angled posteriorly

7. What muscle group is inserted on the pubic ramus and is called paired parasagittal straps in the abdominal wall?
   a. piriformis
   b. coccygeus
   c. obturator fascia
   d. rectus abdominis

463

8. What muscles may be identified in the true pelvis in the transverse plane with cephalic angulation of the transducer at the pubis?
   a. piriformis
   b. coccygeus
   c. obturator internus
   d. rectus abdominis

9. This muscle is best imaged in a transverse plane with caudal angulation at the most superior aspect of the bladder.
   a. levator ani
   b. rectus abdominis
   c. coccygeus
   d. piriformis

10. What muscle group may be seen in the false pelvis along the lateral side walls of the pelvis?
    a. obturator internus
    b. iliopsoas
    c. rectus sheath
    d. psoas major

11. The müllerian duct is important to development of the
    a. fallopian tube
    b. ovary
    c. female internal reproductive organs
    d. uterine canal

12. Bilateral support for the uterus is provided by the
    a. broad ligament
    b. round ligament
    c. uterosacral ligaments
    d. endometrial ligament

13. The ligament that occupies space between the layers of another ligament and occurs in front of and below the fallopian tube is the
    a. broad ligament
    b. uterosacral ligament
    c. round ligament
    d. tubal ligament

14. The texture of the myometrium of the uterus may be described as
    a. heterogeneous
    b. homogeneous with smooth borders
    c. heterogeneous with smooth borders
    d. homogeneous with irregular borders

15. The vessels seen in the periphery of the uterus are called the
    a. arcuate
    b. uterine
    c. ovarian
    d. tubal

16. The best way to measure the cervical-fundal length of the normal uterus is
    a. TA, longitudinal
    b. TV, sagittal
    c. TV, coronal
    d. TA, transverse

17. The normal length of the young adult uterus should measure
    a. 3 to 5 cm
    b. 2 to 3 cm
    c. 5 to 6 cm
    d. 6 to 9 cm

18. The endometrium changes during the menstrual cycle. When the three-line sign appears, this is the
    a. secretory phase
    b. early proliferative phase
    c. midproliferative phase
    d. late proliferative phase

19. The endometrial thickness is measured
    a. from inner to inner border
    b. from anterior to posterior layers
    c. from outer to outer layer, including fluid
    d. from inner to inner on TA only

20. The normal measurement of the endometrium should be _____ in a menstrual woman.
    a. 10 to 12 mm
    b. 1 to 2 mm
    c. 4 to 6 mm
    d. 4 to 12 mm

21. The structure that lies above the utero-ovarian ligaments, the round ligaments, and the tubo-ovarian vessels is the
    a. ovary
    b. fallopian tube
    c. broad ligament
    d. uterine artery

22. The ovary produces two hormones; estrogen is secreted by the _____, whereas progesterone is secreted by the _____.
    a. follicles, corpus luteum
    b. secretory, proliferative
    c. follicles, corpuscle
    d. corpus luteum, nabothian

23. The release of an egg from the ruptured mature follicle is
    a. menstruation
    b. corpus luteum
    c. ovulation
    d. follicle-stimulating hormone (FSH)

24. The ovary is located lateral to the _____ and anteromedial to the _____.
    a. round ligament, broad ligament
    b. uterus, internal iliac vessels
    c. external iliac vessels, piriformis
    d. obturator internus, internal iliac vessels

25. The posterior component of the pelvic cavity is occupied by all of the following except the
    a. rectum
    b. cervix
    c. colon
    d. ileum

26. Which statement is false regarding the ureter?
    a. It crosses the pelvic inlet anterior to the bifurcation of the common iliac artery.
    b. It runs in front of the internal iliac artery and posterior to the ovary.
    c. It runs forward and lateral under the base of the broad ligament.
    d. It runs forward and lateral to the vagina to enter the bladder.

27. The uterus is supported by the
    a. levator ani muscles and pelvic fascia
    b. obturator internus muscles
    c. iliacus muscles
    d. piriformis muscles

28. The ligaments of the uterus include
    a. broad, suspensory, round, ovarian
    b. broad, round, ovarian
    c. broad, fundal, round
    d. broad, fundal, piriformis

29. The texture of the ovary is
    a. less echogenic than the uterus
    b. more echogenic than the uterus
    c. more hypoechoic than the uterus
    d. less hypoechoic than the uterus

30. The failure of fusion that has two vaginas, two cervices, two uterine bodies is
    a. bicornuate uterus
    b. didelphys uterus
    c. bicornis unicollis uterus
    d. arcuatus uterus

31. The transvaginal technique may be contraindicated in all of the following except
    a. premenarche patients
    b. obese patients
    c. sexually inactive patients
    d. patients who refuse or cannot tolerate the examination

32. The Doppler indices used to evaluate the pelvic vessels include all of the following except
    a. A/B ratio
    b. Pourcelot resistive index
    c. Bernoulli's equation
    d. pulsatility index

33. The uterine vessels are found in the
    a. obturator internus
    b. broad ligaments
    c. piriformis
    d. aorta

34. The ovarian arteries and veins are found in the
    a. broad ligaments
    b. suspensory ligaments
    c. round ligaments
    d. oval ligaments

35. The three divisions of the fallopian tube are
    a. intramural, isthmus, ampullary
    b. intramural, ampullary, follicular
    c. isthmus, ampullary, follicular
    d. follicular, fimbriae, luteal

36. When only the body and the fundus of the uterus are flexed posteriorly, it is
    a. anteflexed
    b. anteverted
    c. retroflexed
    d. retroverted

37. The end of the fallopian tube that is open to the peritoneal cavity is called the
    a. isthmus
    b. frondosum
    c. ampulla
    d. fimbria

38. Hydrometra would appear sonographically as
    a. a sonolucent tubular structure in the adnexa
    b. an echogenic thickening of the endometrium
    c. a sonolucent fluid collection in the uterine canal
    d. a sonolucent fluid collection in the uterus, cervix, and vagina

39. The human chorionic gonadotropin (hCG) levels in gestational trophoblastic disease
    a. decrease in time
    b. increase at a markedly higher rate than in a normal pregnancy
    c. increase at a subnormal rate
    d. remain at an even level throughout the course of the disease

40. The hormone responsible for estrogen stimulation is
    a. FSH
    b. luteinizing hormone (LH)
    c. cortisone
    d. progesterone

41. Polycystic ovaries usually have cysts that are
    a. around the periphery of the ovary
    b. throughout the ovary
    c. large and septated
    d. infected

42. Sonographic evaluation of the pelvis in the patient with a suspected mass has several objectives. Which of the following is NOT one?
    a. to confirm the presence of a mass
    b. to determine its origin
    c. to provide a pathologic diagnosis
    d. to characterize its internal echoarchitecture

43. Which of the following is usually a preponderantly cystic mass?
    a. hydrosalpinx
    b. teratoma
    c. ovarian abscess
    d. mucinous cystadenoma

44. Teratomas are
    a. complex masses
    b. cystic masses
    c. always malignant
    d. lethal

45. The most common site of an ectopic pregnancy is
    a. the isthmus of the fallopian tube
    b. the abdomen
    c. the ovary
    d. the ampullary portion of the fallopian tube

46. A fluid collection in the endometrium that simulates the gestational sac of an early pregnancy is called
    a. decidual reaction
    b. endometritis
    c. pseudogestational sac
    d. hydrometra

47. Which of the following is NOT an adnexal structure?
    a. ovarian ligaments
    b. ovaries
    c. uterus
    d. broad ligaments

48. A dermoid is
    a. a large cystic mass with prominent septations
    b. a benign teratoma in which ectodermal elements are preponderant
    c. the most common large cystic mass, which may contain a lattice of internal thin-walled septations
    d. the largest of the functional cysts, associated with trophoblastic disease

49. The total sum of the measurement of the largest pocket of amniotic fluid in four quadrants is called the
    a. amniotic fluid volume
    b. amniotic fluid index
    c. amniotic pocket volume
    d. amniotic quadrant volume

50. A parovarian cyst is a
    a. large cystic mass with prominent septations
    b. benign teratoma in which ectodermal elements are preponderant
    c. the largest of the functional cysts, associated with trophoblastic disease
    d. cyst that arises from the broad ligament

51. Theca lutein cysts are
    a. large cystic masses with prominent septations
    b. benign teratomas in which ectodermal elements are preponderant
    c. the most common large cystic masses, which may contain a lattice of internal thin-walled septations
    d. the largest of the functional cysts, associated with trophoblastic disease or hyperstimulation of the hCG

52. Biparietal diameter can be used for fetal dating as early as
    a. 6 weeks
    b. 8 weeks
    c. 10 weeks
    d. 12 weeks

53. BPD measurement should be taken from the following borders:
    a. outer to outer
    b. outer to inner
    c. inner to inner
    d. inner to outer

54. A brachycephalic head describes a head that is
    a. round
    b. elongated
    c. abnormal
    d. small

55. The crown-rump length (CRL) measurement is the longest length of the embryo
    a. excluding the limbs
    b. including the limbs
    c. including the yolk sac
    d. including the femur

56. An intrauterine growth–restricted fetus is one that
    a. is always born with genetic defects
    b. has an abnormal heart rate
    c. is RH sensitive
    d. is born at or below the 10th percentile of weight for gestational age

57. The abdominal circumference should be taken at the level of
    a. the fetal stomach and the portal vein
    b. the fetal heart and ribs
    c. the fetal kidneys
    d. the umbilical cord insertion site

58. A(n) _____ is formed when an oocyte unites with a sperm cell.
    a. oocyte
    b. zygote
    c. corpus albicans
    d. morula

59. When the uterus empties itself of all products of conception, it is referred to as a(n)
    a. blighted ovum
    b. complete abortion
    c. impending abortion
    d. missed abortion

60. What is the approximate hCG level when a gestational sac is first observed (transabdominally)?
    a. 800 mIU/ml
    b. 1200 mIU/ml
    c. 1800 mIU/ml
    d. 2100 mIU/ml

61. All of the following statements regarding hydatidiform mole are true except
    a. A previous mole results in increased risk for recurrence.
    b. It is associated with markedly elevated hCG levels.
    c. The sonographic appearance is similar to that of a degenerating myoma.
    d. Although considered "tumors" of trophoblastic tissue, they are incapable of metastasizing.

62. Causes of polyhydramnios include all of the following except
    a. congenital abnormalities
    b. heart failure
    c. gastrointestinal anomalies
    d. amniotic bands

63. Higher than normal levels of hCG are seen in which of the following conditions?
    a. multiple gestation
    b. corpus luteum cyst
    c. ectopic pregnancy
    d. anembryonic gestation

64. Postmenopausal ovaries are difficult to recognize sonographically for all of the following reasons except
    a. They are no longer responsive to pituitary gonadotropins.
    b. They are smaller than premenopausal ovaries.
    c. The parenchymal tissue becomes hypoechoic as a result of atrophy.
    d. The blood supply to the ovaries is diminished.

65. Fusion of the amnion and the chorion normally occurs between
    a. 3 and 5 weeks
    b. 5 and 8 weeks
    c. 8 and 10 weeks
    d. 14 and 16 weeks

66. In the 8th to 9th week of gestation, the fetal heart rate on a transvaginal sonogram should measure
    a. 90 beats per minute
    b. 120 beats per minute
    c. 160 beats per minute
    d. 200 beats per minute

67. The most inaccurate measurement for fetal growth assessment is
    a. femur length
    b. biparietal diameter
    c. abdominal circumference
    d. head circumference

68. The fetal renal pelvis should be followed in utero if the measurement exceeds
    a. 1 to 2 mm
    b. 2 to 3 mm
    c. 4 to 5 mm
    d. 5 to 10 mm

69. If you are scanning a first-trimester pregnancy, documentation should be made of
    a. BPD
    b. crown-rump length
    c. head circumference
    d. abdominal circumference

70. To determine situs solitus, the following structures should be identified except
    a. stomach on left
    b. aorta on left, IVC right and anterior
    c. aorta on left, IVC right and posterior
    d. apex to left

71. A solid mass may exhibit all of the following except
    a. distal acoustic shadows
    b. distal acoustic enhancement
    c. irregular, poorly defined walls
    d. a heterogeneous interior

72. What type of cyst is commonly associated with pregnancy?
    a. a theca lutein cyst
    b. a parovarian cyst
    c. a corpus luteum cyst
    d. a follicular cyst

73. If an anterior abdominal wall mass is seen just to the right of the umbilical cord, the most likely diagnosis is
    a. gastroschisis
    b. omphalocele
    c. hernia
    d. limb–body wall defect

74. Trophoblastic disease, which extends outside the uterus and spreads to the lungs or brain, is called
    a. choriocarcinoma
    b. hydatidiform mole
    c. endometrioma
    d. lung-gestational molar

75. In what anatomic site does fertilization of the ovum usually occur?
    a. the vagina
    b. the uterine cavity
    c. the ovary
    d. the fallopian tube

76. A 22-year-old gravid patient presents with oligohydramnios. Which of the following would be least likely?
    a. anencephaly
    b. postterm pregnancy
    c. renal agenesis
    d. premature rupture of the membranes

77. A patient is GPA 8,2,1. How many abortions has she had?
    a. four
    b. eight
    c. two
    d. one

78. A near-term gravid patient lying face up for longer than 15 minutes sometimes will become ill with fainting and nausea. She is probably experiencing
    a. supine hypotensive syndrome
    b. supine hypertensive syndrome
    c. morning sickness
    d. hyperemesis gravidarum

79. Separation of the chorionic and amniotic membranes is normal
    a. after 24 weeks of gestation
    b. before 24 weeks of gestation
    c. after 16 weeks of gestation
    d. before 16 weeks of gestation

80. Which of the following is the appropriate description of gastroschisis?
    a. normal insertion of the umbilical cord, with herniation of the bowel occurring most often on the right side of the umbilicus
    b. herniation of the thoracic and abdominal contents, including the bowel and liver or spleen, with herniation at the base of the umbilical cord
    c. herniation of the umbilical cord
    d. herniation of bowel to the left of the umbilicus, containing spleen covered by peritoneum

81. A leiomyoma that deforms the endometrial cavity and may cause irregular or heavy menstrual bleeding is known as a
    a. pedunculated fibroid
    b. subserosal fibroid
    c. submucosal fibroid
    d. intramural fibroid

82. Calcifications of fibroids may be secondary to all of the following except
    a. diabetes mellitus
    b. hypertension
    c. hypotension
    d. chronic renal failure

83. If the endometrium measures more than 14 mm without hormone replacement therapy, the sonographer should think of
    a. endometrial hyperplasia
    b. adenomyosis
    c. endometritis
    d. endometrioma

84. Clear evidence for endometrial carcinoma is
    a. light bleeding during the secretory phase
    b. myometrial invasion
    c. calcification of the arcuate arteries
    d. gestational trophoblastic disease

85. The most common cause of tubal obstruction is
    a. endometrioma
    b. hydrometrocolpos
    c. adenomyosis
    d. pelvic inflammatory disease

86. The function of the ovary is to
    a. produce testosterone
    b. produce follicles
    c. mature oocytes until ovulation
    d. manufacture corpus luteum

473

87. The normal follicle may enlarge to _____ before ovulation.
    a. 8 cm
    b. 24 mm
    c. 39 mm
    d. 78 mm

88. Increased levels of hCG may cause
    a. hemorrhagic cysts to develop
    b. teratomas
    c. theca lutein cysts
    d. polycystic ovaries

89. Cysts smaller than _____ are not likely to be malignant.
    a. 2 cm
    b. 3 cm
    c. 4 cm
    d. 5 cm

90. Another name for a chocolate cyst is
    a. dermoid tumor
    b. endometrioma
    c. hemorrhagic cyst
    d. adenoma

91. Cysts with thick septations and solid elements most likely are
    a. filled with blood
    b. filled with fluid
    c. malignant
    d. benign

92. The most common mass in young girls is
    a. polycystic ovary
    b. teratoma
    c. pelvic inflammatory disease
    d. Brenner tumor

93. Which statement regarding torsion of the ovary is false?
    a. The ovary becomes edematous, measuring more than 4 cm.
    b. Fluid is often found in the pelvis.
    c. Doppler shows increased blood surrounding the periphery of the ovary.
    d. The ovary is usually hypoechoic.

94. All of the following causes may mimic a pelvic mass except
    a. pelvic kidney
    b. omental cysts
    c. retroflexed ureter
    d. diverticular abscess

95. In an early gestation, the gestational sac
    a. represents the fluid-filled amniotic cavity
    b. surrounds the decidua capsularis and decidua parietalis
    c. can be visualized transvaginally by 4 weeks and transabdominally by 6 weeks
    d. cannot be correlated with hCG

96. The placenta develops from
    a. the portion of the trophoblast attached to the myometrium, the decidua basalis
    b. the portion of the trophoblast attached to the decidua capsularis
    c. the amnion before fusion with the chorionic cavity
    d. the double decidual sac

97. The echogenic secondary yolk sac is
    a. the first structure to be seen within the gestational sac
    b. not visualized in an ectopic gestation
    c. seen transabdominally at ±4 weeks after the LMP
    d. usually between 5 and 7 mm in diameter

98. During the first trimester, the developing embryo grows approximately _____ every day
    a. 2 to 3 mm
    b. 4 to 5 mm
    c. 1 to 2 mm
    d. 2 to 3 mm

99. On transvaginal imaging, by the end of the first trimester, the choroid plexus
    a. is not present and cannot be imaged
    b. can be imaged as a hyperechoic structure in the lateral ventricle
    c. can be imaged as a hypoechoic structure in the lateral ventricle
    d. is seen as a linear echogenic structure in the gestational sac

100. A corpus luteum of pregnancy
    a. is a functional cyst of the ovary
    b. precedes the formation of a follicular cyst
    c. becomes a corpus luteum cyst only if fertilization does not take place
    d. is found with a hydatidiform mole

101. The sonographer finds the cul-de-sac to contain a small amount of clear fluid. This is MOST likely to be evidence of
    a. a normal situation
    b. an ectopic pregnancy
    c. pelvic inflammatory disease
    d. vesicouterine reflux

102. A patient with a positive serum hCG test presents with some bleeding. The LMP indicates 5 to 6 weeks of gestation. Sonography does not reveal a fetal pole. The MOST likely diagnosis is a(n)
    a. hydatidiform mole
    b. complete spontaneous abortion
    c. ectopic pregnancy
    d. normal intrauterine gestation, but too early to detect the fetal pole

103. In a patient with a complete spontaneous abortion, the MOST likely finding is a(n)
    a. empty gestational sac with no evidence of decidua
    b. embryo with no evidence of a heartbeat
    c. complex mass in the cul-de-sac
    d. empty uterus with a decidual reaction

104. A patient presents with a closed cervical os and a distorted gestational sac in the lower uterine segment. This MOST likely represents a(n)
    a. blighted ovum
    b. complete spontaneous abortion
    c. threatened abortion
    d. inevitable abortion

105. With respect to ectopic pregnancies, which of the following is TRUE?
    a. An adnexal mass can usually be palpated.
    b. Implantation in the interstitial portion of the tube is a common occurrence.
    c. Cornual ectopic pregnancies may have dangerous prognoses.
    d. Ectopic pregnancies cannot be carried past the first trimester.

106. A succenturiate placenta is a(n)
    a. early matured placenta
    b. small placenta
    c. accessory lobe of the placenta
    d. benign tumor of the placenta

107. If a sonographer is unable to demonstrate the fetal urinary bladder, it is important to rescan the area in approximately
    a. 5 to 10 minutes
    b. 15 to 45 minutes
    c. 2 hours
    d. 24 hours

108. The normal fetal heart rate in the second and third trimesters generally ranges between
    a. 100 and 120 beats per minute
    b. 120 and 140 beats per minute
    c. 120 and 160 beats per minute
    d. 160 and 200 beats per minute

109. The fetal umbilical cord contains
    a. two arteries and one vein
    b. two arteries and two veins
    c. one artery and one vein
    d. one artery and two veins

110. Measurement of the cerebellum is BEST made at the level of the
    a. thalamus, hippocampus, midbrain, cavum septi pellucidi
    b. vermis, midbrain, cisterna magna
    c. sphenoid, temporal bone, pituitary stalk
    d. foramen magnum, pons, fourth ventricle

111. When measuring the ventricular system of the fetal head, the MOST accurate level to use is the
    a. frontal horn
    b. lateral ventricle parallel to the falx
    c. lateral ventricular atrium
    d. cisterna magna

112. A percentage of fetal blood from the IVC is shunted from
    a. left atrium to right atrium
    b. right atrium to left atrium
    c. ductus venosus to left atrium
    d. right atrium to ductus arteriosus

113. Visualization of a four-chambered heart within the fetal thorax enables determination of all of the following except
    a. position of the heart and size of the chambers
    b. mobility of the atrioventricular valves
    c. mobility of the semilunar valves
    d. visualization of the ventricular inflow tract

114. With respect to ultrasound of the fetal thorax, which of the following is TRUE?
    a. The diaphragm presents as a linear echoic band.
    b. Increased thickness of skin at the ventral aspect of the thorax usually indicates pathology.
    c. The long axis of the fetal heart is usually perpendicular to the long axis of the body.
    d. Visualization of fluid in the pleural space is normal.

115. An embryo presents with an outpouching from the anterior abdominal wall into the base of the umbilical cord. This is MOST likely to be
    a. gastroschisis
    b. omphalocele
    c. normal herniation of the fetal gut
    d. umbilical hernia

116. Which of the following statements is TRUE with regard to fetal bowel?
    a. Peristalsis can be seen in the small bowel, but not in the large bowel.
    b. Peristalsis can be seen in the large bowel, but not in the small bowel.
    c. The presence of echogenic meconium in the large bowel early in the second trimester is normal.
    d. Echogenic meconium may be distinguished from an amniotic bleed.

117. Which of the following statements is TRUE regarding the fetal bladder?
    a. If the bladder appears distended, pathology is always indicated.
    b. The fetus voids approximately once per hour.
    c. If the bladder is not seen, pathology is indicated.
    d. The sonographer should wait 10 minutes to rescan the fetal bladder.

118. Deoxygenated fetal blood enters the placenta through the
    a. umbilical vein
    b. umbilical artery
    c. spiral artery
    d. uterine artery

119. The most common tumor of the placenta is the
    a. choriocarcinoma
    b. subplacental hematoma
    c. chorioangioma
    d. placenta percreta

120. A single umbilical artery may indicate anomalies of all of the following systems except
    a. cardiovascular
    b. hepatobiliary
    c. central nervous
    d. genitourinary

121. Placenta previa is MOST likely to present in association with which of the following?
    a. increased maternal age, increased parity, or previous abortion
    b. second-trimester bleeding
    c. a distance from presenting part to maternal sacrum less than 1.5 cm
    d. a placenta extending to and covering the fundus

122. Regarding BPD measurement as a predictor of gestational age, which of the following is TRUE?
    a. BPD is more accurate than femur length in the late third trimester.
    b. BPD is more accurate than femur length in the second trimester.
    c. BPD is routinely measured at the level of the ventricles.
    d. BPD is more accurate than HC in the second trimester.

123. The largest transverse section of the abdomen is MOST likely found at the location of the
    a. umbilicus and stomach
    b. confluence of the umbilical and portal veins and stomach
    c. stomach and middle portal vein
    d. fetal kidneys

124. IUGR is best defined as a fetus
    a. that is below the 10th percentile in weight
    b. whose mother has hypertension
    c. at high risk of perinatal morbidity
    d. with known systemic disease

125. The type of twinning that occurs when two ova are fertilized is
    a. monozygotic twinning
    b. dizygotic twinning
    c. monochorionic and monoamniotic twinning
    d. monochorionic and diamniotic twinning

126. Which of the following complications is NOT associated with multiple gestations?
    a. IUGR of one or both twins
    b. increased incidence of preeclampsia
    c. increased third-trimester bleeding
    d. postterm labor

127. In a twin pregnancy, visualization of a septum greater than 1 mm in width is MOST likely to represent which type of twinning?
    a. dichorionic
    b. monochorionic
    c. diamniotic
    d. monoamniotic

128. Which of the following is LEAST LIKELY to be found in the fetus of a diabetic mother?
    a. IUGR
    b. microsomia
    c. skeletal and CNS anomalies
    d. cardiac anomalies

129. The presence of hypertension in the second or third trimester is NOT likely to increase the risk of
    a. fetal hydrops
    b. IUGR
    c. placental abruption
    d. toxemia

130. With the PUBS procedure, it is best to involve percutaneous sampling of the
    a. umbilical vein near the cord insertion at the placenta
    b. umbilical vein near the cord insertion at the umbilicus
    c. umbilical artery near the cord insertion at the placenta
    d. umbilical vessels within the placenta

131. Which of the following is MOST likely to cause postpartum hemorrhage?
    a. obesity
    b. increased age or parity
    c. prolonged labor
    d. delayed uterine involution

132. Prolonged severe oligohydramnios is MOST likely to lead to which of the following conditions?
    a. femur dysplasia
    b. pulmonary hypoplasia
    c. postterm pregnancy
    d. single umbilical artery

133. The Spalding sign is most often associated with
    a. fetal hydrops
    b. IUGR
    c. fetal demise
    d. pleural effusion

134. The term *fetus papyraceus* refers to a condition wherein the fetus
    a. is reabsorbed, leaving no detectable sign
    b. lacks normal bone structure
    c. lacks red blood cells, rendering it white as paper
    d. dies, but persists as a flattened structure with bones

479

135. A malformation that is characterized by the fourth ventricle defect of a retrocerebellar cyst communicating with the fourth ventricle is
    a. choroid plexus cyst
    b. Dandy-Walker malformation
    c. hydranencephaly
    d. holoprosencephaly

136. The MOST accurate method for evaluating hydrocephalus is to measure the diameter of the
    a. atrium of the lateral ventricle through the choroid plexus
    b. superior lateral ventricle from the falx to the lateral margin of the ventricle
    c. fourth ventricle at the level of the cerebellum
    d. frontal horns at the level of the thalami

137. A complex mass appearing on either side of the fetal neck is most likely a
    a. meningomyelocele
    b. cephalocele
    c. cystic hygroma
    d. choroid plexus cyst

138. A spinal defect containing meninges and neural tissue is most likely to be a
    a. cephalocele
    b. spina bifida
    c. meningocele
    d. meningomyelocele

139. The "lemon" and "banana" signs are usually associated with
    a. Arnold-Chiari malformation
    b. Dandy-Walker malformation
    c. duodenal atresia
    d. renal agenesis

140. Sonographic visualization of a fluid-filled mass behind the left atrium and ventricle in the lower thorax most likely represents
    a. cystic adenomatoid formation
    b. congenital diaphragmatic hernia
    c. pleural effusion
    d. pericardial effusion

141. Oligohydramnios after week 16 of gestation most likely indicates which of the following?
    a. unilateral renal agenesis
    b. bilateral renal agenesis
    c. dominant polycystic renal disease
    d. unilateral multicystic renal disease

142. Which of the following is NOT likely to be seen as a fluid-filled mass in the RUQ?
    a. congenital duplication cyst
    b. choledochal cyst
    c. urachal cyst
    d. ascites

143. A fetus with findings of a narrow bell-shaped thorax, curved and shortened long bones, and a cloverleaf skull is most likely to have
    a. osteogenesis imperfecta
    b. achondroplasia
    c. VACTERL syndrome
    d. thanatophoric dysplasia

144. Failure of the atrioventricular valves to separate into mitral and tricuspid valves is part of
    a. tetralogy of Fallot
    b. atrioventricular canal defect
    c. hypoplastic heart syndrome
    d. Ebstein's anomaly

145. Sonographic findings of oligohydramnios, absent kidneys, IUGR, and pulmonary hypoplasia are most consistent with
    a. Meckel-Gruber syndrome
    b. Potter's syndrome
    c. amniotic band syndrome
    d. limb–body wall syndrome

146. Uterine contractions *throughout* pregnancy may be confused with
    a. leiomyoma
    b. Braxton Hicks
    c. Breus' mole
    d. hemangioma

147. Ovarian hyperstimulation syndrome may be associated with
    a. polycystic ovaries
    b. theca lutein cysts
    c. corpus luteum cysts
    d. mesenteric cysts

148. An allantoic duct cyst is most likely to be associated with which of the following intrauterine structures?
    a. gallbladder
    b. cystic duct
    c. umbilical cord
    d. hepatic vein

149. When placental tissue is seen to extend beyond the external uterine wall into the bladder, this condition is
    a. placenta previa
    b. placenta percreta
    c. placenta increta
    d. placenta accreta

150. What usually happens to the hCG levels in 48 hours in the presence of an ectopic pregnancy?
    a. hCG levels drop.
    b. hCG levels rise at a subnormal rate.
    c. hCG levels double.
    d. hCG levels rise at a markedly high rate.

151. A fluid collection in the endometrium that simulates the gestational sac of an early pregnancy is called
    a. decidual reaction
    b. endometritis
    c. pseudogestational sac
    d. hydrometra

152. In a nonstimulated cycle, the maximum normal size of the dominant follicle before ovulation is
    a. 5 mm
    b. 15 mm
    c. 25 mm
    d. 35 mm

153. Ovarian hyperstimulation syndrome typically occurs
    a. after the patient has received hCG and may be pregnant
    b. before the patient has received hCG
    c. after failed induction of ovulation
    d. after the patient has received intrauterine artificial insemination

154. The cervical os is usually about _____ cm long.
    a. 1 to 2
    b. 3 to 4
    c. 5 to 7
    d. 6 to 8

155. The cephalic index is defined as the ratio of biparietal diameter to
    a. femur length
    b. occipitofrontal diameter
    c. abdominal circumference
    d. binocular distances

156. The date of the last menstrual period indicates
    a. the date when fertilization occurred
    b. the date when menstrual bleeding ended
    c. the date when ovulation occurred
    d. the date when menstrual bleeding began

157. Which of the following is not a sonographic finding of a hydatidiform mole?
    a. theca lutein cysts
    b. grapelike clusters throughout the uterus
    c. homogeneous uterine texture
    d. low-impedance, high-flow Doppler pattern

158. How early can the site of the placenta be identified on sonography?
    a. 8 weeks
    b. 14 weeks
    c. 16 weeks
    d. 20 weeks

159. Amniotic band syndrome consists of
    a. adhesions of torn amniotic membranes wrapped around fetal parts and producing congenital amputations
    b. complications of placental abruption
    c. a syndrome that occurs after the fetus swallows too much fluid
    d. a and c

160. A 30-year-old gravid patient, 32 weeks by dates, now presents with painless vaginal bleeding that has lasted for 5 days. The first condition to rule out by sonography is
    a. ectopic pregnancy
    b. placenta previa
    c. ovarian cyst
    d. hydatidiform mole

161. The kidneys should be scanned transversely at a level
    a. superior to the hepatic veins
    b. inferior to the bladder
    c. superior to the falciform ligament
    d. inferior to the stomach

162. Ovulation occurs
    a. always after intercourse
    b. approximately on the 7th day of the menstrual cycle
    c. around the 14th day of the menstrual cycle
    d. approximately on the 2nd day of the menstrual cycle

163. The most common cause of painless vaginal bleeding in the second and third trimesters of pregnancy is
    a. trauma
    b. ectopic pregnancy
    c. placental abruption
    d. placenta previa

164. A growth-restricted fetus will show a Doppler pattern in the umbilical cord that is
    a. high resistance
    b. low resistance
    c. normal
    d. indicative of increased diastolic flow

165. The amount of amniotic fluid present increases the most during the
    a. embryonic period
    b. third trimester
    c. second trimester
    d. first trimester

166. What references should be used to document the biparietal diameter?
    a. thalamus, cavum septi pellucidi, falx
    b. thalamus, peduncles
    c. peduncles, cerebellum
    d. falx, cavum septi pellucidi, fourth ventricle

167. The age of conceptus from fertilization is called
   a. menstrual age
   b. embryonic period
   c. conceptional age
   d. zygotic period

168. The term that describes the transformed endometrial lining of the uterus during pregnancy is
   a. chorion
   b. decidua
   c. chorion laeve
   d. decidua basalis

169. The thin decidua overlying the portion of the gestational sac facing the endometrial cavity is the
   a. decidua capsularis
   b. decidua
   c. decidua basalis
   d. decidua vera

170. The formula used to calculate gestational age from CRL is
   a. GA = CRL + 6.5
   b. GA = CRL + 2.3
   c. GA = CRL + 5.6
   d. GA = CRL + 4.2

171. What occurs when there is death of the embryo or fetus, but the gestational parts remain in utero?
   a. incomplete or missed abortion
   b. spontaneous abortion
   c. blighted ovum
   d. ectopic pregnancy

172. Oligohydramnios means the AFI is
   a. less than 12 cm
   b. more than 9 cm
   c. less than 8 cm
   d. less than 5 cm

173. A bicornuate uterus may be identified by
   a. two cervices
   b. two vaginas
   c. two cornua
   d. two urethras

174. In a four-chamber view of the heart, the right side may be differentiated from the left by
   a. flap of the foramen ovale opening to the right
   b. foramen ovale, moderator band, apical position of tricuspid valve
   c. thebesian valve, eustachian valve, papillary muscles
   d. lack of trabeculations at the apex of the ventricle

175. The renal pyramids appear as _____ areas throughout the renal medulla.
    a. hyperechoic
    b. anechoic
    c. hypoechoic
    d. echogenic

176. A diabetic mother may have an increased incidence of delivering a fetus with
    a. neural tube or cardiac defect
    b. Potter's syndrome
    c. trisomy 18
    d. cystic hygroma

177. Hydrops fetalis is characterized by
    a. cystic masses within the lungs
    b. edema, ascites, pleural or pericardial effusion
    c. dilated ventricles
    d. pericardial effusion

178. When measuring AFI, the sonographer should use color Doppler to
    a. separate umbilical cord and uterine wall from fluid
    b. make sure the placenta does not have a tear
    c. look for a rupture in the membrane
    d. record cardiac activity

179. Evaluation of a(n) _____ would be required if intrauterine growth restriction in all its forms were to be detected.
    a. weight chart
    b. head circumference chart
    c. growth profile
    d. abdominal circumference

180. The biophysical profile documents all of the following except
    a. fetal breathing
    b. gross fetal movements
    c. AFI
    d. fetal position

181. Which broad muscle covers the anterior surface of the iliac fossa?
    a. piriformis
    b. iliacus
    c. obturator internus
    d. psoas

182. The broad ligament encloses all of the following except
    a. ovaries
    b. uterus
    c. uterine tubes
    d. bladder

183. The thickened fold of mesentery that supports and stabilizes the position of each ovary is the
    a. ligamentum teres
    b. fibrous ligament
    c. broad ligament
    d. round ligament

184. The pouch located between the uterus and the rectum is
    a. rectouterine
    b. rectovesicular
    c. Morison's
    d. uterine

185. The muscle that originates from the ilium and sacrum and passes through the great sciatic notch to insert on the greater trochanter is the
    a. obturator internus
    b. obturator externus
    c. piriformis
    d. coccygeus

Pediatric Review

Select the answer that best completes the following questions or statements.

1. The neural plate develops at
   a. 4.5 menstrual weeks
   b. 6 menstrual weeks
   c. 9 menstrual weeks
   d. 12 menstrual weeks

2. The conus medullaris is located at approximately the level of
   a. T12-L1
   b. L1-L2
   c. L2-L3
   d. L3-L4

3. What are the common clinical findings in a patient with appendicitis?
   a. RLQ pain, fever, nausea and vomiting
   b. nausea and projectile vomiting
   c. right flank pain and bile stasis
   d. abdominal pain radiating to the right shoulder

4. Early in development, the brain segments into three primary vesicles:
   a. prosencephalon, forebrain, midbrain
   b. prosencephalon, mesencephalon, rhombencephalon
   c. hindbrain, midbrain, rhombencephalon
   d. forebrain, midbrain, prosencephalon

5. What are the outgrowths on either side of the diencephalon?
   a. choroid plexus
   b. cerebral hemispheres
   c. midbrain
   d. pons

6. What structure invaginates into the lateral ventricles?
   a. pia
   b. forebrain
   c. choroid plexus
   d. subarachnoid

7. Extrahepatic obstruction in the neonate includes all except
   a. choledochal cyst
   b. biliary atresia
   c. hepatitis
   d. spontaneous perforation of the bile ducts

8. Dysgenesis of the fourth ventricle results in
   a. corpus callosum malformation
   b. cystic dilatation of the lateral ventricle
   c. Dandy-Walker malformation
   d. hypospadias

9. Define the measurement used to determine whether appendicitis is present.
   a. an outer diameter greater than 10 mm with compression
   b. an outer diameter less than 5 mm with compression
   c. an outer diameter greater than 12 mm without compression
   d. an outer diameter greater than 6 mm with compression

10. What structure forms between the corpus callosum and fornices?
    a. septum pellucidum
    b. Dandy-Walker
    c. 4th ventricle
    d. Sylvian fissure

11. The normal size of the lateral ventricle as measured in the axial plane should be less than
    a. 4 mm
    b. 10 mm
    c. 8 mm
    d. 6 mm

12. The cisterna magna gradually decreases with gestational age.
    a. True
    b. False

13. What pitfalls should be avoided when determining lateral ventricular size? (Choose two answers.)
    a. developing fetal cortical mantle
    b. choroid plexus
    c. echogenic subarachnoid space
    d. echogenic white matter

14. Approximately 30% of fetuses identified with hydrocephalus are associated with
    a. calcified cortex
    b. spina bifida
    c. subarachnoid hemorrhage
    d. agenesis of the corpus callosum

15. Which statement is false regarding the choroid plexus?
    a. The choroid plexus fills the lateral ventricle from side to side during the second trimester.
    b. With the development of hydrocephalus, the choroid plexus in the far ventricle separates from the medial wall of the lateral ventricle.
    c. Its texture is heterogeneous.
    d. The choroid plexus in the near ventricle separates from the lateral wall of the lateral ventricle.

16. The most characteristic finding of absence of the corpus callosum is
    a. complete or partial agenesis of the cerebellar vermis
    b. dilatation and superior displacement of the third ventricle

c. enlargement of the fourth ventricle

d. hydrocephalus

17. What term is used for any cavitation or CSF-filled cyst in the brain?

a. hydranencephaly

b. schizencephaly

c. porencephaly

d. encephalocele

18. What bony parts contribute to formation of the vertebral arch?

a. two pedicles, two laminae, one spinous process, two transverse processes, two superior and two inferior articular processes

b. one pedicle, two laminae, one spinous process, two transverse processes, two superior and two inferior articular processes

c. one pedicle, two laminae, one spinous process, one transverse process, two superior and two inferior articular processes

d. two pedicles, two laminae, two spinous processes, two transverse processes, one superior and one inferior articular process

19. A vein of Galen aneurysm is best imaged with color Doppler as

a. disturbed flow within the structure

b. disturbed flow surrounding the structure

c. disturbed flow posterior to the structure

d. absence of flow within the structure

20. Which phrase describes intussusception in the infant?

a. occurs when bowel prolapses into more distal bowel and is propelled in an antegrade fashion

b. occurs when one segment of bowel twists around another

c. occurs in the presence of appendicitis

d. occurs in utero only

21. What percentage of premature infants may have intracranial hemorrhage?

a. 30

b. 40

c. 80

d. 90

22. What clinical criterion is used to determine whether an infant has pyloric stenosis?

a. jaundice

b. frequent urination

c. fever

d. projectile vomiting

23. What soft tissue structure is seen to form a bridge of gray matter across the third ventricle when it is abnormal?

a. mass intermedia

b. thalamus

c. hypothalamus

d. cerebral peduncle

24. The lateral ventricles drain into the third ventricle via what structure?
    a. aqueduct of Sylvius
    b. medulla oblongata
    c. cerebellar vermis
    d. foramen of Monro

25. What measurements are used to evaluate a patient with pyloric stenosis?
    a. length greater than 16 mm, thickness greater than 4 mm
    b. length less than 16 mm, thickness greater than 4 mm
    c. length greater than 12 mm, thickness greater than 2 mm
    d. length greater than 13 mm, thickness greater than 6 mm

26. What connects the third and fourth ventricles?
    a. cerebral aqueduct
    b. aqueduct of Sylvius
    c. foramen of Monro
    d. foramen of nucleus

27. What anatomic landmark within the brain is used to find the middle cerebral arteries?
    a. vein of Galen
    b. aqueduct of Monro
    c. caudate nucleus
    d. Sylvian fissure

28. What is the most common age and gender for pyloric stenosis to occur?
    a. female, age birth to 3 months
    b. female, age 1 to 5 months
    c. male, age 3 to 6 weeks
    d. male, age 1 to 3 months

29. Name the four segments of the lateral ventricles.
    a. frontal horn, body, occipital and temporal horns
    b. anterior, medial, lateral, posterior
    c. anterior, body, frontal, temporal horn
    d. anterior, body, occipital, frontal horn

30. What is the "pseudokidney" or "sandwich" sign?
    a. the sign of a pelvic kidney
    b. sonographic finding in a patient with appendicitis
    c. sonographic finding in a patient with intussusception
    d. hydroureter with a pelvic kidney

31. Name the fontanelle through which the neonatal brain may be scanned in the coronal plane.
    a. posterior fontanelle
    b. occipital fontanelle
    c. temporal fontanelle
    d. anterior fontanelle

32. The layer of meninges closely adhering to the brain tissue is the
    a. dura mater
    b. pia mater
    c. arachnoid
    d. choroid plexus

33. A subependymal hemorrhage is found at what site?
    a. supraependymal germinal matrix
    b. subependymal choroid plexus
    c. subarachnoid plexus
    d. thalamic-caudate groove

34. In the pediatric ultrasound examination of the abdomen, all of the following are true except
    a. the right hepatic lobe should not extend more than 1 cm below the xiphoid process
    b. the common bile duct should measure less than 2 mm in infants up to 1 year of age
    c. the length of the gallbladder should not exceed the length of the kidney
    d. the texture of the pancreas is hypoechoic when compared with the liver

35. What is the most common site for a choroid plexus hemorrhage?
    a. anterior horn
    b. occipital horn
    c. lateral horn
    d. temporal horn

36. Where does the germinal matrix lie?
    a. between the midbrain and the forebrain
    b. superior to the caudate nucleus in the floor of the lateral ventricle
    c. lateral to the cerebral peduncles
    d. inferior to the cisterna magna

37. Which phrase defines acute periventricular leukomalacia?
    a. hemorrhagic germinal matrix with cavitation
    b. echogenic formations in the epidural cavity
    c. increased echogenicity in the subarachnoid space
    d. multiple foci or coagulation necrosis in periventricular white matter

38. Which two complications are seen in patients with periventricular leukomalacia? (Choose two answers.)
    a. anomalous myelination of the immature brain
    b. hydrocephalus
    c. agenesis of the corpus callosum
    d. abnormal neurologic development

39. Which is the best definition for hydrocephalus?
    a. marked separation of the anterior horns and bodies of the lateral ventricles
    b. enlargement of the ventricular system
    c. decreased production of cerebrospinal fluid
    d. displacement of the inferior part of the cerebellum through the foramen magnum

40. Which detail regarding ventriculitis is false?
    a. common complication of purulent meningitis in newborns
    b. caused by hematogenous spread of the infection to the choroid plexus
    c. ventricular shunt decreases the risk
    d. leads to compartmentalization of the ventricular cavities

41. The hip bones represent the fusion of all the following except
    a. ilium
    b. femur
    c. ischium
    d. pubis

42. Agenesis of the corpus callosum may indicate what malformation?
    a. Dandy-Walker malformation
    b. Arnold-Chiari malformation
    c. vein of Galen malformation
    d. choroid plexus cyst

43. When the hip is laterally and posteriorly displaced to the extent that the femoral head has no contact with the acetabulum and the normal U configuration cannot be obtained on ultrasound, this condition is
    a. frank dislocation
    b. dysplasia
    c. subluxation
    d. normal

44. The _____ nerve is the largest nerve in the body.
    a. cranial
    b. diaphragmatic
    c. sciatic
    d. optic

45. Passage of cerebrospinal fluid between the third and lateral ventricles is accomplished via the
    a. foramen of Magendie
    b. aqueduct of Sylvius
    c. foramen of Luschka
    d. foramen of Monro

46. What is the function of the hippocampus?
    a. taste
    b. smell
    c. memory
    d. motor control

47. Cerebrospinal fluid circulates between the
    a. pia mater and arachnoid
    b. dura mater and arachnoid
    c. pia mater and cerebral cortex
    d. dura mater and periosteum

48. The upper and lower vertebral notches of adjacent vertebrae meet to form the
    a. transverse foramina
    b. central canal
    c. intervertebral foramina
    d. apophyseal joints

49. The most inferior portion of the spinal cord, located at approximately the level of the first or second lumbar vertebra, is called the
    a. cauda equina
    b. filum terminale
    c. sacral plexus
    d. conus medullaris

50. The "ball on a spoon" refers to
    a. ilium and gluteus minimus
    b. femoral head and acetabulum
    c. ischium and pubis
    d. pectineus and iliacus

Answers

CHAPTER 1 FOUNDATIONS OF SONOGRAPHY

Exercise 1

1. G
2. C
3. B
4. I
5. E
6. H
7. D
8. A
9. F
10. J

Exercise 2

							R									
		P			C		E						A			
	C	O	M	P	R	E	S	S	I	O	N		T			
		W			Y		O						T			
		E			S		L						E			
		R			T		U						N			
			D		A		T	R	A	N	S	D	U	C	E	R
			E		L		I						A			
			C				O						T			
R	E	S	I	S	T	A	N	C	E				I			
			B										O			
W	A	V	E				F	R	E	Q	U	E	N	C	Y	
			L													

Exercise 3

1. B
2. D
3. A
4. C
5. A

Exercise 4

1. H
2. M
3. D
4. T
5. C
6. K
7. F
8. N
9. Q
10. E
11. L
12. I
13. A
14. P
15. G
16. O
17. J
18. B
19. S
20. R

Exercise 5

1. compression
2. electrical, mechanical
3. frequency
4. wavelength
5. shorter
6. decreases
7. doubles
8. Curie

9. impede
10. faster
11. 1540
12. sound
13. incidence
14. perpendicular
15. width
16. azimuthal
17. high

EXERCISE 5

1. a. vertical, b. horizontal
2. B
3. low resistance

CHAPTER 2 ESSENTIALS OF PATIENT CARE FOR THE SONOGRAPHER

Exercise 1

1. I	5. J	9. G	13. M
2. C	6. B	10. L	14. O
3. A	7. K	11. H	15. N
4. P	8. E	12. F	16. D

Exercise 2

1. pulse, respiratory rate, blood pressure, body temperature
2. arrhythmias
3. radial
4. in the high 90s (95% or more)
5. 20
6. systolic, diastolic
7. true
8. The bag should be placed low enough to permit adequate draining of the bladder.

Exercise 3

1. a, c, d
2. leg
3. a,b, d, e

Exercise 4

1. hand washing
2. blood, all body fluids, broken skin, mucous membranes), dried blood and/or dried bloody fluids
3. No. Wash your hands after touching blood, body fluids, or contaminated items—*whether or not gloves are worn.*
4. After seeing each patient, thoroughly clean the transducer and equipment with the steriseptic cleaner.
5. MRSA

Exercise 5

1. Patients have the right to
   • be treated with respect
   • make a treatment choice
   • refuse treatment
   • obtain their medical records
   • privacy of their medical records
   • informed consent
   • make decisions about end-of-life care
2. Patient responsibilities include the following:
   • Maintain healthy habits.
   • Be respectful to providers.
   • Be honest with providers.
   • Comply with treatment plans.
   • Prepare for emergencies.
   • Make decisions responsibly.
3. HIPAA
4. a. privacy, b. security c. administrative simplification

CHAPTER 3 ERGONOMICS AND MUSCULOSKELETAL ISSUES IN SONOGRAPHY

Exercise 1

1. L	5. A	8. B	11. G
2. E	6. I	9. N	12. J
3. H	7. F	10. M	13. D
4. C			14. K

Exercise 2

1. exertions
2. postures
3. static
4. motion
5. grip
6. environmental

Exercise 3

1. Bad ergonomics. The sonographer is leaning over the patient, placing strain on the spine and pressure on the right leg. The right arm is outstretched, placing strain on the shoulder.
2. Good ergonomics. The sonographer is sitting level with the patient. The right arm is at the same level as the patient's abdomen, resting on the chair arm. The sonographer's back is straight and legs are slightly elevated on the legs of the chair.
3. Bad ergonomics. The sonographer is leaning slightly forward into the patient, causing strain on the back and neck. The cord is draped across the neck, causing more strain on the neck/shoulder area. The patient should be raised higher, or the sonographer chair should be lowered to be on the same level as the patient.

CHAPTER 4 ANATOMIC AND PHYSIOLOGIC RELATIONSHIPS WITHIN THE ABDOMINAL-PELVIC CAVITY

Exercise 1

1. B	3. A	5. D
2. C	4. E	

Exercise 2

	D							S							C	
V	I	S	C	E	R	A		S	U	P	E	R	F	I	C	I	A	L
	A			N				P					N		U
	P		D		T		L	E	G				F		D
	H		O		E		R		L				E		A
	R		R		P	R	O	X	I	M	A	L	R		L
	A		S		I		O		T				I
	G		A		O		R		E				O
	M		L		R		R		R				R
						M	E	D	I	A	L
									L

Exercise 3

1. I	5. G	9. E	13. L
2. D	6. C	10. N	14. H
3. J	7. B	11. F	
4. A	8. M	12. K	

Exercise 4

1. B	5. D	9. N	13. E
2. F	6. K	10. O	14. I
3. J	7. C	11. L	15. M
4. A	8. G	12. H	

Exercise 5

1. lumbar	5. celiac	9. abdominal
2. pelvic	6. inguinal	10. thoracic
3. femoral	7. costal	
4. popliteal	8. brachial	

Exercise 6

1. diaphragm, abdominal wall, pelvis
2. hypochondrium
3. inferior
4. anterior, left
5. right
6. diaphragm
7. right
8. linea alba
9. rectus abdominis
10. part of the large intestine, rectum, urinary bladder, and reproductive organs
11. vesicouterine
12. rectouterine
13. fallopian
14. coccygeus, levator ani
15. psoas, iliopsoas
16. piriformis
17. parietal, visceral
18. greater
19. lesser
20. epiploic foramen
21. falciform

Exercise 7

1. subphrenic	4. right
2. Morison's pouch	5. hernia
3. peritoneal recesses	

Exercise 8

1. R	6. P	11. R
2. P	7. R	12. R
3. R	8. R	13. R
4. P	9. P	
5. P	10. R	

CHAPTER 5 COMPARATIVE SECTIONAL ANATOMY OF THE ABDOMINAL-PELVIC CAVITY

Exercise 1

1. C
2. A
3. D
4. B

Exercise 2

1. Inferior	6. Medial
2. Superior	7. Inner
3. Lateral	8. Inferior
4. Anterior	9. Inferior
5. Anterior	10. Posterior

Exercise 3

1. right hypochondrium	2. epigastrium	3. left hypochodrium
4. right lumbar region	5. umbilical region	6. left lumbar region
7. right iliac fossa	8. hypogastrium	9. left iliac fossa

Exercise 4

a. 1. Falciform ligament
   2. ligamentum venosum
   3. inferior vena cava
   4. right lobe of liver
   5. lung
   6. stomach
   7. esophagus
   8. spleen
   9. abdominal aorta
b. 1. Caudate lobe
   2. inferior vena cava
   3. aorta
   4. adrenal gland
   5. rectus abdominus muscle
   6. pancreas
   7. kidney
c. 1. Portal vein
   2. hepatic veins
   3. left lobe liver
   4. pancreas
   5. splenic vein
   6. transverse colon
   7. crus of diaphragm
d. 1. Duodenum
   2. gallbladder
   3. common bile duct
   4. peritoneal cavity
   5. psoas major muscle
   6. left lobe liver
   7. gastroduodenal artery
   8. superior mesenteric vein
   9. superior mesenteric artery
e. 1. Gallbladder
   2. duodenum
   3. superior mesenteric vein
f. 1. External iliac artery
   2. external iliac vein
   3. iliopsoas muscle
g. 1. Bladder
   2. obturator internus muscle
   3. seminal vesicles
   4. rectum
   5. pectineus muscle
   6. iliopsoas muscle
   7. levator ani muscle
   8. coccygeus muscle
h. 1. Iliopsoas muscle
   2. obturator externus muscle
   3. obturator internus muscle
   4. bladder
   5. vagina
   6. rectum
i. 1. Caudate lobe
   2. right kidney
   3. perirenal fat
   4. psoas major muscle
   5. gallbladder
   6. liver
   7. transverse colon

j. 1. Head of pancreas
   2. gastroduodenal artery
   3. costodiaphragmatic recess
   4. right kidneuy
   5. superior duodenum
k. 1. Head of pancreas
   2. pyloric antrum
   3. left lobe of liver
   4. diaphragm
   5. right renal artery
   6. inferior vena cava
   7. bladder
   8. prostate
l. 1. Pancreas
   2. esophagus
   3. splenic vein
   4. superior mesenteric artery
   5. aorta
   6. prostate
m. 1. Diaphragm
   2. heart
   3. fundus of stomach
   4. pancreas
   5. spleen
   6. left kidney
   7. quadratus lumborum muscle
   8. iliacus muscle

CHAPTER 6 BASIC ULTRASOUND IMAGING: TECHNIQUES, TERMINOLOGY, AND TIPS

Exercise 1

1. I	4. H	7. F	10. D
2. E	5. A	8. K	11. G
3. C	6. J	9. B	

Exercise 2

1. left
2. left, right
3. scanning table
4. rib
5. 6 to 8
6. above the baseline, below the baseline
7. systolic
8. hepatic veins
9. a. supine b. prone c. right lateral decubitus d. left lateral decubitus

Exercise 3

1. L	4. D	7. I	10. E
2. C	5. A	8. B	11. K
3. F	6. G	9. H	12. J

Exercise 4

1. B
2. C
3. a. hypoechoic b. anechoic c. echogenic d. isoechoic e. hyperechoic
4. D
5. A

Exercise 5

1. 1.a. Curved array. b. Linear array, c. Sector array
2. echogenic
3. left
4. left
5. hypoechoic

CHAPTER 7 IMAGING AND DOPPLER ARTIFACTS

Exercise 1

1. C	6. B	11. E	16. R
2. F	7. I	12. J	17. O
3. A	8. L	13. N	18. Q
4. D	9. K	14. H	
5. G	10. M	15. P	

Exercise 2

1. slice thickness
2. speckle
3. reverberation
4. comet-tail
5. ring-down
6. mirror-image
7. refraction
8. grating lobe duplication
9. range ambiguity
10. shadowing
11. edge shadows
12. enhancement
13. banding
14. aliasing
15. high gain produces a mirror image

CHAPTER 8 THE VASCULAR SYSTEM

Exercise 1

1. A	3. E	5. D	7. H
2. F	4. B	6. C	8. G

Exercise 2

1. A	5. A	9. A
2. B	6. C	10. D
3. B	7. C	11. B
4. A	8. A	12. C

Exercise 3

1. C	4. I	7. G
2. F	5. B	8. E
3. A	6. D	9. H

Exercise 4

R														
E		H					N		H					
S	P	E	C	T	R	A	L	B	R	O	A	D	E	N	I	N	G
I	P	I				N		P						
S	A	P				R		A						
T	T	S		I	N	D	E	X	A	T				
I	O				S		O							
V	F	S	C	L	E	R	O	S	I	S	P	S	E	U	D	O
E	U				S		E							
	G				T		T							
	A	N	E	U	R	Y	S	M	I		A			
	L				V		L							
					E									

499

Exercise 5

1. D	5. B	9. I
2. J	6. A	10. H
3. C	7. F	
4. G	8. E	

Exercise 6

	A	B	C	D
1	Left gastric artery	Left gastric	Phrenic veni	Left branch of portal v.
2	Suprarenal artery	Aorta	Suprarenal vein	Left gastric vein
3	Splenic artery	Celiac trunk	Inferior vena cava	Short gastric v.
4	Abdominal aorta	Splenic	Common iliac vein	Splenic v.
5	Superior mesenterior artery	Common hepatic	Internal iliac vein	Left gastroepiploic v.
6	Common iliac arteries	Right gastric	External iliac vein	Inferior mesenteric v.
7	External iliac artery	Gastroduodenal	Middle sacral vein	Superior mesenteric v.
8	Inferior phrenic artery	Supraduodenal	Right testicular or ovarian vein	Portal vein
9	Celiac trunk	Proper hepatic	Right renal vein	Right branch of portal v.
10	Common hepatic artery	Cystic	Hepatic veins	
11	Left renal artery	Right hepatic		
12	Testicular or ovarian artery	Middle hepatic		
13	Middle sacral artery	Left hepatic		

Exercise 7

1. right
2. celiac
3. left renal vein
4. superior mesenteric artery
5. smaller
6. right
7. gastroduodenal
8. portal
9. splenic
10. hepatic

Exercise 8

1. To distinguish the common bile duct from the hepatic artery, look for absence of flow in the common duct; to distinguish the hepatic artery from the splenic artery, look for direction of flow; to differentiate aneurysm from pancreatic pseudocyst, look for slow flow in the aneurysm; to differentiate dilated intrahepatic bile ducts and prominent hepatic artery, again look for absence of flow in the bile duct.
2. The patient should be instructed to hold his or her breath; this causes the patient to perform a slight Valsalva maneuver toward the end of inspiration, which dilates the inferior vena cava. The patient may be rolled from a supine position to steep left lateral position to better visualize the IVC.
3. diastolic
4. The pulsatile aorta is easily differentiated from the inferior vena cava because the IVC travels in a horizontal course with its proximal portion curving slightly anterior as it pierces the diaphragm to empty into the right atrial cavity. The aorta, on the other hand, follows the curvature of the spine, with its distal portion lying more posterior, before bifurcating into the iliac vessels.
5. parallel
6. low
7. continuous
8. periportal
9. umbilical

Exercise 9

1. arteriosclerosis, atherosclerosis
2. intense back pain, hematocrit
3. outer, outer
4. anterior, anterolateral
5. pseudoaneurysm
6. The typical patient is 40 to 60 years old and hypertensive; males are predominant over females. The patient usually is known to have an aneurysm, and sudden, excruciating chest pain radiating to the back may develop because of a dissection. Patients may go into shock very quickly. The sonographer should look for a dissection "flap" or a recent channel with or without frank aneurysmal dilatation.
7. **Type I** dissection begins at the root of the aorta and may extend the entire length of the arch, descending to the aorta and into the abdominal aorta. **Type II** may occur secondary to cystic medial necrosis (weakening of the arterial wall) or hypertension. **Type III** begins at the lower end of the descending aorta and extends into the abdominal aorta.

8. Masses that can simulate a pulsatile abdominal mass are retroperitoneal tumors, fibroid uterus, and para-aortic nodes.

Exercise 10

1. a. Coronal - patient is slightly oblique with the transducer to the right of the midline.
   b. inferior vena cava
   c. abdominal aorta
   d. right renal artery
   e. left renal artery
   f. right iliac artery
2. a. common hepatic artery
   b. splenic artery
3. The left renal artery
4. Luminal flap from aortic dissection
5. a. common bile duct
   b. pancreatic duct

Exercise 3

6. Tumor mass in inferior vena cava
7. Main portal vein
8. Right hepatic artery

CHAPTER 9 THE LIVER

Exercise 1

1. C	5. M	9. B	13. E
2. A	6. D	10. F	14. L
3. N	7. H	11. J	
4. G	8. I	12. K	

Exercise 2

1. H	5. J	8. C	11. B
2. E	6. I	9. K	
3. D	7. F	10. G	
4. A			

Crossword puzzle solution with the following words: NEO (vertical), HEPATOCELLULAR, ALT (vertical), ABSCESS, METASTATIC, TARGET LESION, INTRAHEPATIC, EXTRAHEPATIC (vertical), ALKPHOS (vertical), CAUDATE (vertical).

Exercise 4

	A	B	C	D
1	Coronary ligament	Gallbladder	Medial left lobe	Falciform ligament
2	Left triangular ligament	Right lobe	Pyloric area	Inferior vena cava
3	Left lobe	Diaphragmatic surface	Ligamentum teres	Coronary ligaments
4	Falciform ligament	Coronary ligament	Hepatic arteries	Bare area
5	Ligamentum teres	Bare area	Left lobe	Right lobe
6	Inferior margin	Inferior vena cava	Portal vein	Right triangular lig.
7	Gallbladder	Caudate lobe	Gastric impression	Hepatic duct
8	Costal surface	Left triangular ligament	Esophageal impression	Cystic duct
9	Right lobe	Left lobe	Ligamentum venosum	Renal impression
10	Right triangular ligament	Falciform ligament	Caudate lobe	Colic impression
11	diaphragm		Inferior vena cava	Gallbladder
12			Coronary ligament	Medial left lobe
13			Bare area	Portal vein
14			Right triagngular lig.	Hepatic artery
15			Right lobe	Ligamentum teres
16			Renal impression	Attachment of lesser omentum
17			Duodenal impression	Left lobe
18			Colic impression	Gastric impression
19			Cystic duct	Left triangular lig.
20			Gallbladder	Caudate lobe
21				

Exercise 5

1. Riedel's
2. Glisson's
3. main lobar
4. falciform
5. teres
6. venosum
7. right, middle, left
8. metabolism
9. bilirubin
10. detoxification
11. glucose
12. edema
13. bilirubin
14. jaundice

Exercise 6

1. D
2. A
3. C
4. B
5. B

Exercise 7

1. hepatopetal, hepatofugal
2. near field
3. sector or annular
4. lipid
5. coarse, decreased
6. hepatic adenomas, hyperplasia

7. neoplasm
8. spleen, kidney
9. portal hypertension
10. recanalized
11. decreased
12. smaller
13. Budd-Chiari

Exercise 8

1. fatty infiltration of different grades.
2. hepatitis with "starry" sky pattern
3. extrahepatic mass
4. adenoma
5. abscess
6. metastatic tumor

CHAPTER 10 THE GALLBLADDER AND THE BILIARY SYSTEM

Exercise 1

1. C
2. L
3. M
4. A
5. F
6. O
7. G
8. B
9. I
10. E
11. D
12. J
13. N
14. H
15. K

Exercise 2

1. E	5. L	9. D	13. N
2. C	6. O	10. M	14. B
3. K	7. A	11. G	15. H
4. I	8. J	12. P	16. F

Exercise 3

A.
1. Right hepatic duct
2. cystic duct
3. gallbladder
4. ampulla of Vater
5. Sphincter of Oddi
6. Left hepatic duct
7. common hepatic duct
8. Duct of Santorini
9. Duct of Wirsung
10. Unicnate process

B.
1. Gallbladder
2. Liver

3. Distal region of bile duct
4. Small intestine
5. Intrahepatic bile ducts
6. Left and right hepatic ducts
7. Hilum region of bile duct
8. Extrahepatic region of bile duct

Exercise 4

1. bile
2. common bile
3. Vater
4. Oddi
5. cystic
6. cholesterol
7. Courvoisier's
8. anterior, right
9. anterior, left

Exercise 5

							D												
							E	C	H	O	G	E	N	I	C				P
							C												O
							U					H							S
		F				O	B	L	I	Q	U	E							T
F		O					I					P							E
I	N	S	P	I	R	A	T	I	O	N		A	N	T	E	R	I	O	R
B		S					U					T							I
R		A					S					I							O
O												C							R
U																			
S	O	N	O	L	U	C	E	N	T										

Exercise 6

1. right upper abdominal quadrant
2. right
3. 3
4. WES
5. emphysematous
6. choledochal
7. adenomyomatosis
8. Mirizzi
9. cholangitis
10. Caroli's

Exercise 7

1. Hartman's pouch
2. Adenoma
3. acute cholecystitis
4. gangrenous gallbladder
5. wall echo shadow
6. gallstones
7. Caroli's disease
8. stone in common bile duct with dilated intrahepatic ducts

Exercise 1

1. E	5. K	9. L	12. G
2. I	6. J	10. C	13. F
3. B	7. D	11. N	14. H
4. M	8. A		

Exercise 2

A crossword-style grid with the following answers filled in:

- HEMATOPOIESIS
- POLY
- CULLING
- HEMOGLOBIN
- LYMPH
- MALPIGHIAN CORPUSCLES
- SPLENIC SINUS (vertical)
- PHAGOCYTOSIS (vertical)
- ERYTHROCYTE (vertical)
- RED PULP (vertical)

Exercise 3

1. K	5. I	9. H	13. F
2. O	6. A	10. B	14. L
3. G	7. C	11. M	15. E
4. N	8. D	12. J	

Exercise 4

A. 1. Transverse colon
2. small bowel
3. quadratus lumborum muscle
4. left kidney
5. spleen
6. splenic artery
7. splenic vein
8. pancreas
9. fundus of stomach
10. heart
11. diaphragm

B. 1. Suprarenal gland
2. gastrosplenic ligament
3. lienorenal ligament
4. splenic artery
5. spleen
6. hilum
7. phrenicocolic ligament
8. transverse mesocolon
9. kidney
10. Jejunum
11. Superior mesenteric artery and vein
12. duodenum
13. pancreas
14. Portal vein
15. Inferior vena cava
16. Celiac trunk
17. stomach

Exercise 5

1. lymphoid
2. intraperitoneal
3. inferior
4. accessory
5. hematocrit
6. sepsis
7. leukocytosis
8. sickle cell
9. candidiasis

Exercise 6

1. granuloma
2. splenic abscess
3. splenic infarct
4. splenic hematoma
5. splenic cyst

CHAPTER 12 THE PANCREAS

Exercise 1

1. E	5. O	9. H	13. I
2. A	6. N	10. D	14. B
3. G	7. K	11. C	15. F
4. J	8. L	12. M	

Exercise 2

Crossword puzzle (completed):
- ILEUS (across)
- AMYLASE (across)
- ISLETS OF LANGERHANS (across)
- INSULIN (across)
- SERUM (down)
- GLUCAGONS (down)
- ACINI CELLS (down)
- ENDOCRINE (down)
- EXOCRINE (down)
- ENZYME (down)

Exercise 3

1. I	4. A	7. C	10. G
2. L	5. D	8. B	11. F
3. J	6. H	9. K	12. E

Exercise 4

A.
1. Gastroduodenal artery
2. Head of the pancreas
3. Transverse colon
4. Right kidney
5. Right adrenal gland
6. Right lobe of liver
7. Inferior vena cava
8. Hepatic artery
9. Diaphragm
10. Left portal vein
11. Duodenum
12. Left portal vein
13. Cystic duct

B.
1. Aorta
2. Celiac axis
3. Splenic artery and vein
4. Spleen
5. Magna pancreatic artery
6. Dorsal pancreatic artery
7. Superior mesenteric artery and vein
8. Aorta
9. Inferior vena cava
10. Duodenum
11. Common hepatic artery
12. Main portal vein
13. Left gastric artery
14. Inferior vena cava

Exercise 5

1. retroperitoneal
2. hyperechoic
3. anterior
4. superior mesenteric
5. splenic
6. Wirsung
7. gastroduodenal
8. common bile
9. anterior

Exercise 6

1. exocrine, endocrine
2. diabctcs mellitus
3. acini
4. Oddi
5. Langerhans
6. amylase, lipase
7. lipase
8. glucose

Exercise 7

1. pancreatitis
2. Morison's
3. Grey Turner's
4. phlegmon
5. pancreatic
6. lesser sac
7. enzymes
8. adenocarcinoma

Exercise 8

1. right hepatic artery
2. common bile duct, right hepatic artery
3. acute pancreatitis
4. dilated pancreatic duct
5. pseudocyst of pancreas
6. serous cystadenoma
7. adenocarcinoma of pancreas

Exercise 1

1. F	6. C	11. T	16. P
2. H	7. M	12. I	17. K
3. B	8. A	13. Q	18. L
4. J	9. N	14. O	19. R
5. D	10. E	15. S	20. G

Exercise 2

Exercise 3

1. J	4. B	7. C	10. D
2. H	5. A	8. G	11. K
3. L	6. F	9. I	12. E

Exercise 4

A. 1. salivary glands
2. esophagus
3. stomach
4. pancreas
5. small intestine
6. descending colon
7. sigmoid colon
8. rectum
9. anus
10. appendix
11. cecum
12. ascending colon
13. transverse colon
14. duodenum
15. gallbladder
16. liver
17. pharynx

B. 1. Fundus
2. Body
3. Antrum
4. Duodenum
5. Pyloric sphincter
6. Oblique muscle layer
7. Circular muscle layer
8. Longitudinal muscle
9. Ring of muscle
10. Esophagus

C. 1. Esophageal hiatus of diaphragm
2. stomach
3. short gastric arteries
4. spleen
5. splenic artery
6. left gastroepiploic artery
7. right gastroepiploic artery
8. pancreas
9. superior pancreatiocoduodenal artery
10. gastroduodenal artery
11. common hepatic artery
12. celiac trunk
13. left hepatic artery
14. aorta
15. left gastric artery

Exercise 5

1. antrum, pyloric
2. anterior
3. Vater
4. mesentery
5. peristalsis
6. gastrin

7. bacteria
8. blood
9. anemia

Exercise 6

1. gastroesophageal
2. antrum
3. Several measurements can be taken to determine if the mass is the fluid-filled stomach or another mass arising from adjacent organs: give the patient a carbonated drink to see bubbles in the stomach; ask the clinician to place a nasogastric tube for drainage; watch for a change in the shape or size of the "stomach" mass with ingestion of fluids; alter the patient's position by scanning in an upright or left or right lateral decubitus position; watch for peristalsis; or ask the patient to drink water to see the swirling effect.
4. keyboard

Exercise 7

1. bezoars
2. polyp
3. leiomyoma
4. appendicitis
5. compression
6. target
7. mucocele
8. Crohn's

Exercise 8

1. Antrum of stomach
2. Keyboard sign of the small villae
3. appendocolith
4. Appendicitis

CHAPTER 14 PERITONEAL CAVITY AND ABDOMINAL WALL

Exercise 1

1. A
2. E
3. C
4. B
5. D

Exercise 2

Exercise 3

A. 1. Left subphrenic space
   2. stomach
   3. spleen
   4. left kidney
   5. liver
   6. pancreas
   7. right subphrenic space
   8. falciform ligament

B. 1. Stomach
   2. spleen
   3. colon
   4. left kidney
   5. Gerota's fascia
   6. posterior pararenal space
   7. anterior pararenal space
   8. right kidney
   9. perirenal space
   10. liver

C. 1. Falciform ligament
   2. stomach
   3. pancreas
   4. spleen
   5. left kidney
   6. Morison's pouch
   7. right kidney
   8. right subhepatic space
   9. liver
   10. left subhepatic space
D. 1. Lung
   2. diaphragm
   3. lesser omentum
   4. lesser sac
   5. pancreas
   6. duodenum
   7. mesentery
   8. rectouterine pouch
   9. anal cana
   10. vagina
   11. urethra
   12. public symphysis
   13. bladder
   14. uterovesical space
   15. uterus
   16. small intestine
   17. greater omentum
   18. transverse colon
   19. transverse mesocolon
   20. stomach
   21. liver
   22. subphrenic space
E. 1. Costal cartilage
   2. rib
   3. rectus abdominis
   4. transversus abdominia
   5. linea alba
   6. accurate line
   7. inguinal ligament
   8. inguinal canal
   9. iliac crest
   10. internal oblique
   11. internal intercostal
   12. external intercostal

Exercise 4

1. coronary
2. posteromedially
3. inferior
4. ventrally
5. inferior
6. left

Exercise 5

1. omentum
2. peritoneum
3. parietal, visceral
4. lesser

5. epiploic
6. pelvis
7. lesser
8. greater
9. falciform
10. rectus

Exercise 6

1. Douglas
2. (a) through the portal system; (b) by way of ascending cholangitis of the common bile duct; (c) via the hepatic artery secondary to bacteremia; (d) by direct extension from an infection; and (e) by implantation of bacteria after trauma to the abdominal wall
3. bilomas
4. carbuncle
5. acute

Exercise 7

1. urachal
2. urinoma
3. ovaries
4. sandwich
5. lymphocele
6. hematomas
7. hernia

Exercise 8

1. ascites
2. biloma
3. lymphocele
4. Urachal Cyst

CHAPTER 15 THE URINARY SYSTEM

Exercise 1

1. D	4. B	7. E	10. G
2. H	5. A	8. C	11. L
3. J	6. I	9. F	12. K

Exercise 2

1. E	5. K	9. D	13. I
2. M	6. H	10. J	14. P
3. G	7. O	11. B	15. C
4. N	8. A	12. L	16. F

Exercise 3

1. E	3. B	5. F	7. D
2. A	4. G	6. H	8. C

Exercise 4

A. 1. Glomerulus
   2. Ascending loop
   3. Capsule
   4. Cortex
   5. Minor calyces
   6. Major calyx
   7. Renal artery

8. Renal vein
9. Pelvis
10. Ureter
11. Medullary rays
12. Perinephric fascia
13. Perinephris fat
14. Interlobar artery
15. Renal papilla
16. Pyramid
17. Collecting tubule
18. Descending loop
B. 1. Inferior vena cava
2. Aorta
3. Left adrenal gland
4. Spleen
5. Stomach
6. Pancreas
7. Descending colon
8. Jejunum
9. Ureter
10. Superior mesenteric artery
11. Small intestin
12. Right colic flexure
13. Duodcnum
14. Liver
15. Right adrenal gland
C. 1. Left gastric artery
2. Splenic artery
3. Left renal artery
4. Left renal vein
5. Left kidney
6. Superior mesenteric artery
7. Aorta
8. Inferior vena cava
9. Right kidney
10. Right renal vein
11. Right renal artery
12. Hepatic artery

Exercise 5

1. wastes
2. downward
3. true
4. Gerota's
5. pyramids
6. corpuscle, tubule
7. urine
8. glomerulus, Bowman's
9. (a) where the ureter leaves the renal pelvis, (b) where it is kinked as it crosses the pelvic brim, and (c) where it pierces the bladder wall
10. superior mesenteric

Exercise 6

1. retroperitoneum
2. electrolytes
3. carbon dioxide
4. vascular
5. hematuria, pus
6. acidic, alkaline
7. specific gravity
8. low
9. hematocrit
10. elevation

Exercise 7

1. parenchyma
2. arcuate
3. cortex, hypoechoic
4. columns of Bertin
5. crura
6. apex, base
7. dromedary hump
8. junctional parenchymal defect
9. horseshoe, lower
10. ureterocele

Exercise 8

1. renal hilum
2. abnormal
3. adenoma
4. angiomyolipoma
5. lipoma
6. corticomedullary
7. acute tubular necrosis
8. hydronephrosis
9. ureterovesical
10. bladder
11. color Doppler
12. pyonephrosis
13. infarction
14. pain
15. hydronephrosis, superior

Exercise 9

1. graft rejection
2. hypcracute
3. acute
4. cadaveric, donor-relative
5. anuria
6. high-velocity

Exercise 10

1. The renal veins arise from the inferior vena cava in this image.
2. The column of Bertin.
3. Dromedary hump
4. Junctional parenchymal defect.
5. Renal sinus lipomatosis.
6. Extra renal pelvis.
7. Renal cyst
8. Wilms' tumor.
9. Medullary sponge kidney

CHAPTER 16 THE RETROPERITONEUM

Exercise 1

1. D	4. E
2. A	5. C
3. B	

Exercise 2

1. D	3. F	5. C	7. H
2. A	4. E	6. B	8. G

509

Exercise 3

A. 1. Anterior perirenal space
   2. retroperitoneal space
   3. posterior perirenal space
   4. perirenal space
B. 1. Skin
   2. pancreas
   3. lateroconal fascia
   4. descending colon
   5. posterior renal fascia
   6. sscending colon
   7. anterior renal fascia
   8. duodenum
   9. peritoneum
   10. transversalis fasica

Exercise 4

1. pararenal, perirenal, and pararenal
2. perirenal
3. pararenal
4. pararenal
5. superior, medial
6. anterior, posterior

Exercise 5

1. Addison's
2. aldosterone
3. glucocorticoids
4. cortisone
5. masculine
6. catecholamines

Exercise 6

1. b,c,d,e
2. a
3. hypertension
4. urinoma

Exercise 7

1. adrenal gland
2. enlarged lymph nodes.
3. adrenal metastatic tumor
4. neuroblastoma.

CHAPTER 17 ABDOMINAL APPLICATIONS OF ULTRASOUND CONTRAST AGENTS

Exercise 1

1. I	5. G	8. J	11. F
2. D	6. K	9. A	12. H
3. M	7. C	10. L	13. E
4. B			

Exercise 2

1. acoustic emission
2. contrast-enhanced sonography
3. color flow imaging
4. gray-scale harmonic imaging
5. harmonic imaging
6. induced acoustic emission
7. mechanical index
8. power Doppler imaging
9. ultrasound contrast agents

Exercise 3

1. C	4. C	7. D	9. E
2. B	5. E	8. B	10. D
3. E	6. C		

Exercise 4

1. scatterers
2. gray-scale
3. first, second
4. microbubbles
5. reticuloendothelial
6. second
7. oscillate
8. signal-to-noise
9. perfusion
10. small
11. low

CHAPTER 18 ULTRASOUND-GUIDED INTERVENTIONAL TECHNIQUES

Exercise 1

1. E	4. J	7. C	9. B
2. A	5. G	8. D	10. F
3. H	6. I		

Exercise 2

1. alpha-fetoprotein
2. fine-needle aspiration
3. international normalized ratio
4. prostate-specific antigen
5. prothrombin time
6. partial thromboplastin time

Exercise 3

1. malignancy
2. PTT
3. benign, malignant, infectious
4. core
5. thin
6. free
7. risks
8. A member of the biopsy team should ask the patient to recite his or her full name. The patient's ID or history number is confirmed, along with the type and location of the procedure. This is documented usually at the bottom of the consent form. The word "timeout" may also be typed on the screen and an image documented to be part of the ultrasound examination. This is helpful because there will be a preprocedural image; the "timeout" image, which documents date and time; and then needle tip documentation images.

9. postprocedural pain or discomfort, vasovagal reaction, hematomas
10. respiration
11. Move the needle up and down in a bobbing motion. Bob or jiggle the stylet inside the needle. Angle the transducer in a superior and inferior motion. This is helpful when the needle is bent out of the plane of the sound beam. Use harmonics or compound imaging. A last resort is to remove the needle and start again, while closely watching displacement of the tissue as the needle advances.
12. lower
13. same

CHAPTER 19 EMERGENT ABDOMINAL ULTRASOUND PROCEDURES

Exercise 1
1. D	3. H	5. C	7. B
2. A	4. F	6. G	8. E

Exercise 2
A. 1. falciform ligament
  2. stomach
  3. pancreas
  4. spleen
  5. left kidney
  6. Morison's pouch
  7. right kidney
  8. right subhepatic space
  9. liver
  10. left subhepatic space
B. 1. lesser omentum
  2. greater sac
  3. stomach
  4. aorta
  5. lesser sac
  6. gastrosplenic ligmanet
  7. spleen
  8. lienorenal ligament
  9. left kidney
  10. inferior vena cava
  11. portal vein
  12. bile duct
  13. hepatic artery
  14. liver
  15. falciform ligament

Exercise 3
1. blunt
2. intraperitoneal
3. FAST
4. hemorrhage
5. four, pericardial
6. dependent
7. acute cholecystitis
8. acute
9. urolithiasis
10. hydronephrosis
11. cephalic

12. decreased
13. ascending
14. systemic
15. chest
16. Valsalva

Exercise 4
1. FAST scan
2. Morison's pouch
3. Fluid surrounds the splenic capsule
4. Subcapsular hematoma of the spleen
5. Fluid in pouch of Douglas
6. Right ventricular collapse

CHAPTER 20 SONOGRAPHIC TECHNIQUES IN THE TRANSPLANT PATIENTS

Exercise 1
1. D	3. F	5. A	7. B
2. E	4. G	6. C	

Exercise 2
1. liver
2. Hepatitis C, alcohol
3. hepatocellular
4. chronic
5. Glucose

Exercise 3
1. Continuous
2. Elevated
3. Rejection
4. Abscesses
5. Stenosis
6. edema
7. hepatic
8. Biliary
9. Obstruction
10. Seromas
11. Lymphocele
12. Biloma
13. Gas

Exercise 4
1. Parallel
2. Elevated
3. Bleeding
4. Symptomatic
5. Bladder
6. Calculi
7. Thrombus
8. Acute
9. Stenosis
10. Pseudoaneurysm
11. Lymphocele

Exercise 5
1. "blob"
2. Pancreatitis

511

3. Venous
4. Pseudoaneurysm
5. Fluid

Exercise 6

1. Grayscale ultrasound shows a hypoechoic wedge shaped area along the periphery.
2. large hematoma
3. Renal vein thrombosis.
4. Lymphocele.

Exercise 2

CHAPTER 21 THE BREAST

Exercise 1

1. A		4. B
2. C		5. F
3. E		6. D

Exercise 3

1. O	6. D	11. H	16. G
2. K	7. J	12. C	17. E
3. B	8. N	13. F	
4. M	9. A	14. L	
5. Q	10. P	15. I	

Exercise 4

A. 1. Acini
2. Dense connective tissue
3. Loose connective tissue
4. Cooper's ligament
5. Major duct
6. Duct orifice
7. Nipple
8. Areola
9. Cooper's ligament
10. Subcutaneous layer
11. Rib
12. Retromammary layer
13. Pectoralis major muscle
14. Pectoralis fascia

B. 1. Main lymphatic drainage
2. Periareolar lymphatics
3. Sternum
4. Internal mammary nodes
5. Pectoralis major
6. Pectoralis minor
7. Interpectoral nodes
8. Axillary vein
9. Pectoralis minor
10. Pectoralis major

Exercise 5

1. sweat
2. subcutaneous, mammary, retromammary
3. echogenic
4. hypoechoic
5. upper outer
6. acini
7. pectoralis
8. adipose or fatty
9. axillary

Exercise 6

1. fluid
2. ductal
3. milk
4. acini
5. estrogen
6. progesterone
7. prolactin

Exercise 7

1. dense
2. menstrual cycle
3. irregular
4. fibroadenomas
5. intracapsular
6. linguine
7. malignancies
8. benign, malignant
9. horizontally
10. parallel
11. vertical
12. vascularity

Exercise 8

1. fibrocystic
2. intraductal
3. cancer
4. mobile
5. fibrocystic
6. encapsulated
7. terminal
8. in situ

Exercise 9

1. Cooper's ligament
2. Fatty breast
3. Enlarged lymph nodes
4. Simple cyst
5. Fibroadenoma
6. Ruptured implant
7. malignant

CHAPTER 22 THE THYROID AND PARATHYROID GLANDS

Exercise 1

1. C	5. B	9. M	12. A
2. I	6. J	10. H	13. F
3. L	7. G	11. K	
4. D	8. E		

Exercise 2

1. B	3. C	5. F	7. G
2. H	4. A	6. D	8. E

Exercise 3

1. F	5. D	9. E	12. C
2. H	9. I	10. A	13. B
3. J	7. L	11. G	
4. K	8. M		

Exercise 4

A.
1. Thyroid cartilage
2. cricoid cartilage
3. pyramidal lobe
4. isthmus
5. parathyroid gland
6. trachea
7. inferior thyroid vein
8. common carotid artery
9. middle thyroid vein
10. internal jugular vein
11. superior thyroid vein
12. superior thyroid artery

B.
1. Thyroid gland
2. sternohyoid
3. omohyoid
4. sternothyroid
5. sternocleidomastoid m.
6. minor neurovascular bundle
7. esophagus
8. longus colii
9. vertebral body
10. inferior thyroid artery
11. common carotid artery
12. internal jugular vein
13. recurrent laryngeal nerve
14. parathyroid gland
15. trachea

Exercise 5

1. carotid, jugular
2. strap
3. posterior medial
4. calcium-sensing
5. parathyroid hormone (PTH)
6. decreases
7. kidney
8. hypercalcemia
9. adenoma

Exercise 6

1. metabolism
2. calcitonin
3. iodine
4. hypothalamus
5. hypothyroidism
6. nuclear
7. goiter
8. multinodular
9. Graves'
10. adenoma
11. papillary
12. homogeneous
13. longus colli

Exercise 7

1. esophagus.
2. The peripheral hypoechoic halo
3. malignant (punctate calcifications)

CHAPTER 23 THE SCROTUM

Exercise 1

1. F	6. H	10. P	14. G
2. A	7. Q	11. E	15. M
3. J	8. B	12. K	16. I
4. L	9. N	13. O	17. D
5. C			

Exercise 2

1. D	4. E
2. A	5. B
3. C	

Exercise 3

1. F	4. I	7. H
2. B	5. C	8. D
3. E	6. G	9. A

Exercise 4

1. scrotum
2. head
3. vas deferens
4. tunica albuginea
5. mediastinum
6. hydroceles
7. pampiniform

Exercise 5

1. rupture
2. echogenic
3. epididymo-orchitis
4. increased
5. torsion
6. clapper
7. adolescents
8. absence
9. albuginea
10. varicoceles
11. hydrocele

Exercise 6

1. testis mediastinum
2. dilatation of the rete testis
3. The arrow is pointing to the stalk connecting the cyst to the epididymal head.
4. Hydrocele

CHAPTER 24 THE MUSCULOSKELETAL SYSTEM

Exercise 1

1. E	4. K	7. I	10. C
2. H	5. F	8. L	11. G
3. B	6. A	9. D	12. J

Exercise 2

1. D	4. J	7. E	9. C
2. F	5. H	8. G	10. I
3. A	6. B		

Exercise 3

A. 1. bipennate
   2. unipennate
   3. multipennate
   4. circumpennate
B. 1. Deltoid
C. 1. Gastrocnemius
D. 1. Aponeurosis
   2. trapezius
   3. infraspinatus
   4. teres major
   5. rhomboids
   6. external oblique
E. 1. Acromjoclavicular joint
   2. subscapularis
   3. biceps tendon

Exercise 4

1. fibers
2. muscle
3. multipennate, circumpennate
4. tendon
5. synovial
6. shoulder, hand, wrist, ankle
7. ligaments
8. bursa
9. nine
10. paratenon
11. epitendineum
12. parallel
13. origin, insertion
14. hyperechoic, hypoechoic
15. friction
16. communicating

Exercise 5

1. F	3. C	5. D
2. E	4. A	6. B

Exercise 6

1. internal
2. left, right
3. biceps
4. anteromedially
5. supraspinatus
6. glenoid labrum
7. superficial, posterior
8. carpal, flexor
9. radial
10. Achilles
11. partial
12. full-thickness
13. flattens
14. double-effusion
15. synovial
16. halo
17. distraction
18. compression

514

Exercise 7

1. supraspinatus tendon
2. tendon inflammation and focal areas of tendinitis
3. **A,** Tenosynovitis of the extensor tendons of the hand displays the characteristic anechoic fluid *(star)* surrounding the tendon (T). **B,** The fluid within the tendon sheath creates a halo effect *(arrows)* around the tendon on the transverse image.
4. intramuscular hematoma
5. The right median nerve is notably flattened; the left median nerve is mildly flattened.

CHAPTER 25 NEONATAL AND PEDIATRIC ABDOMEN

Exercise 1

1. H	5. K	9. F	12. I
2. E	6. D	10. M	13. C
3. A	7. B	11. N	14. L
4. G	8. J		

Exercise 2

1. 1
2. 1mm, 2mm, 4mm, 7mm
3. kidney
4. hepatitis, biliary atresia, choledochal cyst
5. choledochal cyst
6. intrahepatic
7. hemangioendothelioma
8. hepatomegaly
9. hepatoblastoma
10. pyloric canal
11. male
12. projectile
13. 3.5
14. perforation
15. noncompressible
16. localized pain
17. intussusception
18. target or donut

Exercise 3

1. Fluid collections within the pancreas
2. Splenomegaly with inhomogeneous texture
3. Choledochal cyst
4. Infantile hemangioma with focal areas of calcification
5. Appendicitis
6. Intussusception

CHAPTER 26 NEONATAL AND PEDIATRIC ADRENAL AND URINARY SYSTEM

Exercise 1

1. R	7. N	13. A	19. O
2. J	8. P	14. D	20. I
3. K	9. B	15. Q	21. L
4. W	10. C	16. G	22. S
5. E	11. T	17. U	23. M
6. V	12. H	18. F	

Exercise 2

1. renunculi
2. column of Bertin
3. lobes
4. pyramids
5. fat
6. pyramids
7. liver
8. arcuate
9. junctional
10. superior

Exercise 3

1. hydronephrosis
2. UPJ (ureteropelvic junction)
3. proximal
4. posterior
5. ascites
6. ureterocele
7. prune belly
8. multicystic
9. noncommunicating
10. recessive
11. Wilms'
12. neuroblastoma
13. adrenal
14. hemorrhage

Exercise 4

1. Severe diffuse right hydroureter with primary reflexing megaureter.
2. Adrenal gland.
3. Major obstruction is present with loss of the renal parenchyma
4. Duplex kidney with associated ectopic ureterocele
5. Multicystic dysplastic kidney disease
6. Infantile autosomal recessive polycystic kidney disease
7. Wilms' tumor with extension into the IVC
8. Adrenal hemorrhage

CHAPTER 27 NEONATAL ECHOENCEPHALOGRAPHY

Exercise 1

1. I	6. M	11. C	16. L
2. O	7. G	12. Q	17. F
3. D	8. A	13. J	18. N
4. K	9. R	14. B	
5. E	10. H	15. P	

Exercise 2

1. G	5. J	9. B	13. K
2. D	6. C	10. M	14. O
3. A	7. H	11. E	15. N
4. L	8. F	12. I	

Exercise 3

A. 1. Anterior fontanelle
   2. Coronal suture
   3. Sagittal suture
   4. Posterior fontanelle
   5. Lambdoid suture
B. 1. Foramen of Monro
   2. Trigone
   3. Cerebral Aqueduct (Aqueduct of Sylvius)
   4. Median aperture (Foramen of Magendie)
   5. Fourth Ventricle
   6. Temporal horn of lateral ventricle
   7. Third Ventricle
   8. Anterior horn of lateral ventricle
C. 1. Subarachnoid space
   2. Quadrigeminal cistern
   3. Lateral aperture (foramen of Luschka)
   4. Cisternal Magna
   5. Central canal
   6. Pontine cistern
   7. Interpeduncular cistern
   8. Suprasellar cistern
   9. Choroid plexus
D. 1. Frontal lobe
   2. Anterior horn of lateral ventricle
   3. Temporal lobe
   4. Sylvian fissure
   5. Corpus callosum

Exercise 4

1. fourth ventricle
2. fontanelles
3. anterior
4. dura mater
5. tentorium cerebelli
6. lateral
7. corpus callosum
8. thalamus, nucleus
9. aqueduct of Sylvius
10. Luschka
11. choroid plexus
12. Sylvian fissure
13. thalamus
14. medulla oblongata
15. cerebellar peduncles

Exercise 5

1. coronal
2. anteriorly
3. posteriorly
4. echogenic
5. higher
6. fourth

Exercise 6

1. Chiari
2. hydrocephalus
3. holoprosencephaly

4. fourth
5. cisterna magna
6. corpus callosum
7. hydrocephalus
8. communicating
9. aqueductal stenosis
10. subependymal-intraventricular
11. germinal matrix
12. posterior
13. echogenic
14. hypoxia
15. periventricular
16. echolucencies
17. ventriculitis
18. ependymitis

Exercise 7

1. Corpus callosum
2. Hydrocephalus
3. Germinal Matrix Hemorrhage
4. Acute PVL
5. Lobar holoprosencephaly
6. Dandy Walker abnormality

CHAPTER 28 THE NEONATAL HIP

Exercise 1

1. E   3. A   5. F
2. B   4. D   6. C

Exercise 2

1. D   3. A   5. B
2. F   4. C   6. E

Exercise 3

A. 1. Acetabulum
   2. Head of femur
   3. Acetabular fossa
   4. Pad of fat
   5. Ligament of head of femur
   6. Capsule
   7. Synovial membrane
   8. Acetabular labrum
B. 1. Synovial sheath
   2. Ligament of head of femur
   3. Arterial supply from obturator artery
   4. Arterial supply from circumflex femoral arteries
   5. Epiphyseal line
   6. Iliac crest
   7. Acetabulum
   8. Pubis
   9. Obturator foramen
   10. Ischial tuberosity
   11. Ischium
   12. Ischial spine
   13. Greater sciatic notch
   14. Ilium

Exercise 4

1. sacroiliac
2. ilium, ischium, pubis
3. femur
4. profunda
5. sciatic
6. fascia lata
7. femoral
8. vein, artery
9. sheath
10. pectineus, iliacus
11. hip joint
12. minimus
13. piriformis
14. acetabulum
15. iliofemoral

Exercise 5

1. C	3. A	5. B
2. E	4. F	6. D

Exercise 6

1. psoas, iliacus, rectus
2. medially, laterally
3. medius, minimus
4. piriformis, obturator

Exercise 7

1. 2, 8
2. linear-array
3. hypoechoic
4. echogenic
5. labrum
6. coronal/neutral
7. coronal/flexion
8. femoral head, acetabulum
9. transverse/flexion
10. transverse/neutral

Exercise 8

1. acquired
2. teratogenic
3. developmental displacement of the hip

Exercise 9

1. normal
2. "Ball on a Spoon:
3. "U"
4. "V"
5. Dysplasia

CHAPTER 29 NEONATAL AND INFANT SPINE

Exercise 1

1.B	5.C	8. A	11. G
2.D	6.H	9. L	12. J
3.F	7.M	10. K	13. E
4.I			

Exercise 2

A. 1. Spine
   2. Vertebral foramen
   3. Superior articular facet
   4. Posterior tubercle
   5. Anterior tubercle
   6. Body
   7. Transverse process
   8. Foramen transversarium
   9. Pedicle
   10. Lamina
   11. Lamina
   12. Spine
   13. Transverse process
   14. Superior articular facet
   15. Vertebral foramen
   16. Demifacet for rib head
   17. Body
   18. Pedicle
   19. Facet for rib tubercle
   20. Spine
   21. Lamina
   22. Superior articular process
   23. Pedicle
   24. Body
   25. Vertebral foramen
   26. Transverse process
   27. Inferior articular process
   28. Promontory
   29. Superior articular process
   30. Lateral mass
   31. Transverse process of coccyx
   32. Anterior sacral foramina
B. 1. Dura and arachnoid
   2. Sacral hiatus
   3. Sacrococcygeal membrane
   4. Extradural space
   5. Lower limits of Subarchnoid space
   6. Filum terminale
   7. Subarchnoid space
C. 1. Dura matter
   2. Arachnoid mater
   3. Cauda equine
   4. Internal vertebral vein
   5. Intervertebral
   6. Annulus
D. 1. Gray matter
   2. White matter
   3. Pia mater
   4. Arachnoid mater
   5. Dura mater
   6. Spinal nerve
   7. Posterior root ganglion
   8. Anterior rootlets of spinal nerve

Exercise 3

1. dimple
2. hemangioma, hairy
3. 1 inch

4. dysraphism
5. 8.5
6. mesoderm
7. diastematomyelia
8. myelomeningocele
9. meninges

Exercise 4

1. anteriorly
2. foramen
3. laminae
4. sacroiliac
5. hiatus
6. intervertebral
7. fibrosus, pulposus
8. third
9. medullaris, terminale
10. median
11. cauda equina
12. dura, arachnoid, pia
13. dura
14. arachnoid
15. pia

Exercise 5

1. hypoechoic
2. canal
3. oscillate
4. tethered
5. eccentrically
6. echogenic
7. myelomeningocele
8. meningocele
9. hemangiomas

Exercise 6

1. Tip of the conus medullaris with arrows pointing to the nerve rootlets.
2. DS- dural sac; arrow points to filum terminale
3. Tethered spinal cord
4. Hydromyelia in an infant with diastematomyelia. Acute kyphosis of the spine is seen at the thoracolumbar junction, and a dilated central canal (arrow).

CHAPTER 30 ANATOMIC AND PHYSIOLOGIC RELATIONSHIPS WITHIN THE THORACIC CAVITY

Exercise 1

1. D	3. A	5. C
2. B	4. E	6. F

Exercise 2

1. H	4. B	7. E
2. D	5. A	8. G
3. F	6. I	9. C

Exercise 3

A. 1. Pulmonary trunk
   2. pulmonary valve
   3. conus arteriosus
   4. supraventricular crest
   5. interventricular septum
   6. posterior papillary muscle
   7. moderator band
   8. anterior papillary muscle
   9. tricuspid valve
   10. right atrium
   11. superior vena cava
   12. aorta

B. 1. Crista terminalis
   2. right auricle
   3. membranous septum
   4. petinate muscles
   5. coronary sinus
   6. eustachian valve
   7. inferior vena cava
   8. fossa ovalis
   9. medial cusp of tricuspid valve
   10. interatrial septum
   11. right pulmonary artery
   12. superior vena cava

C. 1. Inferior vena cava
   2. right atrium
   3. anterior cusp
   4. posterior cusp
   5. posterior papillary muscle and chordae
   6. anterior papillary muscle and chordae
   7. partietal band
   8. septal band
   9. medial papillary muscle and chordae
   10. medial cusp
   11. interventricular part
   12. atrioventricular part

D. 1. Ligamentum arteriosum
   2. aortic arch
   3. left pulmonary artery
   4. right pulmonary artery
   5. left pulmonary vein
   6. formaen ovale
   7. right pulmonary veins
   8. left atrium
   9. coronary sinus
   10. mitral valve
   11. aortic valve
   12. conus arteriosus

E. 1. Left atrium
   2. posterior cusp
   3. commissural cusps
   4. posterior papillary muscle
   5. anterior papillary muscle
   6. chordae tendineae
   7. anterior cusp
   8. mitral valve annulus

F. 1. Aortic sinus of Valsalva
   2. ascending aorta
   3. orifice of left coronary artery
   4. left cusp
   5. non-coronary (posterior) cusp
   6. right cusp

7. anterior mitral valve leaflet
8. muscular interventricular septum
9. membranous septum
10. orifice of right coronary artery
G. 1. Left common carotid artery
2. left subclavian artery
3. aortic arch
4. ligamentum venosum
5. left pulmonary artery
6. left pulmonary veins
7. ascending aorta
8. superior vena cava
9. right pulmonary veins
10. right pulmonary artery
11. brachiocephalic trunk
12. right subclavian artery
13. right common carotid artery

Exercise 4

1. E	3. G	5. H	7. F
2. C	4. A	6. B	8. D

Exercise 5

1. oxygenated, waste
2. diaphragm
3. Louis
4. pleural
5. costophrenic
6. left
7. anterior
8. anterior
9. posterior
10. parietal
11. pericardial
12. endocardium
13. myocardium
14. filling
15. lungs
16. superior, inferior
17. interatrial
18. atrioventricular
19. eustachian
20. coronary
21. tricuspid
22. supraventricularis
23. infundibulum
24. mitral
25. chordae
26. apex, base
27. membranous
28. coronary

Exercise 6

1. 70
2. systole, diastole
3. pulmonary
4. increased

5. Valsalva
6. sinoatrial
7. atrioventricular
8. P
9. QRS
10. T
11. Starling
12. preload
13. afterload

Exercise 7

1. laminar
2. turbulent
3. viscosity
4. parabolic
5. flat
6. systole
7. diastole
8. high

CHAPTER 31 HEMODYNAMICS

Exercise 1

1. F		7. L		12. D
2. C		8. B		13. G
3. H		9. I		14. O
4. A		10. N		15. M
5. E		11. P		16. K
6. J				

Exercise 2

1. See Fig 31-1 for the answers
2.

Right Atrium (RA) 1-5mmHg	**Left Atrium** (LA) 2-12mmHg
Right Ventricle (RV): 15-30mmHg in systole 1-7mmHg in diastole	**Left ventricle** (LV): 90-140 in systole 5-12mmHg in diastole
Pulmonary Artery (PA) 15-30mmHg in systole 4-12 in diastole	**Aorta** (Ao) 90-140mmHg in systole 60-90mmHg in diastole

3. 4-8
4. Increases
5. Preload
6. Highest
7. Negative
8. Positive
9. Perpendicular
10. Aliasing
11. Right atrial

Exercise 3

1. mitral valve; pulsed Doppler
2. Aliasing
3. Diastole

CHAPTER 32 ECHOCARDIOGRAPHY: TECHNIQUES, TERMINOLOGY, AND TIPS

Exercise 1

1. E 4. A 6. D
2. C 5. G 7. F
3. B

Exercise 2

			P									
	L		A									
F	O	U	R		C	H	A	M	B	E	R	
	N		A									
	G		S	H	O	R	T		A	X	I	S
			T									U
	A		E									B
	X		R									C
	I		N									O
	S		A	P	I	C	A	L				S
			L									T
												A
	S	U	P	R	A	S	T	E	R	N	A	L

Exercise 3

1. fifth
2. hemodynamic
3. parallel
4. positive
5. Nyquist
6. spectral
7. directly

Exercise 4

1. Parasternal long axis
2. Right parasternal long axis
3. A. Aortic valve B, Mitral Valve C. Left ventricle
4. Aortic root
5. Mitral regurgitation
6. Parasternal short axis
7. Parasternal short axis
8. High parasternal short axis
9. Apical views
10. Subcostal four chamber
11. suprasternal

CHAPTER 33 INTRODUCTION TO CLINICAL ECHOCARDIOGRAPHY: LEFT SIDE VALVULAR HEART DISEASE

Exercise 1

1. B 3. A 5. C
2. D 4. E 6. G

Exercise 2

1. *tendinae*
2. *anterior*
3. *diastole; systole*
4. ventricle, atrium
5. Long
6. *blunting or reversal*
7. *rheumatic*
8. *calcification*
9. *Decreased; elevation*
10. *Acute*
11. *Perpendicular*
12. *Descending*
13. *Subvalvular*
14. *Bicuspid aortic valve*
15. *Calcific*
16. *overestimation; underestimation*

Exercise 3

1. *long*
2. *suprasternal; two; proximal abdominal*
3. *50%*
4. *6*
5. *Dissection*
6. *Systole; larger*

Exercise 4

1. **A**
2. Mid-systolic mitral valve prolapse
3. PISA
4. There is blunting of the systolic component of the pulmonary venous inflow which indicates mitral regurgitation.
5. Mitral stenosis
6. Aortic regurgitation prevents the ALMV from opening in diastole; diastolic flutter is present.
7. Supravalvular aortic stenosis
8. Quadricuspid
9. 68mmHg
10. Aortic dissection

CHAPTER 34 INTRODUCTION TO CLINICAL ECHOCARDIOGRAPHY: PERICARDIAL DISEASE, CARDIOMYOPATHIES, AND TUMORS

Exercise 1

1. L	5. F	9. E	13. K
2. A	6. H	10. J	14. M
3. N	7. I	11. D	
4. C	8. B	12. G	

Exercise 2

1. visceral
2. parietal
3. Posterior
4. Anterior
5. Posterior

Exercise 3

1. Dilated
2. Non-compaction
3. Diastolic
4. Takotsubo
5. Hypertrophic
6. systolic

Exercise 4

1. Adenocarcinoma
2. Carcinoid
3. Myxoma
4. Fibroelastoma
5. Lipomatous
6. Thrombus
7. "dark"
8. subacterial endocarditis

Exercise 5

1. Pericardial effusion
2. Cardiac tamponade
3. There is a thrombus at the apex of the left ventricle
4. Non-compaction
5. Dilated cardiomyopathy (note the "B" bump on the anterior mitral leaflet and the increased distance between the septum and "E" point).
6. Infiltrative cardiomyopathy
7. SAM

CHAPTER 35 FETAL ECHO: NORMAL

Exercise 1

1. E	3. G	5. D	7. H
2. C	4. A	6. B	8. F

Exercise 2

1. F	4. H	7. I	10. A
2. J	5. K	8. B	11. G
3. D	6. E	9. C	

Exercise 3

A.
1. First aortic arch
2. splanchnic mesenchyne
3. fusing heart tubes
4. unfused heart tubes
5. truncus arteriosus
6. common cardinal vein
7. umbilical vein
8. Vitaline vein
9. sinus venosus
10. bulbus cordis
11. first and second arches

B.
1. Septum secundum
2. foramen ovale
3. valve of foramen ovale
4. left atrioventricular canal
5. left auricle
6. right atrium
7. aorta
8. pulmonary trunk
9. interventricular foramen
10. left atrioventricular canal
11. endocardial cushion
12. right atrioventricular canal
13. bulbar ridge
14. 14.right auricle
15. truncal ridge
16. ductus arteriosus
17. aorticopulmonary septum
18. membranous interventricular septum
19. muscular interventricular septum
20. right ventricle

C. 1. Aortic arch
   2. ductus arteriosus
   3. pulmonary trunk
   4. pulmonary veins
   5. left atrium
   6. aorta
   7. umbilical vein
   8. placenta
   9. umbilical arteries
   10. portal vein
   11. portal sinus
   12. ductus venosus
   13. inferior vena cava
   14. right atrium
   15. foramen ovale
   16. superior vena cava

Exercise 4

1. 3rd, 5th
2. yolk
3. cardinal
4. umbilical
5. Endocardial
6. primum
7. foramen
8. bulbus cordis
9. ductus arteriosus
10. dividens
11. arteriosus
12. posterior
13. floor
14. ductus
15. bradycardia, tachycardia

Exercise 5

1. horizontal
2. larger
3. toward
4. moderator band
5. inferior
6. atrioventricular
7. anterior, left
8. inflow, outflow
9. septum, anterior
10. systole, diastole
11. anterior
12. innominate, carotid, left subclavian
13. patent ductus arteriosus

Exercise 6

1. The right lower pulmonary vein is not shown.
2. The left ventricle should be measured at the level of the mitral annulus.
3. The end-diastole stage of the cardiac cycle is shown.
4. The main pulmonary artery with the bifurcation is anterior and to the left of the circular aorta, making this a normal relationship and ruling out transposition of the great vessels.

5. The aortic arch is shown with the head and neck vessels.
6. The structure of the patent ductus arteriosus is shown.

CHAPTER 36 FETAL ECHOCARDIOGRAPHY: CONGENITAL HEART DISEASE

Exercise 1

1. J	5. B	8. I	11. D
2. M	6. H	9. C	12. L
3. F	7. E	10. G	13. K
4. A			

Exercise 2

1. H	4. G	7. J	10. D
2. E	5. A	8. B	11. F
3. I	6. C	9. K	

Exercise 3

1. E	4. H	7. D	10. I
2. K	5. G	8. J	11. C
3. B	6. A	9. F	

Exercise 4

1. ventricular septal defect
2. ostium secundum
3. ostium primum
4. arrhythmias
5. aneurysmal
6. incomplete
7. complete
8. left, right
9. atrialized
10. pulmonary stenosis
11. acyanotic, cyanotic
12. double-outlet right
13. domed
14. bicuspid aortic
15. Subvalvular aortic stenosis
16. Hypoplastic left
17. Transposition of the great arteries
18. Truncus arteriosus
19. pulmonary
20. Rhabdomyoma
21. Cor triatriatum
22. azygous
23. TAPVR—anomalous pulmonary venous return

Exercise 5

1. Premature
2. simultaneously
3. Supraventricular tachyarrhythmias
4. atrial
5. Atrial fibrillation
6. suboptimal
7. atrioventricular block
8. complete

Exercise 6

1. a) 4 o'clock; dilated with a "rounded" shape
   b) the left ventricle is dilated
   c) The ratio of the cardiac circumference is greater than 50% of the thoracic circumference; d) Contractility would be expected to be very low
2. Atrioventricular septal defect is demonstrated (both an atrial and septal component).
3. *A:* Large defect in the center of the heart; the membranous and primum septum defects are seen with the cleft mitral valve. There is a common leaflet from the anterior mitral leaflet to the septal tricuspid leaflet.
   B: The chordal attachments from the medial portion of the cleft mitral leaflet are related to the papillary muscle on the right side of the septal defect.
   C: There is a large defect in the center of the heart with a free-floating common atrioventricular leaflet.
4. Hypoplastic left heart.
5. Truncus arteriosus results when the aorta and pulmonary arteries (PA) fail to complete their rotations and divisions early in development. A single large great artery is shown as it arises from the center of the heart on the long-axis view.
6. Ebstein's anomaly
7. The illustration shows transposition of the great arteries. The aorta is anterior and is emptying the right ventricle, and the pulmonary artery is posterior, arising from the left ventricle.
8. There is a discrete narrowing of the isthmus of the aorta at the level of the left subclavian artery.

CHAPTER 37 EXTRACRANIAL CEREBROVASCULAR EVALUATION

Exercise 1

1. I	6. B	10. D	14. J
2. M	7. N	11. O	15. P
3. E	8. Q	12. K	16. H
4. C	9. A	13. G	17. F
5. L			

Exercise 2

A. 1. Superficial temporal artery
   2. maxillary artery
   3. ascending pharyngeal artery
   4. fascial artery
   5. lingual artery
   6. superior thyroid artery
   7. right common carotid artery
   8. brachiocephic trunk
   9. right subclavian artery
   10. vertebral artery
   11. carotid bulb
   12. internal carotid artery
   13. external carotid artery
   14. occipital artery
   15. posterior auricular artery

Exercise 3

1. left
2. brachiocephalic, left, subclavian
3. innominate
4. medial
5. longer
6. bifurcation
7. smaller
8. ICA
9. posterolateral
10. subclavian
11. extravertebral

Exercise 4

1. interruption
2. ischemic
3. contralateral

Exercise 5

1. ≥20 mmHg
2. low
3. positive
4. continuous, above
5. continuous
6. pulsatile
7. faster
8. lateral

Exercise 6

1. highest
2. subclavian steal
3. multiphasic
4. recurrent

Exercise 7

1. homogeneous, heterogeneous
2. calcified
3. decreased
4. multiple
5. fibromuscular dysplasia

Exercise 8

1. The external carotid artery (ECA) demonstrates a higher resistance flow pattern and shows pulsatility.
2. High resistance
3. A longitudinal view of the internal carotid artery (ICA) demonstrates irregular plaque along the posterior surface.
4. Carotid sonography revealed bilateral common carotid artery dissections due to uncontrolled hypertension.

CHAPTER 38 INTRACRANIAL CEREBROVASCULAR EVALUATION

Exercise 1

1. E	4. A	7. F
2. B	5. H	8. C
3. G	6. I	9. D

Exercise 2

1. E	3. C	5. F	7. G
2. H	4. A	6. B	8. D

Exercise 3

A. 1. Anterior communicating artery
   2. Anterior cerebral artery
   3. Middle cerebral artery
   4. Posterior communicating artery
   5. Posterior cerebral artery
   6. Basilar artery
   7. Vertebral artery
B. 1. Basilar artery
   2. Left vertebral artery
   3. Left subclavian artery
   4. Aortic arch
   5. Right brachiocephalic trunk
   6. Right subclavian artery
   7. Right vertebral artery

Exercise 4

1. carotid, vertebral
2. ophthalmic
3. communicating
4. cerebral
5. cerebral
6. communicating
7. vertebral
8. basilar
9. posterior cerebral
10. circle of Willis

Exercise 5

1. hematocrit
2. flow
3. hyperventilation
4. hypoventilation

Exercise 6

1. transtemporal
2. suboccipital
3. foramen magnum
4. transorbital
5. submandibular

Exercise 7

1. subarachnoid
2. increase
3. ischemia
4. stenoses
5. increased
6. subclavian
7. basilar
8. away, toward

Exercise 8

1. Intracranial arterial narrowing *(arrow)* is seen with increased velocities in the middle cerebral artery.

CHAPTER 39 PERIPHERAL ARTERIAL EVALUATION

Exercise 1

1. N	6. A	11. D	16. O
2. G	7. L	12. B	17. E
3. R	8. S	13. M	18. F
4. C	9. P	14. Q	19. J
5. K	10. H	15. I	

Exercise 2

A. 1. Abdominal aorta
   2. Common iliac artery
   3. Internal iliac artery
   4. External iliac artery
   5. Common femoral artery
   6. Deep femoral artery
   7. Femoral artery
   8. Popliteal artery
   9. Anterior tibial artery
   10. Posterior tibial artery
   11. Peroneal artery
   12. Medial malleolus
   13. Dorsalis pedis artery
B. 1. Left common carotid artery
   2. Left vertebral artery
   3. Subclavian artery
   4. Axillary artery
   5. Brachial artery
   6. Ulnar artery
   7. Radial artery
   8. Radial deep palmar arch
   9. Superficial palmar arch

Exercise 3

1. thoracic, abdominal
2. bifurcation
3. femoral
4. profunda
5. popliteal
6. anterior, peroneal
7. dorsalis
8. peroneal
9. subclavian
10. axillary
11. brachial

Exercise 4

1. claudication, rest
2. distal

Exercise 5

1. 15
2. supine, heart
3. 20%
4. elevated, lower
5. segmental

Exercise 6

1. increase, decrease
2. healing

Exercise 7

1. hemodynamics
2. 60
3. triphasic
4. forward, reversal
5. decreases
6. thrombus
7. neck
8. systole, diastole

Exercise 8

1. The triphasic Doppler flow signal demonstrates a fast upstroke to peak systole, reversal of blood flow during early diastole, and a forward flow component during late diastole.
2. The peak-systolic velocity is 61 cm per second, and the waveform shape is abnormal.
3. Spectral waveforms demonstrated an increase in peak-systolic velocity (PSV) to approximately 300 cm/sec. along with the presence of spectral broadening.
4. A dialysis fistula was created between the cephalic vein and the brachial artery

CHAPTER 40 PERIPHERAL VENOUS EVALUATION

Exercise 1

1. J	5. A	9. E	13. N
2. D	6. H	10. B	14. M
3. F	7. C	11. I	
4. L	8. K	12. G	

Exercise 2

1. F	5. M	8. C	11. B
2. K	6. H	9. E	12. G
3. A	7. L	10. I	13. J
4. D			

Exercise 3

A. 1. Inferior vena cava
   2. Common iliac vein
   3. Internal iliac vein
   4. External iliac vein
   5. Common femoral vein
   6. Junction of great saphenous and femoral veins
   7. Deep femoral vein
   8. Femoral vein
   9. Popliteal vein
   10. Anterior tibial vein
   11. Posterior tibial vein
   12. Peroneal vein
B. 1. Femoral vein
   2. Greater saphenous vein
   3. Dodd perforator
   4. Body perforator
   5. Cockett perforators
C. 1. Femoral vein
   2. Vein of Giacomini

   3. Saphenopopliteal junction
   4. Accessory saphenous vein
   5. Lesser saphenous vein
D. 1. Right external vein
   2. Right internal jugular vein
   3. Right brachiocephalic vein
   4. Superior vena cava
   5. Right atrium
   6. Ulnar vein
   7. Deep palmar network
   8. Radial vein
   9. Brachial veins
   10. Axillary vein
   11. Right subclavian vein
E. 1. Axillary vein
   2. Cephalic vein
   3. Basilic vein
   4. Median cubital vein
   5. Cepahlic vein
   6. Basilic vein

Exercise 4

1. pulmonary
2. thrombotic
3. superficial
4. superficial, deep
5. unidirectional

Exercise 5

1. area, calf
2. distention
3. externally, flexed
4. collapse
5. saphenous
6. reduce
7. posterior
8. superficial

Exercise 6

1. pressure
2. compress
3. conduit
4. incompetent
5. superficial

Exercise 7

1. The image on the right was made with transducer pressure. The vein walls collapse, suggesting no evidence of venous thrombosis in the lesser saphenous, popliteal, or gastrocnemius veins. The popliteal artery (PA) is still visualized and does not collapse.
2. The vein walls completely coapt which suggests no thrombus is present.
3. This is normal phasic flow in the subclavian vein.
4. The vein walls do not coapt, however no intraluminal echoes are seen. This is suggestive of acute thrombus.

CHAPTER 41 NORMAL ANATOMY AND PHYSIOLOGY OF THE FEMALE PELVIS

Exercise 1

1. D	4. G	7. E	9. F
2. I	5. C	8. H	10. B
3. A	6. J		

Exercise 2

1. N	6. J	11. Q	16. M
2. F	7. E	12. H	17. G
3. I	8. R	13. O	18. K
4. D	9. C	14. A	
5. B	10. L	15. P	

Exercise 3

1. D	4. I	7. H	10. C
2. G	5. A	8. E	11. F
3. B	6. L	9. J	12. K

Exercise 4

A. 1. Obturator internus muscle
   2. Femoral nerve
   3. Piriformis muscle
   4. Psoac major muscle
   5. Iliacus muscle
   6. Ischial spine
B. 1. Symphysis pubis
   2. Obturator internus muscle
   3. Levator ani muscles
   4. Coccygeus muscle
   5. Piriformis muscle
   6. Ischial spine
   7. Rectum
   8. Vagina
   9. Urethra
C. 1. Pouch of Douglas
   2. Posterior fornix
   3. Cervix
   4. Rectum
   5. Vagina
   6. Urethra
   7. Urinary bladder
   8. Anterior fornix
D. 1. Ovary
   2. Body
   3. Round ligament
   4. Isthmus
   5. Internal Os
   6. Lateral fornix
   7. Cervix
   8. External Os
   9. Vagina
   10. Transverse perineal muscle
   11. Levator ani muscle
   12. Obturator internus muscle
   13. Cardinal ligament
   14. Uterine artery
   15. Fallopian tube

E. 1. Uterine fundus
   2. Fallopian tube
   3. Fimbriae
   4. Myometrium
   5. Endometrium
   6. Uterine isthmus
   7. Lateral fornix
   8. Vagina
   9. Cerrvix
   10. Ectocervix
   11. Endocervix
   12. Ovarian ligament
   13. Ovary
F. 1. Anteversion
   2. Anteflexion
   3. Retroflexion
   4. Retroversion
   5. Retroversion with retroflexion
G. 1. Ampulla
   2. Isthmus
   3. Interstitial portion
   4. Ovarian ligament
   5. Fimbriae
   6. Infundibulum
   7. Mesosalpinx
H. 1. Internal iliac artery
   2. Tubal branch of uterine artery
   3. Ovarian branch of uterine artery
   4. Infundibulopelvic ligament
   5. Ureter
   6. Uterine artery
   7. Vaginal artery
   8. Internal pudendal artery
   9. Azygos arteries
   10. Cervical branch of uterine artery

Exercise 5

1. vesicouterine
2. rectouterine
3. Douglas
4. Retzius
5. anterior
6. posteriorly
7. ovulation

Exercise 6

1. 28
2. hypothalamus
3. ovum
4. 14
5. follicle
6. follicular
7. luteinizing
8. luteal
9. proliferative
10. secretory

Exercise 7

1. transabdominal
2. transvaginal
3. wider
4. piriformis
5. obturator
6. levator ani
7. perineum
8. psoas, iliacus
9. puborectalis
10. vagina
11. posterior
12. uterus
13. cornua
14. internal
15. isthmus
16. anteverted
17. fallopian
18. infundibulum
19. medial, anterior
20. tunica albuginea
21. medulla
22. radial

CHAPTER 42 THE SONOGRAPHIC AND DOPPLER EVALUATION OF THE FEMALE PELVIS

Exercise 1

1. B	5. L	9. C	13. E
2. O	6. A	10. M	14. I
3. F	7. N	11. G	15. H
4. D	8. J	12. K	

Exercise 2

1. G	4. H	7. I	9. B
2. J	5. C	8. D	10. E
3. A	6. F		

Exercise 3

A. 1. Anterior
   2. Caudal
   3. Posterior
   4. Cranial
   5. Caudal
   6. Posterior
   7. Bowel
   8. Cranial
   9. Anterior
   10. Uterus
B. 1. Right
   2. Cranial
   3. Left
   4. Caudal
   5. Right
   6. Uterus
   7. Caudal
   8. Left
   9. Cranial

Exercise 4

1. displaces, flattens
2. triangular
3. iliac
4. renal
5. anterior, posterior
6. length, width, axial
7. sagittal
8. symmetrical
9. obturator internus
10. levator ani
11. piriformis
12. lateral
13. low
14. decreases
15. myometrium
16. endometrium
17. arcuate
18. internal
19. transabdominal
20. endometrial
21. hyperechoic
22. thin
23. functionalis
24. basalis
25. secretory
26. echogenic
27. fluid
28. follicular
29. Sonohysterography

Exercise 5

1. The fundus is to the left of the image, and the cervix is to the right of the image.
2. The structure in the center of this image is the endometrial cavity.
3. The visible structures are the multiple anechoic follicles.
4. This is a transvaginal scan of the endometrium during the secretory phase. The basalis (B) is at its greatest thickness and echogenicity with posterior acoustic enhancement (arrows).

CHAPTER 43 PATHOLOGY OF THE UTERUS

Exercise 1

1. C	4. D	7. H
2. F	5. I	8. E
3. A	6. B	9. G

Exercise 2

1. B	3. E	5. A
2. D	4. C	6. F

Exercise 3

1. D	4. F	7. E
2. I	5. H	8. G
3. B	6. C	9. A

Exercise 4

1. nabothian
2. polyps
3. stenosis
4. cuff
5. Gartner's
6. imperforate
7. leiomyoma
8. estrogen
9. Submucosal
10. myomas, arcuate
11. adenomyosis
12. arteriovenous
13. hyperplasia
14. sequential
15. polyps
16. Endometritis
17. synechiae
18. carcinoma
19. cancer
20. intrauterine contraceptive

Exercise 5

1. Gartner's duct cyst
2. Adenomyosis
3. cervical polyps
4. submucosal myoma
5. uterine synechiae
6. IUCD is penetrating the uterine wall

CHAPTER 44 PATHOLOGY OF THE OVARIES

Exercise 1

1. S	7. G	13. K	19. F
2. U	8. P	14. C	20. J
3. Q	9. B	15. M	21. D
4. T	10. I	16. H	
5. R	11. E	17. O	
6. L	12. N	18. A	

Exercise 2

A. 1. Uterine fundus
   2. Fallopian tube
   3. fimbriae
   4. Myometrium
   5. Endometrium
   6. Uterine isthmus
   7. Lateral fornix
   8. Vagina
   9. Ectocervix
   10. Endocervix
   11. Ovarian ligament
   12. Ovary

Exercise 3

1. laterally,
2. medially

3. homogeneous
4. peripherally
5. proliferative
6. oophorus
7. follicular
8. luteal
9. corpus luteum
10. complex
11. malignant
12. 10
13. benign
14. diastolic
15. ruptured
16. theca-lutein
17. hyperstimulation
18. polycystic
19. broad
20. endometrial
21. chocolate
22. blood
23. complete
24. edematous
25. benign
26. malignant
27. cystic
28. increased
29. angiogenesis
30. ovaries

Exercise 4

1. Ovarian torsion
2. Ovarian carcinoma.
3. Theca-lutein cysts
4. Endometrioma
5. Mucinous cystadenoma.
6. Hemorrhagic cyst

CHAPTER 45 ADENEXA

Exercise 1

1. N	5. E	9. J	13. F
2. L	6. A	10. D	14. B
3. C	7. M	11. K	15. I
4. G	8. H	12. O	

Exercise 2

1. Curtis
2. mucosa
3. endometritis, salpingitis
4. pyosalpinx
5. pain, vaginal
6. hydrosalpinx
7. echogenic
8. tubo-ovarian
9. peritonitis
10. adenomyosis, endometriosis
11. anechoic, solid

Exercise 3

1. A dilated, inflammed fallopian tube (hydrosalpinx) is found.
2. Pyosalpinx. The dilated fallopian tube fills with pus which is seen as low-level echoes with thick walls.
3. Pyogenic abscess. The low level echoes suggest blood or cellular debris.
4. A large, complex tubo-ovarian abscess is seen lateral to the uterus.

CHAPTER 46 THE ROLE OF ULTRASOUND IN EVALUATING FEMALE INFERTILITY

Exercise 1

1. D	3. E	5. F	7. C
2. B	4. H	6. A	8. G

Exercise 2

1. 12
2. nonhostile
3. intracavitary
4. bicornuate
5. Bicornuate
6. patency
7. dominant
8. 22
9. elevated
10. 12 to14
11. hyperstimulation
12. hyperstimulation
13. heterotopic

Exercise 3

1. Multiple fibroids are demonstrated.
2. Submucosal fibroid with saline infusion sonography.
3. The ovarian follicular phase is shown.
4. Hyperstimulation of the ovary

CHAPTER 47 ROLE OF SONOGRAPHY IN OBSTETRICS

Exercise 1

1. E	6. B	11. D	16. Q
2. I	7. K	12. O	17. P
3. C	8. F	13. M	
4. G	9. H	14. L	
5. A	10. J	15. N	

Exercise 2

1. H	4. D	7. L	10. F
2. E	5. C	8. I	11. J
3. A	6. G	9. K	12. B

CHAPTER 48 CLINICAL ETHICS FOR OBSTETRIC SONOGRAPHY

Exercise 1

1. F	4. A	7. J	10. E
2. B	5. K	8. H	11. C
3. I	6. G	9. D	

Exercise 2

1. morality
2. right, good
3. values
4. autonomy
5. ethics
6. first do no harm
7. nonmaleficence
8. education
9. beneficence
10. minimum
11. privacy
12. competency, knowledge, sonographic
13. autonomy
14. consent
15. veracity
16. Justice
17. timing
18. beneficence

CHAPTER 49 THE NORMAL FIRST TRIMESTER

Exercise 1

1. E	4. I	7. F
2. A	5. G	8. C
3. D	6. B	9. H

Exercise 2

1. K	5. M	9. H	13. A
2. C	6. B	10. D	14. F
3. N	7. J	11. L	
4. G	8. E	12. I	

Exercise 3

A. 1. Morula
   2. Zygote
   3. Fertilization
   4. Ovum
   5. Developing follicle
   6. Blastocyst
   7. Implantation
B. 1. Decidua basalis
   2. Amniotic cavity
   3. Yolk sac
   4. Placenta
   5. Chorion leave
   6. Decidua capsularis
   7. Amniotic cavity
   8. Chorionic cavity
   9. Decidua parietalis
C. 1. Amnion
   2. connecting stalk
   3. Embryonic disc
   4. Yolk sac
   5. Chorion
   6. Chorionic cavity
   7. Amniotic sac
   8. Umbilical cord
   9. Yolk sac

10. Amnion
11. Connecting stalk
12. Yolk sac
13. Chorionic cavity
14. Smooth chorion
15. Amnion
16. Amniotic sac
17. Umbilical cord
18. Yolk sac remnant

Exercise 4

1. gestation
2. embryo
3. fetus
4. 2
5. zygote
6. 7 to 9
7. cardiovascular
8. proportionately
9. plateau
10. 1000 to 2000
11. ectopic
12. double decidual
13. 1
14. yolk
15. 6th
16. 5th through 7th
17. 12th
18. 11th
19. 8th to 11th
20. lateral

Exercise 5

1. length, width, height
2. 12
3. 10 to 15
4. 0.1
5. 3
6. 4
7. 6
8. 8
9. 11th

Exercise 6

1. 5.5 and 6.5
2. two
3. one, two, two
4. one, one

Exercise 7

1. The thickened decidua and the gestational sac are seen in this sagittal image of an early first-trimester 5-week intrauterine gestation.
2. Twin pregnancy
3. Normal herniated bowel
4. The curved arrow points to the amniotic membrane, and the straight arrows are pointing to the umbilical cord.
5. crown-rump length
6. Nuchal translucency

CHAPTER 50 1ST TRIMESTER COMPLICATIONS

Exercise 1

1. I	4. B	7. K	10. D
2. C	5. J	8. G	11. H
3. F	6. E	9. A	

Exercise 2

1. D	4. E	7. F
2. H	5. I	8. A
3. B	6. C	9. G

Exercise 3

1. Choroid plexus
2. Ossification
3. Anencephaly
4. Ventriculomegaly
5. Dandy-Walkert
6. 10 to 12
7. Cystic hygroma
8. Subchorionic
9. Corpus luteum
10. Previous pelvic infections, IUCD, fallopian tube surgery, infertility treatments, and previous ectopic pregnancy
11. Empty, mass
12. pseudogestational sac
13. interstitial pregnancy
14. 90
15. Subchorionic
16. Incomplete
17. Trophoblastic
18. Elevated
19. Snowstorm
20. Theca-lutein

Exercise 4

1. Hydatidiform mole
2. Anencephaly
3. Conjoined twins
4. Cystic hygroma

CHAPTER 51: SONOGRAPHY OF THE 2ND AND 3RD TRIMESTERS

Exercise 1

1. F	5. B	9. G	13. M
2. J	6. O	10. A	14. C
3. N	7. H	11. K	15. I
4. D	8. L	12. E	

Exercise 2

1. human chorionic gonadotropin hCG
2. gravidity
3. parity
4. two, one, no, three

Exercise 3

1. mother

2. cardiac
3. situs
4. 34
5. transverse
6. vertex, breech
7. footling
8. down, up

Exercise 4

1. hypoechoic
2. large, small
3. ossify
4. dura, arachnoid
5. round or oval, smooth
6. falx
7. nervous
8. glomus
9. 10
10. midline
11. third
12. Willis
13. cerebellum
14. magna
15. 3 to 11
16. cerebellum

Exercise 5

1. amniotic
2. one third
3. swallowing
4. periphery
5. sacral
6. three
7. railway
8. equidistant
9. center
10. transverse

Exercise 6

1. longitudinal
2. swallowed
3. pulsations
4. right
5. oxygenation
6. higher
7. bypasses
8. away
9. directly
10. ductus venosus
11. umbilical
12. falciform
13. hepatic
14. foramen
15. venosus
16. left
17. gallbladder
18. stomach
19. 11th, 16th
20. meconium
21. 15th

22. pelvocaliceal
23. 10
24. echogenic
25. once
26. normal
27. abducted
28. 12 to 16, 20th to 22nd
29. 12th
30. soft tissue

Exercise 7

1. bowing,
2. humerus
3. 39th
4. ulna
5. opened
6. 33 to 35

Exercise 8

1. breech position
2. A. choroid plexus
   B. thalamus
   C. cerebellum
   The biparietal diameter should be measured at *the level of the thalamus.*
3. The *f* denotes the frontal bone, the t denotes the tongue, and the c denotes the chin.
4. The right side is closest to the transducer.
5. The *L* is pointing to the labia majora.
6. The scrotum and the penis are demonstrated.
7. The radius is anterior, and the ulna is posterior.

CHAPTER 52 OBSTETRIC MEASUREMENTS AND GESTATIONAL AGE

Exercise 1

1. G	5. D	9. B	12. F
2. J	6. E	10. C	13. K
3. L	7. H	11. I	
4. A	8. M		

Exercise 2

1. E	4. F	7. J	10. A
2. C	5. B	8. H	11. D
3. I	6. K	9. G	

Exercise 3

1. decidua
2. transverse, longitudinal
3. 10
4. 8
5. 6, 8
6. 16
7. 1 to 2
8. crown-rump length
9. 8
10. anembryonic

Exercise 4

1. a. biparietal

531

b. head
c. abdominal
d. femur
2. axial
3. thalamus, pellucidi
4. ovoid
5. leading, leading
6. transverse
7. perpendicular
8. underestimate, overestimate
9. growth
10. liver, umbilical
11. circular
12. femur
13. abdomen
14. elbow

Exercise 5

1. gestational sac
2. A
3. A, spine ; B, stomach ; C, portal vein
4. Femur
5. a, radius ; b, ulna ; hand
6. cerebellum ; formen magnum

CHAPTER 53 FETAL GROWTH ASSESSMENT BY SONOGRAPHY

Exercise 1

1. K	4. C	7. J	10. D
2. E	5. L	8. B	11. A
3. H	6. F	9. G	12. I

Exercise 2

1. 10
2. Symmetrical
3. Asymmetrical
4. small
5. AC

Exercise 3

1. head-sparing
2. head
3. liver
4. oligohydramnios

EXERCISE 4

1. a. cardiac nonstress test
   d. observation of fetal breathing movements
   f. gross fetal body movements
   g. fetal tone
   h. amniotic fluid volume

2. increases, decreases
3. resistance
4. 4000
5. diabetes mellitus

Exercise 5

1. fetal hydrops
2. 30 minutes

3. positive fetal tone
4. Four quadrant amniotic fluid volume
5. Abnormal

CHAPTER 54 SONOGRAPHY AND HIGH RISK PREGNANCY

Exercise 1

1. T	6. P	11. N	16. F	20. G
2. L	7. H	12. I	17. S	21. U
3. D	8. O	13. A	18. C	
4. J	9. R	14. K	19. M	
5. B	10. E	15. Q		

Exercise 2

1. advanced maternal age
2. nuchal
3. quad
4. targeted
5. hydrops
6. antigen
7. cordocentesis
8. thrombocytopenia
9. nonimmune
10. structural
11. macrosomic
12. diabetic
13. small
14. eclampsia
15. lupus
16. Hyperemesis

Exercise 3

1. one-half
2. 20
3. 16 and 20

Exercise 4

1. five
2. gestational
3. Dizygotic,
4. dichorionic, diamniotic
5. monozygotic
6. early, late
7. early
8. 4 to 8
9. mono-, mono-
10. conjoined
11. poly-oli
12. arteriovenous
13. acardiac
14. amniotic
15. smaller
16. reverse

Exercise 5

1. Scalp edema is shown in image *A*. Pleural effusion is shown in image *B*, and abdominal ascites is shown in image *C*.
2. Polyhydramnios is demonstrated.

3. Abdominal ascites is demonstrated. In image *B*, the umbilical vein is denoted with the *v*.
4. Dichorionic, diamniotic twin gestation is demonstrated.
5. Monochorionic, monoamniotic twinning is demonstrated.

CHAPTER 55 PRENATAL DIAGNOSIS OF CONGENITAL ANOMALIES

Exercise 1

1. K	4. G	7. J	10. I
2. B	5. C	8. A	11. D
3. E	6. H	9. F	

Exercise 2

1. 3
2. chorionic villus sampling
3. embryoscopy
4. amniocentesis
5. each
6. cordocentesis
7. alpha-fetoprotein
8. amniotic
9. neural tube defects
10. omphalocele, gastroschisis
11. twice

Exercise 3

1. 46, 22
2. aneuploidy
3. Down
4. 50
5. 25
6. boys
7. sons, daughters
8. multifactorial
9. mosaicism

Exercise 4

1. aneuploidy
2. 3
3. neck, nuchal
4. 3, 4
5. Turner's
6. cystic hygroma
7. coarctation

Exercise 5

1. *A* thickened nuchal fold.
   B, double-bubble sign
   C, endocardial cushion defect with a common atrio-ventricular valve
   D echogenic bowel
2. Image *A* shows a single ventricle characteristic of holoprosencephaly and splaying of the cerebellar hemispheres consistent with a Dandy-Walker malformation. Images *B* and *C* show polydactyly on the right and left hands, respectively, and image *D* demonstrates an omphalocele.
3. Image *A* shows a clenched hand, and image *B* demonstrates an omphalocele. Hydronephrosis was also present (image *C*).

4. Image *A* shows a septated cystic hygroma in the nuchal area; image *B* shows hydrops.

CHAPTER 56 THE PLACENTA

Exercise 1

1. D	3. A	5. C	7. E
2. G	4. H	6. F	8. B

Exercise 2

1. M	5. L	9. C	13. K
2. D	6. B	10. I	14. E
3. O	7. G	11. N	15. H
4. J	8. A	12. F	

Exercise 3

A. 1. Embryo in amniotic sac
   2. Chorionic villi
   3. Yolk sac
   4. Decidua basalis
   5. Uterine cavity
   6. Decidua capsularis
   7. Exocoelomic cavity
   8. Decidua vera
B. 1. Decidua vera
   2. Chorion frondosum
   3. Amniotic sac
   4. Decidua basalis
   5. Uterine cavity
   6. Chorion leave
   7. Decidua capsularis
   8. Yolk sac
C. 1. Trophoblastic layer
   2. Myometrium
   3. Decidua basalis
   4. Decidual septum
   5. Venous sinuses
   6. Spiral arteries
   7. Marginal lake
   8. Amnion
   9. Umbilical arteries and vein
   10. Umbilical cord
   11. Fetal capillaries in villi
   12. Intervillous space

Exercise 4

1. oxygenated, deoxygenated
2. umbilical cord
3. chorionic plate
4. basal
5. spiral
6. hypotension
7. center
8. blood
9. excrete, swallows

Exercise 5

1. subplacental
2. 45 to 50 mm
3. position

533

4. full bladder
5. succenturiate
6. high
7. placentomegaly
8. previa
9. complete
10. transperineal
11. vasa
12. placenta
13. cesarean section
14. increta
15. circumvallate
16. abruption
17. Retroplacental
18. Marginal
19. infarction
20. trophoblastic
21. chorioangioma

Exercise 6

1. Velamentous insertion
2. Placentomegaly
3. Placental lake
4. Placenta previa
5. Circumvallate placenta

CHAPTER 57 THE UMBILICAL CORD

Exercise 1

1. H	6. M	10. K	14. F
2. D	7. A	11. I	15. O
3. C	8. L	12. Q	16. G
4. J	9. B	13. N	17. E
5. P			

Exercise 2

1. oxygen
2. herniate
3. two, one, Wharton's
4. bladder, liver
5. venosus
6. portal, systemic
7. venosum
8. lateral

Exercise 3

1. True
2. False
3. nuchal
4. battledore
5. velamentous
6. prolapse
7. Compression
8. single

Exercise 4

1. Absent cord twists
2. left
3. Omphalocele

4. Gastroschisis
5. Marginal insertion
6. two vessel cord

CHAPTER 58 AMNIOTIC FLUID, FETAL MEMBRANES, AND FETAL HYDROPS

Exercise 1

1. G	4. F	7. D
2. B	5. I	8. A
3. C	6. H	9. E

Exercise 2

1. H	5. I	9. J	13. B
2. F	6. L	10. G	14. C
3. D	7. M	11. K	
4. N	8. E	12. A	

Exercise 3

1. Amniotic fluid
2. amniotic, yolk
3. lungs
4. frondosum
5. 8
6. swallows, produces
7. kidney
8. exchange
9. oligohydramnios
10. 50
11. isolated
12. decreased, increased
13. echo-free

Exercise 4

1. subjective
2. quadrant
3. single
4. 5 to 10, 20 to 24
5. perpendicular
6. maximum
7. oligohydramnios

Exercise 5

1. polyhydramnios
2. nervous
3. depressed
4. oligohydramnios
5. 2, 5
6. IUGR
7. blood
8. compression

Exercise 6

1. amniotic band syndrome
2. birth
3. synechiae

Exercise 7

1. Polyhydramnios

2. Measure largest vertical pocket in each sac.
3. 3D image shows an amniotic band attached to the wall of the gestational sac.
4. Uterine synechiae
5. Fetal ascites

CHAPTER 59 THE FETAL FACE AND NECK

Exercise 1

1. F	5. E	9. H	13. J
2. I	6. K	10. O	14. N
3. L	7. A	11. D	15. C
4. B	8. M	12. G	

Exercise 2

1. J	5. F	9. C	13. E
2. D	6. N	10. K	14. H
3. M	7. G	11. B	
4. I	8. A	12. L	

Exercise 3

A. 1. Optic pit
   2. Branchial arches
   3. Stomodeum
B. 1. Oropharyngeal membrane
   2. Nasal placode
   3. Maxillary prominence
   4. Mandibular prominence
   5. Heart prominence
C. 1. Nasal placode
   2. Lens placode
   3. Nasal pit
   4. Otic pit
   5. Heart prominence
   6. Lower nasal prominence
   7. Stomodeum
   8. Cervical
   9. Auricular hillocks

Exercise 4

1. branchial
2. 6
3. mandibular
4. neural
5. ectoderm
6. medially, upper

Exercise 5

1. congenital
2. chromosomal
3. curvilinear
4. hypertelorism
5. craniosynostosis
6. kleeblattschädel
7. thanatophoric, ventriculomegaly
8. Trigonocephaly
9. Frontal bossing
10. maxillary
11. 21

12. frontonasal
13. Beckwith-Wiedemann
14. microphthalmia, anophthalmia
15. hypotelorism
16. Hypertelorism
17. profile
18. Cleft
19. left

Exercise 6

1. lip
2. dystocia
3. Turner's
4. cystic
5. hydrops
6. goiter

Exercise 7

1. In image *A,* the "l" denotes the lens; in image *B,* the arrows point to the eyelids.
2. In image *A,* the "t" denotes the tongue; in image *B,* the coronal view is demonstrated.
3. Thanatophoric dysplastic fetus with a cloverleaf skull (kleeblattschädel) is demonstrated.
4. The arrow is pointing to the absent nasal bone in a fetus with trisomy 21.
5. Image A: A midline sagittal view of the face in a fetus with holoprosencephaly shows a proboscis *(arrow);* a dorsal sac (sometimes seen with holoprosencephaly) can be seen in the posterior fetal cranium *(open arrow).* Image B: An axial view of the same fetus displays the monoventricle seen with holoprosencephaly. Image C: Coronal view of the same fetus reveals hypotelorism *(arrows).*
6. Unilateral cleft lip with extension into the nasal cavity is demonstrated. The defect extends from the upper lip to the nasal cavity. O, orbit.
7. Cystic hygroma is present in all these images. Image *A* demonstrates a small cystic hygroma. Image *B* shows the large septated compartments seen in a fetus with a large cystic hygroma. Image *C,* a transverse view of the fetal neck, demonstrates the remaining "webbing" from resolution of a cystic hygroma.

CHAPTER 60: THE FETAL NEURAL AXIS

Exercise 1

1. M	5. J	9. G	13. H
2. B	6. N	10. I	14. D
3. L	7. C	11. A	15. K
4. F	8. P	12. O	16. E

Exercise 2

1. forebrain, spinal
2. prosencephalon
3. mesencephalon
4. rhombencephalon
5. anencephaly
6. cephalocele

7. encephalocele
8. meningocele
9. Chiari type II
10. Alobar
11. Semilobar
12. lobar
13. corpus
14. Aqueductal stenosis
15. porencephalic
16. schizencephaly
17. obstruction
18. occipital, frontal
19. 10

Exercise 3

1. An anencephalic fetus; absence of the brain and calvarium is identified. Note the froglike appearance.
2. Acrania
3. Encephalocele
4. Abnormally shaped cerebellum "banana sign" (calipers [+]) in a 21-week fetus with a lumbosacral meningomyelocele. Note the lemon-shaped frontal bones consistent with frontal bossing.
5. Holoprosencephaly
6. Proboscis seen in patient with holoprosencephaly
7. Agenesis of corpus callosum

CHAPTER 61: THE FETAL THORAX

Exercise 1

1. I	4. B	7. K	10. C
2. D	5. J	8. A	11. H
3. G	6. E	9. F	

Exercise 2

1. fluid
2. bell, clavicles
3. smaller
4. hypoplasia
5. effusion, malformation
6. echogenicity
7. liver
8. second, third
9. 20

Exercise 3

1. hypoplasia
2. reduction
3. four-chamber
4. Bronchogenic
5. hydrothorax
6. sequestration
7. thoracic
8. adenomatoid
9. abdominal
10. Bochdalek
11. Morgagni
12. malformations

13. left
14. right
15. hypoplasia
16. extracorporeal membrane oxygenation (ECMO)

Exercise 4

1. The fetal lungs are more echogenic than the fetal liver.
2. The apex of the heart points toward the left side of the abdomen. The heart axis is normal.
3. The fetal lungs are very echogenic compared with the liver. There is pleural effusion and ascites. The fetus has tracheal atresia.
4. The type of cystic adenomatoid shown here is type I CAM.
5. A diaphragmatic hernia is also seen. Displacement of the heart to the right chest is shown in image *A,* as well as a herniated bowel *(arrows).* In the same fetus (image *B*), the liver (L) is shown in close proximity to the heart (h) and bowel (b) because of the absent diaphragm.
6. This image demonstrates a large left-sided hernia. The stomach and bowel are seen within the thoracic cavity.

CHAPTER 62: FETAL ANTERIOR ABDOMINAL WALL

Exercise 1

1. B	4. J	7. E	9. I
2. G	5. H	8. C	10. F
3. D	6. A		

Exercise 2

1. ectoderm, mesoderm, endoderm
2. bowel
3. 10-12th
4. gastroschisis, omphalocele, umbilical hernia
5. distortion
6. omphalocele
7. membrane
8. chromosomal
9. Liver
10. right
11. Small
12. Alpha-fetoprotein
13. without
14. amniotic band
15. Beckwith-Wiedemann
16. exstrophy
17. pentalogy of Cantrell
18. ectopia cordis
19. Limb–body wall

Exercise 3

1. omphalocele
2. cleft distal sternum, anterior ventral wall defect, cardiac defect, diaphragmatic defect, defect of apical pericardium.
3. ectopia cordis
4. Limb-body-wall complex

CHAPTER 63 THE FETAL ABDOMEN

Exercise 1

1. G	4. A	7. E
2. C	5. F	8. B
3. D	6. H	9. I

Exercise 2

1. M	5. L	9. D	12. B
2. E	6. F	10. N	13. G
3. A	7. C	11. I	14. J
4. H	8. K		

Exercise 3

1. foregut
2. esophageal
3. foregut
4. lesser
5. epiploic
6. midgut
7. distal
8. stenosis, atresia
9. umbilical, two
10. hematopoiesis
11. midgut
12. Meckel's

Exercise 4

1. fluid-filled
2. 20, 30
3. portal, umbilical
4. color
5. swallowing
6. meconium
7. hyperechoic
8. peristalsis
9. haustral
10. colon
11. hypoechoic
12. left, right
13. 20

Exercise 5

1. Situs inversus
2. partial situs inversus
3. pseudoascites
4. proximal
5. diameter
6. esophageal
7. absent, hydramnios
8. proximal
9. meconium ileus
10. Anorectal atresia
11. subjective
12. abnormal

Exercise 6

1. *P* is the portal sinus; *PV* is the umbilical portion of the left portal vein; *S* is the stomach; and *sp* is the spine.
2. Partial situs inversus
3. A. Pseudoascites
   B. Ascites
4. Duodenal atresia (double bubble)
5. meconium peritonitis

CHAPTER 64 THE FETAL UROGENITAL SYSTEM

Exercise 1

1. G	4. H	7. D	10. C
2. K	5. J	8. A	11. I
3. F	6. B	9. E	

Exercise 2

1. E	5. C	9. K	13. H
2. L	6. B	10. M	14. D
3. O	7. G	11. F	15. J
4. I	8. N	12. A	

Exercise 3

1. amniotic fluid
2. mesoderm
3. nephrogenic
4. genital
5. metanephros
6. 11th, 12th
7. amniotic fluid
8. placenta
9. pelvis
10. echogenic, right

Exercise 4

1. agenesis
2. divided
3. horseshoe
4. urogenital
5. Exstrophy
6. allantois
7. urachus
8. fistula
9. urachal

Exercise 5

1. 13
2. hyperechoic
3. 25
4. 4, 7
5. 45 to 60
6. hypertrophied
7. urethra
8. large
9. multicystic

10. polycystic
11. hydronephrosis
12. pelvis, vesicoureteric
13. bilateral

Exercise 6
1. amniotic fluid
2. 30
3. incompatible
4. adrenal
5. Ectopic
6. Potter's
7. oligohydramnios
8. cystic
9. noncommunicating
10. large, echogenic
11. ureteropelvic, ureterovesical, megacystis
12. hydronephrosis

Exercise 7
1. pyelectasis, calyces
2. ureteropelvic
3. Ureterovesical
4. ureterocele
5. Bladder, keyhole
6. oligohydramnios, ascites

Exercise 8
1. turtle
2. hamburger
3. pseudohermaphroditism
4. Ovarian cysts
5. Hydrocele
6. cryptorchidism
7. Ambiguous
8. hydrometrocolpos

Exercise 9
1. (A) The kidney in this fetus reflects dilation of ureter, renal pelvis, and calyces. (B) Image of a dilated tortuous ureter. (C) The keyhold sign is noted in this enlarged bladder and urethra.
2. Fetal kidneys are symmetrically enlarged. (Mother has polycystic kidney disease).
3. Unilateral multicystic dysplastic kidney.
4. Bilateral renal enlargement in fetus with Beckwith-Wiedermann syndrome.
5. (A, B) Mild hydronephrosis in right kidney, severe hydronephrosis in left kidney. (C) Moderate hydronephrosis of both kidneys. (D) Bilateral severe hydronephrosis.

CHAPTER 65 THE FETAL SKELETON

Exercise 1
1. E	4. H	7. I
2. C	5. F	8. D
3. A	6. B	9. G

Exercise 2
1. mesoderm
2. somites, mesoderm
3. ectoderm
4. 8th
5. 9th
6. dysplasia

Exercise 3
1. thanatophoric
2. short, cloverleaf
3. achondroplasia
4. bone, hypomineralization
5. brittle, sclera
6. imperfecta
7. hypophosphatasia
8. bowing
9. limbs
10. narrow, atrial septal defect
11. sirenomelia
12. single
13. amniotic band
14. talipes
15. Rocker-bottom

Exercise 4
1. Lethal skeletal dysplasia consistent with thanatophoric dysplasia is visible. Images *A* and *B* show right arm micromelia. The lower extremities were also short. Images *C* and *D* demonstrate a narrow thorax with shortened ribs. The abdomen was protuberant (image *E)* and, compared with the narrow thorax, give the appearance of a "champagne cork" (image *F).*
2. Image *A* shows decreased ossification in the fetal head, which is compressible. Severe micromelia is noted in the femur (image *B*) and humerus (image *C*).
3. Image *A* shows the small thoracic cavity *(arrows)* as compared with the fetal abdomen. Image B shows hypomineralization of the fetal skull.
4. Image *A* shows a normal femur compared with image *B*, in which a femoral fracture is shown. Osteogenesis imperfecta type I or IV is suspected.
5. Image *A* shows rigid legs with hyperextended knees. Image *B* shows the fetal arms contracted and crossed over the chest with clenched fists.
6. A fetus with camptomelic dysplasia and Swyer syndrome shows abnormal plantar flexion of the feet.

CARDIOVASCULAR ANATOMY REVIEW

1. a	10. d	19. b	28. c	37. c
2. a	11. b	20. b	29. b	38. c
3. d	12. b	21. b	30. b	39. b
4. b	13. b	22. b	31. a	40. a
5. b	14. d	23. a	32. c	41. a
6. c	15. a	24. d	33. a	42. b
7. d	16. d	25. c	34. b	43. d
8. b	17. d	26. d	35. c	44. b
9. c	18. d	27. d	36. a	

GENERAL SONOGRAPHY REVIEW

1. d	35. d	69. a	103. a	137. d	171. d
2. b	36. c	70. c	104. c	138. b	172. d
3. c	37. b	71. a	105. d	139. d	173. a
4. c	38. c	72. d	106. a	140. b	174. d
5. a	39. a	73. d	107. d	141. a	175. b
6. c	40. c	74. c	108. d	142. d	176. d
7. a	41. d	75. b	109. d	143. b	177. a
8. b	42. d	76. c	110. a	144. c	178. b
9. c	43. b	77. a	111. a	145. a	179. d
10. a	44. d	78. d	112. b	146. a	180. b
11. d	45. b	79. b	113. a	147. c	181.
12. b	46. a	80. c	114. b	148. b	182.
13. b	47. c	81. d	115. c	149. c	183.
14. b	48. a	82. c	116. a	150. b	184. c
15. b	49. d	83. d	117. a	151. b	185. c
16. b	50. d	84. c	118. c	152. a	186. b
17. c	51. b	85. c	119. b	153. d	187. c
18. b	52. d	86. c	120. b	154. d	188. d
19. b	53. d	87. d	121. b	155. d	189. b
20. a	54. d	88. a	122. c	156. b	190. c
21. d	55. c	89. b	123. d	157. a	191. b
22. b	56. b	90. b	124. c	158. d	192. c
23. b	57. c	91. d	125. d	159. d	193. b
24. b	58. b	92. c	126. a	160. c	194. d
25. a	59. b	93. c	127. c	161. b	195. b
26. c	60. c	94. d	128. a	162. a	196. b
27. b	61. d	95. d	129. d	163. c	197. b
28. c	62. b	96. b	130. c	164. b	198. b
29. a	63. a	97. c	131. a	165. b	199. c
30. c	64. c	98. c	132. c	166. b	200. d
31. a	65. d	99. a	133. a	167. a	
32. b	66. a	100. b	134. c	168. a	
33. c	67. c	101. c	135. d	169. b	
34. c	68. a	102. d	136. b	170. a	

OBSTETRICS AND GYNECOLOGY REVIEW

1. c	6. a	11. c	16. b	21. b	26. c
2. b	7. d	12. a	17. d	22. a	27. a
3. b	8. c	13. c	18. c	23. c	28. a
4. c	9. a	14. b	19. b	24. b	29. b
5. b	10. b	15. a	20. d	25. b	30. b

31. b	57. a	83. a	109. a	135. b	161. d
32. c	58. b	84. b	110. b	136. a	162. c
33. b	59. b	85. d	111. c	137. c	163. d
34. c	60. c	86. c	112. b	138. d	164. a
35. a	61. d	87. b	113. c	139. a	165. c
36. c	62. d	88. c	114. c	140. b	166. a
37. d	63. a	89. d	115. c	141. b	167. c
38. c	64. c	90. b	116. a	142. c	168. b
39. b	65. d	91. c	117. b	143. d	169. d
40. a	66. c	92. b	118. b	144. b	170. a
41. a	67. c	93. c	119. c	145. b	171. a
42. c	68. d	94. c	120. b	146. a	172. d
43. a	69. b	95. c	121. a	147. b	173. c
44. a	70. c	96. a	122. b	148. c	174. b
45. d	71. b	97. a	123. b	149. b	175. c
46. c	72. c	98. c	124. a	150. b	176. a
47. c	73. a	99. b	125. b	151. c	177. b
48. b	74. a	100. a	126. d	152. c	178. a
49. b	75. d	101. a	127. a	153. a	179. c
50. d	76. a	102. d	128. b	154. b	180. d
51. d	77. d	103. d	129. a	155. b	181. b
52. d	78. a	104. c	130. a	156. d	182. d
53. b	79. d	105. c	131. c	157. c	183. c
54. a	80. a	106. c	132. b	158. a	184. a
55. a	81. c	107. b	133. c	159. a	185. c
56. d	82. c	108. c	134. d	160. b	

PEDIATRIC REVIEW

1. a	10. a	19. a	28. c	37. d	46. c
2. b	11. b	20. a	29. a	38. a, d	47. a
3. a	12. b	21. b	30. c	39. b	48. c
4. b	13. a, c	22. d	31. d	40. c	49. d
5. b	14. b	23. a	32. b	41. b	50. b
6. c	15. c	24. d	33. d	42. b	
7. c	16. b	25. a	34. a	43. a	
8. c	17. c	26. b	35. b	44. c	
9. d	18. a	27. d	36. b	45. d	